MODERN MANAGEMENT OF KERATOCONUS

MODERN MANAGEMENT OF KERATOCONUS

Edited by

Brian S Boxer Wachler MD
Boxer Wachler Vision Institute
Los Angeles
California, USA

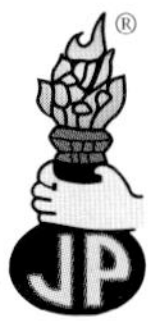

JAYPEE BROTHERS MEDICAL PUBLISHERS (P) LTD

New Delhi • Ahmedabad • Bengaluru • Chennai • Hyderabad • Kochi • Kolkata • Lucknow • Mumbai • Nagpur

Published by

Jitendar P Vij
Jaypee Brothers Medical Publishers (P) Ltd
B-3 EMCA House, 23/23B Ansari Road, Daryaganj, **New Delhi** 110 002 India
Phones: +91-11-23272143, +91-11-23272703, +91-11-23282021, +91-11-23245672
Rel: +91-11-32558559 Fax: +91-11-23276490 +91-11-23245683
e-mail: jaypee@jaypeebrothers.com, Visit our website: www.jaypeebrothers.com

Branches

- 2/B, Akruti Society, Jodhpur Gam Road Satellite
  Ahmedabad 380 015, Phones: +91-79-26926233, Rel: +91-79-32988717, Fax: +91-79-26927094
  e-mail: ahmedabad@jaypeebrothers.com
- 202 Batavia Chambers, 8 Kumara Krupa Road, Kumara Park East
  Bengaluru 560 001, Phones: +91-80-22285971, +91-80-22382956, +91-80-22372664, Rel: +91-80-32714073
  Fax: +91-80-22281761, e-mail: bangalore@jaypeebrothers.com
- 282 IIIrd Floor, Khaleel Shirazi Estate, Fountain Plaza, Pantheon Road
  Chennai 600 008, Phones: +91-44-28193265, +91-44-28194897, Rel: +91-44-32972089
  Fax: +91-44-28193231, e-mail:chennai@jaypeebrothers.com
- 4-2-1067/1-3, 1st Floor, Balaji Building, Ramkote, Cross Road
  Hyderabad 500 095, Phones: +91-40-66610020, +91-40-24758498, Rel: +91-40-32940929
  Fax:+91-40-24758499, e-mail: hyderabad@jaypeebrothers.com
- Kuruvi Building, 1st Floor, Plot/Door No. 41/3098, B & B1, St. Vincent Road
  Kochi 682 018 Kerala, Phones: +91-484-4036109, +91-484-2395739
  Fax: +91-484-2395740, e-mail: kochi@jaypeebrothers.com
- 1-A Indian Mirror Street, Wellington Square
  Kolkata 700 013, Phones: +91-33-22651926, +91-33-22276404, +91-33-22276415, Rel: +91-33-32901926
  Fax: +91-33-22656075, e-mail: kolkata@jaypeebrothers.com
- Lekhraj Market III, B-2, Sector-4, Faizabad Road, Indira Nagar
  Lucknow 226 016, Phones: +91-522-3040553, +91-522-3040554, e-mail: lucknow@jaypeebrothers.com
- 106 Amit Industrial Estate, 61 Dr SS Rao Road, Near MGM Hospital, Parel,
  Mumbai 400 012, Phones: +91-22-24124863, +91-22-24104532, Rel: +91-22-32926896
  Fax: +91-22-24160828, e-mail: mumbai@jaypeebrothers.com
- "KAMALPUSHPA" 38, Reshimbag, Opp. Mohota Science College, Umred Road
  Nagpur 440 009, Phone: Rel: +91-712-3245220, Fax: +91-712-2704275, e-mail:
  nagpur@jaypeebrothers.com

Modern Management of Keratoconus

First Edition: **2008**

ISBN 978-81-8448-209-6

Typeset at JPBMP typesetting unit

Printed at Ajanta Offset

Dedication

Typically, the editor writes the Dedication. Because this book is about helping patients, I thought it would best if an extra special patient wrote the Dedication for this book; Kenny Atkins was the first reported patient in the United States to have Intacs for keratoconus.

— Brian S Boxer Wachler, MD

When I started college I became an Ocean Lifeguard. At school, I found it was becoming harder to focus on textbooks. At first I thought it was just the chlorine – I swam competitively, and at the time we didn't wear goggles for pool workouts. One day a teacher noticed that when I was reading in class I was reading with only one eye. I had my eyes checked and I was diagnosed with astigmatism in one eye and I started wearing glasses while studying. Those glasses for reading books became prescription sunglasses at work, as lifeguarding became my chosen profession. I found it hard to focus in the afternoon as the Southern California sun set lower in the sky.

Prescription sunglasses were expensive and easily scratched. When running out for a rescue, I would often lose them as I threw them on the beach. I tried soft lenses, but the wind blowing sand into my eyes made this very uncomfortable. The lenses often slid up behind my eyes and even floated away when I swam with them. I went for several weeks at a time without correction because of the irritation. By late afternoon I would see double images of objects far away, such as a boat on the horizon.

When laser eye surgery became available, I was excited about the chance to retire my prescription sunglasses and buy ones "off the shelf." However, I was discouraged to learn that I had keratoconus in one eye and was not a candidate for LASIK. I was very frustrated with my problem.

I came across an article and some studies by Dr Boxer Wachler. I was optimistic after my first meeting with him in 1999. Dr. Boxer Wachler explained a new procedure that involved inserting Intacs between the layers of the cornea that would help correct its irregular shape and subsequently my vision. At that time, the procedure had not been reported on a patient with keratoconus in the United States, but he felt the procedure was ready to be attempted. Since my condition was primarily in one eye, I was a good candidate and I welcomed the opportunity.

A week after surgery, the vision in that eye improved to a great degree. I was able to see nearly equally with both eyes and it was unnecessary to wear glasses or contacts at work. After a few months I noticed that I was relying more and more on the corrected eye!

It has now been about eight years since I had Intacs and I still do not wear corrective lenses. I am able to pick objects out of the glare on the horizon and street signs on the freeway well before I need to turn. The freedom I have gained and the confidence I now have in my vision has proven invaluable to me and my ability to continue in my profession. The ability to see well in lifeguarding is critical, and I no longer have the worry that I might miss something that could result in someone's pain, suffering or their life. I owe this self assuredness to Dr Boxer Wachler and to Intacs.

I feel fortunate to have been at the right place at the right time in history. I can appreciate the saying, "Nothing ventured, nothing gained." I am glad that my pioneering experience helped pave the way for the thousands of other patients who have subsequently benefited from innovative advancements for keratoconus. I am pleased to dedicate this book to the thousands of future patients who will benefit from these innovations.

—Kenny Atkins, first reported Intacs for keratoconus patient in the United States

Contributors

Dianne Anderson, OD, FAAO
Chicago, Illinois, USA

Brian S Boxer Wachler, MD
Boxer Wachler Vision Insitute, Los Angeles, California, USA

Colin CK Chan, MD, FRANZCO
The Eye Institute, Sydney, Australia

Paulo Ferrara, MD
Clinica de Olhos Dr Paulo Ferrara, Belo Horizonte – MG, Brazil

Carl Garbus, OD, FAAO
Family Vision Care Optometry, Los Angeles, California, USA

Shawn Jalali, MD
Boxer Wachler Vision Insitute, Los Angeles, California, USA

Robert Joyce, OD
San Diego, California, USA

A John Kanellopoulos, MD
Laservisiongr Institute, Athens, Greece

M Cristina Kenney, MD, PhD
Department of Ophthalmology, Eye Institute, University of California at Irvine, Irvine, California, USA

Carlo F Lovisolo, MD
Quattroelle Eye Centers, Milan, Italy

Jes Mortensen, MD
The Eye Department, Orebro University Hospital, Orebro, Sweden

J Bradley Randleman, MD
Department of Ophthalmology, Emory University and Emory Vision, Atlanta, Georgia

Michael K Smolek, PhD
Physiological Optics and Computer-Aided Diagnostics Laboratories, LSU Health Sciences Center, LSU Eye Center of Excellence, New Orleans, LA

R Doyle Stulting MD, PhD
Department of Ophthalmology, Emory University and Emory Vision, Atlanta, Georgia

Acknowledgements

The editor would like to express his deep gratitude to Selina his wife whose unwavering support was critical for this book.

He would also like to acknowledge the dedications of all the contributors who spent countless hours on their chapters to provide the invaluable information contained within.

The editor would like to specifically acknowledge Joseph Colin, MD and Theo Seiler, MD, PhD and his group for their pioneering work in the field. Without their efforts, there would be no foundation upon which to build this book.

Contents

SECTION 1
Understanding Keratoconus and Keratoectasia

SECTION 2
Diagnosing Keratoconus and Keratoectasia

SECTION 3
Cornea Rehabilitation Treatments

SECTION 4
Cornea Replacement Treatments

SECTION 5
Contact Lenses

SECTION 6
Toward the Ultimate Goal of Reducing Need for Glasses and Contact Lenses

Section 1

Understanding Keratoconus and Keratoectasia

Michael K Smolek, *PhD*

1 What is Keratoconus?

Introduction

Keratoconus is a non-inflammatory, degenerative disease that compromises the structural integrity of the collagen matrix within the corneal stroma. The hallmark characteristic is the development of a localized, cone-shaped ectasia (bulge or hernia) that is accompanied by thinning of the stroma in the area of the cone **(Figure 1-1)**. This leads to increased irregular astigmatism as well as a steeper corneal curvature. While the spherocylindrical components of the refractive error can be corrected in the patient's refractive prescription, it is the residual irregular astigmatism that cannot be easily corrected. This causes retinal image blur and poor visual acuity. Keratoconus can cause mild to severe loss of vision. Even with advanced cases, patients do not "go blind" as there will always be the perception of light. The legal definition of blindness is visual acuity of 20/200 or worse, and some patients may meet this criterion.

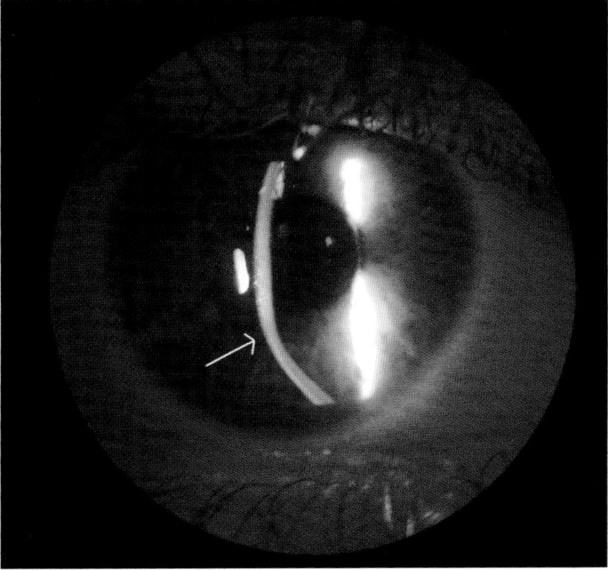

FIGURE 1-1: Keratoconus. Note the protruding cornea (arrow) (Courtesy: Brian S Boxer Wachler, MD).

Incidence

The incidence of keratoconus in the general population (the number of new cases reported annually) is approximately 2 per 100,000 (0.002%) according to a well-designed United States study that collected data over a 48-year period.[1] Other studies undertaken in the United Kingdom and Finland report similar incidences of 2.2 and 1.4 cases per 100,000, respectively.[2,3]

The prevalence of keratoconus (i.e. the number of all existing cases) has been reported to be 54.5 per 100,000 (~0.05%) in the general population.[1] However, the prevalence of keratoconus diagnosed among refractive surgery candidate populations is at least 5.7% in locations where refractive surgery was relatively new to the geographic area.[4,5] This 100-fold higher prevalence over the general population has been attributed to keratoconus patients self-selecting laser vision correction procedures for treatment of their poor visual acuity. Prevalence has been shown to drop to 1 to 1.5% for an established surgical practice in which the initial interest in refractive surgery had diminished over time.[6,7] Nevertheless, the prevalence value for a typical refractive surgery clinic is still 20 times higher than the prevalence of keratoconus found in the general population. With 1 out of every 100 surgical candidates potentially having keratoconus or exhibiting keratoconus-like signs, it is clear that clinicians must use a well-established screening protocol for ruling out keratoconus to reduce the risk of unidentified patients undergoing LASIK or PRK who may develop LASIK-induced keratoconus (keratoectasia).

It is a general rule that whatever test for keratoconus is performed in one eye, it should always be done in the fellow eye and the results compared. Normal corneas tend to be very similar in appearance due to the midline, mirror-image symmetry of the body.[8] Keratoconus often arises first in one eye before arising in the fellow eye. This lapse in keratoconus development gives rise to a different appearance of signs in fellow eyes and this is a useful indicator of the disease.[5] Keratoconus may remain latent at a subclinical state or be completely uninvolved in the fellow eye for up to 6% of cases.[9]

Conclusion

Keratoconus is a corneal condition that leads to blurred vision. Even though it is relatively uncommon, keratoconus causes significant distortions in vision. It is seen more frequently in refractive surgery practices and careful attention must be paid to identify such patients in order to preclude them from LASIK.

References

1. Kennedy RH, Bourne WM, Dyer JA. A 48-year clinical and epidemiological study of keratoconus. Am J Ophthalmol 1986; 101:267-73.
2. Pearson Arm Soneji B, Sarvananthan N, et al. Does ethnic origin influence the incidence or severity of keratoconus? Eye 2000;14:625-8.
3. Ihalainen A. Clinical and epidemiological features of keratoconus: genetic and external factors in the pathogenesis of the disease. Acta Ophthalmol Suppl 1986;178:1-64.
4. Agossou K, Saragoussi JJ, Assouline M, David T, Abenhaim A, Pouliquen Y. Characteristics of corneal topography in candidates for surgery for myopia. [French] Journal Francais d Opthalmologie 1995;18:688-93.
5. Wilson SE, Klyce SD. Screening for corneal topographic abnormalities before refractive surgery. Ophthalmology 1994;101:147-52.
6. Ambrosio R Jr, Klyce SD, Wilson SE. Corneal topographic and pachymetric screening of keratorefractive patients. J Refract Surg 2003;19:24-9.
7. Stephen D Klyce. Personal communication. April 15, 2007.
8. Smolek MK, Klyce SD, Sarver EJ. Inattention to nonsuperimposable midline symmetry causes wavefront analysis error. Arch Ophthalmol 2002; 120:439-47.
9. Rabinowitz YS, Nesburn AB, McDonnell PJ. Videokeratography of the fellow eye in unilateral keratoconus. Ophthalmology 1993;100:181-6.

M Cristina Kenney, *MD, PhD*

2 Causes of Keratoconus

Degradative Enzymes and Their Inhibitors

The characteristic stromal thinning and loss of Bowman's layer found in keratoconic corneas are associated with increased degradative enzyme activities and a decline in the enzyme inhibitors **(Figure 2-1)**. Over 2 decades ago, it was noted that early changes in keratoconic corneas included active degradation of the basal epithelial layer and increased gelatinase activities.[1-3] Later, investigators reported that keratoconic corneas had increased levels of lysosomal enzymes (acid esterase, acid phosphatase, acidic lipase), cathepsins and matrix metalloproteinase-2 (MMP-2).[4-10] Moreover, the conjunctiva also showed increased lysosomal enzyme activities.[11] More recently, Collier and co-workers showed that MT1-MMP (MMP-14), the membrane-type metalloproteinase that activates MMP-2, is also elevated in keratoconic corneas.[12]

In addition to higher levels of degradative enzymes, the inhibitors for these enzymes, such as α_1-proteinase inhibitor, α_2-macroglobulin, tissue inhibitor of metalloptoteinase-1 (TIMP-1), and TIMP3 are decreased in keratoconic corneas.[7,13-17] The α_1-proteinase inhibitor is capable of blocking trypsin, chymotrypsin, elastase and plasmin; the α_2-macroglobulin blocks trypsin, chymotrypsin, papain, collagenase, elastase, thrombin, plasmin and kallikrein; the TIMP-1 inhibits matrix metalloproteinases but also can inhibit apoptosis and affect cell growth. It is now generally accepted that the imbalance of degradative enzymes and their inhibitors plays a major role in the loss of Bowman's layer and stromal thinning in keratoconic corneas.

Abnormal Stromal Matrix

Studies to identify the biochemical differences in keratoconus have helped us understand the matrix content of these thinned, unusually pliable corneas. Keratoconic corneas have decreased total protein and sulfated proteoglycan levels, collagen crosslinking, and variable total collagen content [18-21] **(Figure 2-1)**. However, many of these changes are also found in general wound healing and are not specific for keratoconus.

Immunohistochemical studies showed that keratoconic corneas have decreased levels of fibronectin, laminin, entactin, type IV collagen and type XII collagen associated with the epithelial basement membranes. [22-24] In anterior stromal scar regions, keratoconic corneas have non-specific fibrotic changes such as elevated levels of type III collagen, tenascin-C, fibrillin-1, and keratocan.[22,23,25,26] The changes in the extracellular matrix within

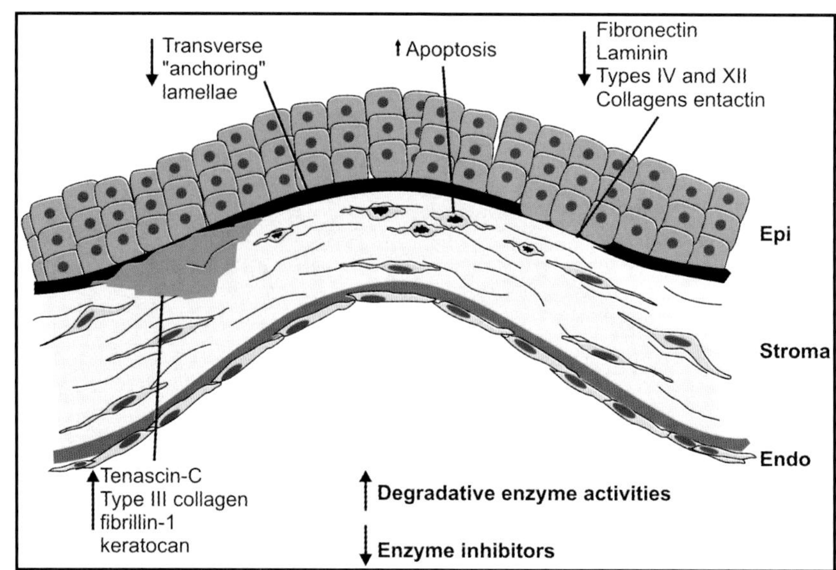

FIGURE 2-1: Schematic of abnormalities associated with keratoconus corneas. Epi, epithelium; Stroma, corneal stroma; Endo, endothelium.

the keratoconic corneas are complex because the abnormalities are not uniform. There are areas with normal matrix patterns while areas of active, thinning disease have deposits of fibrotic matrix components that are similarly found in wound healing and other diseases.

There is a school of thought that stromal lamellar slippage plays a significant role in keratoconus thinning and anterior protrusion. Confocal microscopy and X-ray scattering have given us a better understanding of the structural matrix changes in keratoconic corneas.[27,28] The stromal lamellae in keratoconic corneas are distributed unevenly which suggests interlamellar and intralamellar slippage.[29] In addition, while normal corneas have interwoven lamellae that transversely insert into Bowman's layer for approximately 120 μm, the keratoconic corneas lack these "anchoring" lamellae.[27] As it has been suggested that the anterior interweaving lamellae are critical for maintaining the corneal shape,[30, 31] the loss of these "anchoring" lamellae could theoretically cause corneal lamellar slippage, stretching, and warpage. Further studies are required to understand the biomechanical importance of these anterior interweaving lamellae.

Transcription Factors and Signal Transduction Pathways

Newer molecular techniques have allowed evaluation of transcription factors and signal transduction pathways in keratoconic corneas. Two transcription factors, Sp1 and Krüppel-like factor 6 (KLF6), are elevated in keratoconic corneas and can repress the promoter activity of the α_1-proteinase inhibitor, leading to lower protein levels.[32-34] This is significant since as mentioned earlier, the α_1-proteinase inhibitor is reportedly decreased in these corneas.[13] More recently, keratoconic corneas were shown to have elevated levels of the Sp3 repressor short proteins.[35] When the Sp3 protein is overexpressed in culture, the expression of nerve growth factor receptor, $\text{TrkA}^{\text{NGFR}}$ a protein essential for corneal sensitivity, is decreased.[35] Confocal microscopy shows that these corneas have a significantly lower density of nerves and that the nerves present have increased diameter.[36-38] This is consistent with the clinical findings of enlarged nerves in keratoconic corneas. Furthermore, the nerves that cross through Bowman's layer into the epithelium are associated with high levels of cathepsin B and G, degradative enzymes that can contribute to the anterior stromal destruction.[39] It is not clear if the nerve abnormalities of keratoconic corneas are the underlying etiology or a biological response to other factors. Further work is needed in this area.

Application of gene array analysis to keratoconic corneas demonstrated low levels of alpha-enolase and beta-actin.[40] Suggested molecular markers for keratoconus are the absence of aquaporin 5, a water channel protein, in the keratoconic epithelial cells [41] and the unambiguous expression of DSG3 in the epithelium.[42] These molecular studies showed abnormal expression of numerous genes but no specific overall pathways have been elucidated with this approach.

Genetics of Keratoconus

It is likely that both genetics and environment contribute to the development of keratoconus. [43] Keratoconus is found in identical twins and multigenerational families.[44-49] The prevalence of keratoconus is 3.34% in families with first degree relatives having the disease and this is 15 to 67 times higher than the general population.[50] Keratoconus can also be associated with other ocular diseases. It is described in patients with Leber's congenital amaurosis, cataracts, granular corneal dystrophy, Avellino corneal dystrophy and posterior polymorphism dystrophy.[51-60] Some patients with keratoconus have associated systemic syndromes. For example, keratoconus is found in 0.5 to 15% of trisomy 21 (Down syndrome) patients [61-63] and is associated with Ehlers-Danlos syndrome[64, 65] and osteogenesis imperfecta.[66-68]

Most families with keratoconus show autosomal dominant inheritance with variable penetration. [69, 70] There are at least 10 different chromosomes associated with keratoconus (21, 20q12, 20p11-q11, 18p, 17, 16q, 15q, 13, 5q14.3-q21.1, 3p14-q13, 2p24).[71-77] Over 50 candidate genes have been excluded in keratoconus populations.[76, 78, 79] In the Japanese population, there are three HLA antigens, HLA-A26, B40 and DR9, associated with early onset keratoconus.[80] Our genetic study showed an intronic 7 base deletion in the superoxide dismutase 1 (SOD1) gene that segregated within a keratoconus family.[81] The SOD1 gene is on chromosome 21 and patients with trisomy 21 (Down syndrome) have a higher than normal incidence of keratoconus. Human VSX 1 is a homeobox gene initially associated with a patient that had both keratoconus and posterior polymorphism dystrophy.[57] Novel mutations were reported in the VSX1 gene in a series of individual keratoconic patients.[82] Expression of VSX1 occurs during corneal myofibroblast differentiation during wound healing [83] and may play a role in the stromal repair process in keratoconus. However, most recently, a study of sporadic keratoconic subjects reported a single mutation of Asp144Glu, a non-disease causing polymorphism and concluded that VSX1 was not related to the development of keratoconus.[84]

With this complex genetic picture, it is very likely that keratoconus has multiple genes involved and these may be related to a final common pathway that causes a general KC phenotype. Further work will be required to establish the genetic component of keratoconus.

Apoptosis in Keratoconus

Apoptosis is a biological process of programmed cell death commonly associated with caspase dependent cascade and occurs during development, diseases and wound healing. It is reported that 60% of keratoconic corneas have apoptotic stromal keratocytes compared to 35% in other corneal dystrophies and none in normal corneas.[85,86] Apoptosis occurs in the anterior stroma and other layers of keratoconic corneas[86-88] **(Figure 2-1)**. The loss of keratocyte density was even greater in the keratoconic patients that wore contact lenses.[89] This is consistent with studies that show chronic, repetitive injury to the corneal epithelium stimulates stromal apoptosis.[90,91] In addition, keratoconic corneas have elevated levels of leukocyte common antigen related protein (LAR),[92] a transmembrane phosphotyrosine phosphatase, that stimulates apoptosis, and decreased levels of

TIMP1, a protein that inhibits apoptosis.[93] In addition to blocking enzyme activities, TIMP1 and TIMP3 can also modulate apoptosis in corneal cells.[94] Finally, chronic irritation due to vigorous eye rubbing and moderate to severe atopy may lead to oxidative damage and apoptosis.

Cathepsins represent a caspase-independent pathway for apoptosis. Keratoconic corneas express elevated levels of cathepsin G, cathepsin B and cathepsinV/L2. [5, 15, 39, 95] In addition, human corneal fibroblasts also express RNA levels for cathepsin K and cathepsin D. Oxidative stress causes rupture of lysosomes, release of mitochondrial cytochrome C and apoptosis.[96] Cathepsins mediate apoptosis by triggering mitochondrial dysfunction, cleaving Bid and releasing cytochrome C.[97-100] Moreover, isolated mitochondria exposed to purified cathepsin D have increased ROS/RNS production.[96] Pepstatin A, an inhibitor of cathepsin D, decreases caspase-9 and caspase-3 activation and lowers apoptosis.[101] Therefore, in addition to their significant ability to degrade extracellular matrix, cathepsins may play a significant role in the apoptosis found in these corneas.

Oxidative Damage in Keratoconus Corneas

Keratoconic corneas show signs of oxidative damage with increased levels of inducible nitric oxide synthase (iNOS), nitrotyrosine (a marker for peroxynitrite, $ONOO^{\bullet}$), malondialdehyde (MDA), glutathione S-transferase activity, and lower than normal levels for extracellular superoxide dismutase (SOD3, EC-SOD) and aldehyde dehydrogenase class 3, (ALDH3A1) **(Table 2-1)**, important enzymes critical for the removal of harmful oxidants.[102-105] These types of antioxidant abnormalities are associated with increased levels of superoxide radicals ($O_2^{\bullet}$), hydrogen peroxide (H_2O_2) and hydroxyl radicals ($OH^{\bullet}$), commonly referred to as reactive oxygen species (ROS), and cytotoxic aldehydes **(Figure 2-2)**. These elements can react with proteins, DNA and lipids to cause alterations in the cellular structure and function of the cell **(Figures 2-3 and 2-4)**.

The mitochondrial DNA (mtDNA) in keratoconic corneas is damaged extensively compared to age-matched normal corneas.[106] There is an important relationship between oxidative stress, ROS formation and mitochondria. The mitochondria have unique circular mtDNA that is inherited from the mother. In addition, producing energy through oxidative phosphorylation (OXPHOS), mitochondria are also a significant endogenous source of ROS. Compared to nuclear DNA, mtDNA is particularly susceptible to damage because it lacks introns and has an inefficient mtDNA repair system along with a high transcription rate. The mtDNA codes for 13 OXPHOS proteins, 22 tRNAs and 2 rRNAs,[107] so when mtDNA is damaged, OXPHOS is decreased and ROS formation is increased resulting in additional mtDNA damage.[108, 109] The resultant mitochondrial dysfunction can alter

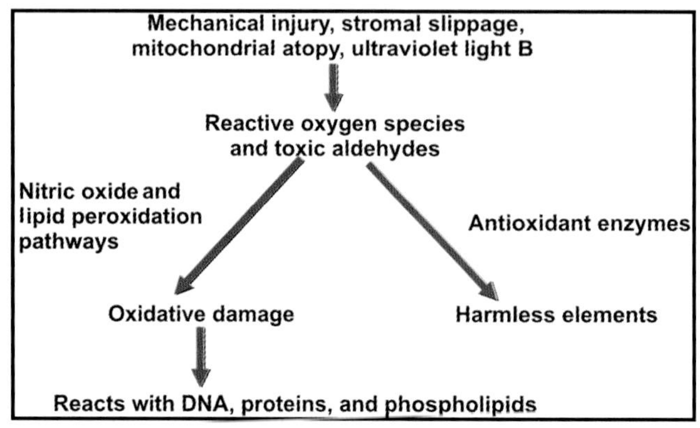

FIGURE 2-2: Mechanisms of oxidative damage that ultimately can decrease cell function and lead to cell death.

Table 2-1: Altered antioxidant and lipid peroxidation enzymes in keratoconus corneas

Enzyme	*KC corneas*
ALDH3[102,103]	↓
Catalase[95]	↑
Inducible NOS (iNOS)[105]	↑
Peroxynitrite[105]	↑
EC-SOD (SOD3)[104]	↓
Glutathione S transferase[102]	↑
SOD1 (ZnCu-SOD)[81]	↓

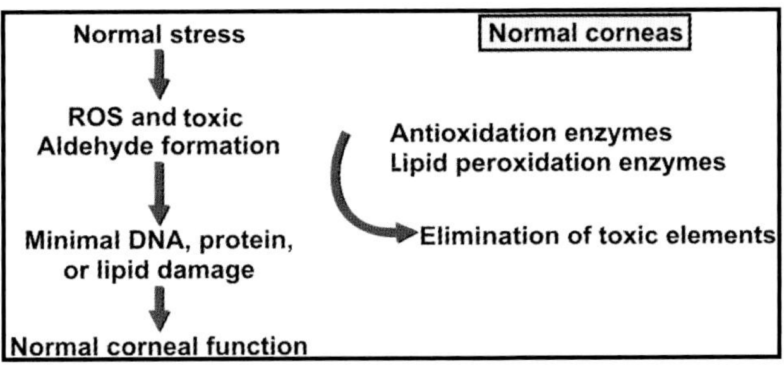

FIGURE 2-3: Elimination of ROS and aldehydes by antioxidant and lipid peroxidation enzymes occurs in normal corneas.

gene expression, cause apoptosis and promote loss of cell viability.[110-112] This mtDNA damage may play a role in keratoconus pathogenesis.

Keratoconic corneas have (i) oxidative, cytotoxic by-products from both the lipid peroxidation and nitric oxide pathways; [105,113] (ii) abnormalities in levels and activities for corneal antioxidant enzymes which are responsible for elimination of ROS and toxic aldehydes; [95,102-104] (iii) defects in the SOD1 gene, an antioxidant enzyme; [81] and (iv) increased mtDNA damage.[106] Furthermore, many of these characteristics of oxidative stress are also found in cultured KC cells. [114] These cultured keratoconus corneal cells have an inherent, hypersensitive

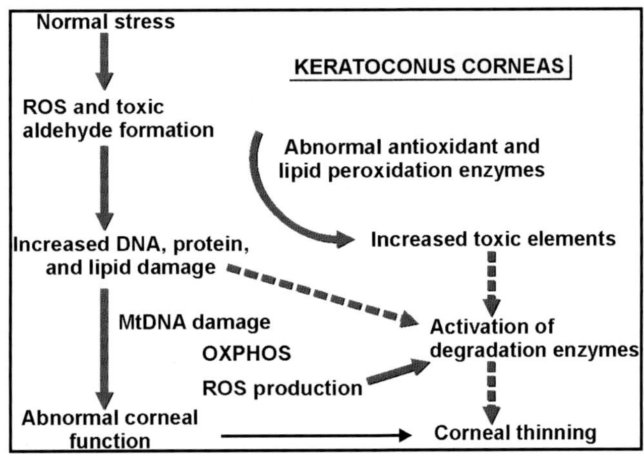

FIGURE 2-4: Increased levels of ROS and aldehydes cause damage to DNA, proteins and lipids along with abnormal corneal cell function and activation of degradative enzymes in KC corneas.

response to oxidative stressors that involves mitochondrial dysfunction and DNA damage. This innate hypersensitivity may play a role in the development and progression of keratoconus.

Oxidative Stress as a Final Common Pathway for Keratoconus

While some investigators suggest that there is a single, prime causative defect at work in keratoconic corneas, we feel it is more likely multiple pathways all related to a "final common pathway" causing keratoconus. This is supported by the fact that at least 10 different chromosomes are associated with keratoconus and multiple molecular abnormalities have been reported.

When analyzing molecular and genetic studies, it is evident that there are multiple defects that seem on the surface not to be connected to each other. Our working hypothesis is that the overlying final common pathway of keratoconus is related to the oxidative stress pathway. In other words, different keratoconic patients may have multiple genes and biochemical events involved but each would be traced back to abnormalities within or related to the oxidative stress pathway. We believe that keratoconic corneas have underlying defects in their ability to process ROS and thereby undergo oxidative damage. This triggers a series of "downstream" events that ultimately lead to corneal thinning and loss of vision. Understanding these mechanisms will help guide future therapies for this debilitating corneal disorder.

Conclusion

Keratoconic corneas have increased levels of numerous enzymes capable of degrading a wide variety of corneal extracellular matrices. Moreover, these degradative enzymes are associated with oxidative stress. The mechanisms that regulate the enzyme-inhibitor interactions are not understood at this time.

Acknowledgments and Grant Support: Discovery Eye Foundation, Schoellerman Charitable Foundation, Guenther Foundation, Iris and B. Gerald Cantor Foundation, Research to Prevent Blindness Foundation, and the National Keratoconus Foundation.

References

1. Teng CC. Electron microscope study of the pathology of keratoconus. I Am J Ophthalmol 1963;55:18-47.
2. Rehany U, Lahav M, Shoshan S. Collagenolytic activity in keratoconus. Ann Ophthalmol 1982;14(8):751-4.
3. Kao WW, Vergnes JP, Ebert J, et al. Increased collagenase and gelatinase activities in keratoconus. Biochem Biophys Res Commun 1982;107(3):929-36.
4. Sawaguchi S, Yue BY, Sugar J, Gilboy JE. Lysosomal enzyme abnormalities in keratoconus. Arch Ophthalmol 1989;107(10):1507-10.
5. Zhou L, Sawaguchi S, Twining SS, et al. Expression of degradative enzymes and protease inhibitors in corneas with keratoconus. Invest Ophthalmol Vis Sci 1998;39(7):1117-24.
6. Kenney MC, Chwa M, Lin B, et al. Identification of cell types in human diseased corneas. Cornea 2001;20(3):309-16.
7. Kenney MC, Chwa M, Opbroek AJ, Brown DJ. Increased gelatinolytic activity in keratoconus keratocyte cultures. A correlation to an altered matrix metalloproteinase-2/tissue inhibitor of metalloproteinase ratio. Cornea 1994;13(2):114-24.
8. Smith VA, Hoh HB, Littleton M, Easty DL. Over-expression of a gelatinase A activity in keratoconus. Eye 1995;9 (Pt 4):429-33.
9. Parkin BT, Smith VA, Easty DL. The control of matrix metalloproteinase-2 expression in normal and keratoconic corneal keratocyte cultures. Eur J Ophthalmol 2000;10(4):276-85.
10. Smith VA, Easty DL. Matrix metalloproteinase 2: involvement in keratoconus. Eur J Ophthalmol 2000;10(3):215-26.
11. Fukuchi T, Yue BY, Sugar J, Lam S. Lysosomal enzyme activities in conjunctival tissues of patients with keratoconus. Arch Ophthalmol 1994;112(10):1368-74.
12. Collier SA, Madigan MC, Penfold PL. Expression of membrane-type 1 matrix metalloproteinase (MT1-MMP) and MMP-2 in normal and keratoconus corneas. Curr Eye Res 2000;21(2):662-8.
13. Sawaguchi S, Twining SS, Yue BY, et al. Alpha-1 proteinase inhibitor levels in keratoconus. Exp Eye Res 1990;50(5):549-54.

14. Brown D, Chwa MM, Opbroek A, Kenney MC. Keratoconus corneas: increased gelatinolytic activity appears after modification of inhibitors. Curr Eye Res 1993;12(6):571-81.
15. Whitelock RB, Fukuchi T, Zhou L, et al. Cathepsin G, acid phosphatase, and alpha 1-proteinase inhibitor messenger RNA levels in keratoconus corneas. Invest Ophthalmol Vis Sci 1997;38(2):529-34.
16. Kenney MC, Chwa M, Alba A, et al. Localization of TIMP-1, TIMP-2, TIMP-3, gelatinase A and gelatinase B in pathological human corneas. Curr Eye Res 1998;17(3):238-46.
17. Smith VA, Matthews FJ, Majid MA, Cook SD. Keratoconus: matrix metalloproteinase-2 activation and TIMP modulation. Biochim Biophys Acta 2006;1762(4):431-9.
18. Yue BY, Sugar J, Benveniste K. Heterogeneity in keratoconus: possible biochemical basis. Proc Soc Exp Biol Med 1984;175(3):336-41.
19. Critchfield JW, Calandra AJ, Nesburn AB, Kenney MC. Keratoconus: I. Biochemical studies. Exp Eye Res 1988;46(6):953-63.
20. Yue BY, Baum JL, Silbert JE. The synthesis of glycosaminoglycans by cultures of corneal stromal cells from patients with keratoconus. J Clin Invest 1979;63(4):545-51.
21. Sawaguchi S, Yue BY, Chang I, et al. Proteoglycan molecules in keratoconus corneas. Invest Ophthalmol Vis Sci 1991;32(6):1846-53.
22. Kenney MC, Nesburn AB, Burgeson RE, et al. Abnormalities of the extracellular matrix in keratoconus corneas. Cornea 1997;16(3):345-51.
23. Zhou L, Yue BY, Twining SS, et al. Expression of wound healing and stress-related proteins in keratoconus corneas. Curr Eye Res 1996;15(11):1124-31.
24. Cheng EL, Maruyama I, Sundar Raj N, et al. Expression of type XII collagen and hemidesmosome-associated proteins in keratoconus corneas. Curr Eye Res 2001;22(5):333-40.
25. Tuori A, Virtanen I, Aine E, Uusitalo H. The expression of tenascin and fibronectin in keratoconus, scarred and normal human cornea. Graefes Arch Clin Exp Ophthalmol 1997;235(4):222-9.
26. Wentz-Hunter K, Cheng EL, Ueda J, et al. Keratocan expression is increased in the stroma of keratoconus corneas. Mol Med 2001;7(7):470-7.
27. Morishige N, Wahlert AJ, Kenney MC, et al. Second-harmonic imaging microscopy of normal human and keratoconus cornea. Invest Ophthalmol Vis Sci 2007;48(3):1087-94.
28. Hayes S, Boote C, Tuft SJ, et al. A study of corneal thickness, shape and collagen organisation in keratoconus using videokeratography and X-ray scattering techniques. Exp Eye Res 2007;84(3):423-34.
29. Meek KM, Tuft SJ, Huang Y, et al. Changes in collagen orientation and distribution in keratoconus corneas. Invest Ophthalmol Vis Sci 2005;46(6):1948-56.
30. Bron AJ. The architecture of the corneal stroma. Br J Ophthalmol 2001;85(4):379-81.
31. Muller LJ, Pels E, Vrensen GF. The specific architecture of the anterior stroma accounts for maintenance of corneal curvature. Br J Ophthalmol 2001;85(4):437-43.
32. Whitelock RB, Li Y, Zhou LL, et al. Expression of transcription factors in keratoconus, a cornea-thinning disease. Biochem Biophys Res Commun 1997;235(1):253-8.
33. Li Y, Zhou L, Twining SS, et al. Involvement of Sp1 elements in the promoter activity of the alpha1-proteinase inhibitor gene. J Biol Chem 1998;273(16):9959-65.
34. Chiambaretta F, Nakamura H, De Graeve F, et al. Kruppel-like factor 6 (KLF6) affects the promoter activity of the alpha 1-proteinase inhibitor gene. Invest Ophthalmol Vis Sci 2006;47(2):582-90.
35. de Castro F, Silos-Santiago I, Lopez de Armentia M, et al. Corneal innervation and sensitivity to noxious stimuli in trkA knockout mice. Eur J Neurosci 1998;10(1):146-52.
36. Simo Mannion L, Tromans C, O'Donnell C. An evaluation of corneal nerve morphology and function in moderate keratoconus. Cont Lens Anterior Eye 2005;28(4):185-92.
37. Mannion LS, Tromans C, O'Donnell C. Corneal nerve structure and function in keratoconus: a case report. Eye Contact Lens 2007;33(2):106-8.
38. Patel DV, McGhee CN. Mapping the corneal sub-basal nerve plexus in keratoconus by in vivo laser scanning confocal microscopy. Invest Ophthalmol Vis Sci 2006;47(4):1348-51.
39. Brookes NH, Loh IP, Clover GM, et al. Involvement of corneal nerves in the progression of keratoconus. Exp Eye Res 2003;77(4):515-24.
40. Srivastava OP, Chandrasekaran D, Pfister RR. Molecular changes in selected epithelial proteins in human keratoconus corneas compared to normal corneas. Mol Vis 2006;12:1615-25.
41. Rabinowitz YS, Dong L, Wistow G. Gene expression profile studies of human keratoconus cornea for NEIBank: a novel cornea-expressed gene and the absence of transcripts for aquaporin 5. Invest Ophthalmol Vis Sci 2005;46(4):1239-46.
42. Nielsen K, Heegaard S, Vorum H, et al. Altered expression of CLC, DSG3, EMP3, S100A2, and SLPI in corneal epithelium from keratoconus patients. Cornea 2005;24(6):661-8.
43. Edwards M, McGhee CN, Dean S. The genetics of keratoconus. Clin Experiment Ophthalmol 2001;29(6):345-51.
44. Parker J, Ko WW, Pavlopoulos G, et al. Videokeratography of keratoconus in monozygotic twins. J Refract Surg 1996;12(1):180-3.
45. Bechara SJ, Waring GO, 3rd, Insler MS. Keratoconus in two pairs of identical twins. Cornea 1996;15(1):90-3.

46. Zadnik K, Mannis MJ, Johnson CA. An analysis of contrast sensitivity in identical twins with keratoconus. Cornea 1984;3(2):99-103.
47. Schmitt-Bernard C, Schneider CD, Blanc D, Arnaud B. Keratographic analysis of a family with keratoconus in identical twins. J Cataract Refract Surg 2000;26(12):1830-2.
48. McMahon TT, Shin JA, Newlin A, et al. Discordance for keratoconus in two pairs of monozygotic twins. Cornea 1999;18(4):444-51.
49. Valluri S, Minkovitz JB, Budak K, et al. Comparative corneal topography and refractive variables in monozygotic and dizygotic twins. Am J Ophthalmol 1999;127(2):158-63.
50. Wang Y, Rabinowitz YS, Rotter JI, Yang H. Genetic epidemiological study of keratoconus: evidence for major gene determination. Am J Med Genet 2000;93(5):403-9.
51. Elder MJ. Leber congenital amaurosis and its association with keratoconus and keratoglobus. J Pediatr Ophthalmol Strabismus 1994;31(1):38-40.
52. Stoiber J, Muss WH, Ruckhofer J, et al. Recurrent keratoconus in a patient with Leber congenital amaurosis. Cornea 2000;19(3):395-8.
53. Dharmaraj S, Leroy BP, Sohocki MM, et al. The phenotype of Leber congenital amaurosis in patients with AIPL1 mutations. Arch Ophthalmol 2004;122(7):1029-37.
54. Yoshida H, Funabashi M, Kanai A. Histological study of the corneal granular dystrophy complicated by keratoconus. Folia Ophthalmol Jpn 1980;31:218-23.
55. Wollensak G, Green WR, Temprano J. Keratoconus associated with corneal granular dystrophy in a patient of Italian origin. Cornea 2002;21(1):121-2.
56. Igarashi S, Makita Y, Hikichi T, et al. Association of keratoconus and Avellino corneal dystrophy. Br J Ophthalmol 2003;87(3):367-8.
57. Heon E, Greenberg A, Kopp KK, et al. VSX1: a gene for posterior polymorphous dystrophy and keratoconus. Hum Mol Genet 2002;11(9):1029-36.
58. Godel V, Blumenthal M, Iaina A. Congenital Leber amaurosis, keratoconus, and mental retardation in familial juvenile nephronophtisis. J Pediatr Ophthalmol Strabismus 1978;15(2):89-91.
59. Flanders M, Lapointe ML, Brownstein S, Little JM. Keratoconus and Leber's congenital amaurosis: a clinicopathological correlation. Can J Ophthalmol 1984;19(7):310-4.
60. Hameed A, Khaliq S, Ismail M, et al. A novel locus for Leber congenital amaurosis (LCA4) with anterior keratoconus mapping to chromosome 17p13. Invest Ophthalmol Vis Sci 2000;41(3):629-33.
61. Krachmer JH, Feder RS, Belin MW. Keratoconus and related noninflammatory corneal thinning disorders. Surv Ophthalmol 1984;28(4):293-322.
62. Walsh SZ. Keratoconus and blindness in 469 institutionalised subjects with Down syndrome and other causes of mental retardation. J Ment Defic Res 1981;25 (Pt 4)243-51.
63. Shapiro MB, France TD. The ocular features of Down's syndrome. Am J Ophthalmol 1985;99(6):659-63.
64. Kuming BS, Joffe L. Ehlers-Danlos syndrome associated with keratoconus. A case report. S Afr Med J 1977;52(10):403-5.
65. Robertson I. Keratoconus and the Ehlers-Danlos syndrome: a new aspect of keratoconus. Med J Aust 1975;1(18):571-3.
66. Hyams SW, Kar H, Neumann E. Blue sclerae and keratoglobus. Ocular signs of a systemic connective tissue disorder. Br J Ophthalmol 1969;53(1):53-8.
67. Zimmermann DR, Fischer RW, Winterhalter KH, et al. Comparative studies of collagens in normal and keratoconus corneas. Exp Eye Res 1988;46(3):431-42.
68. Woodward EG, Morris MT. Joint hypermobility in keratoconus. Ophthalmic Physiol Opt 1990;10(4):360-2.
69. Rabinowitz YS, Maumenee IH, Lundergan MK, et al. Molecular genetic analysis in autosomal dominant keratoconus. Cornea 1992;11(4):302-8.
70. Rabinowitz YS, Zu H, Yang Y, Wang J, Rotter S, Pulst S. Keratoconus: non-parametric linkage analysis suggests a gene locus near to the centromere on chromosome 21. Investigative Ophthalmology and Visual Science 1999;40 (Suppl):2975.
71. Rabinowitz YS ZH, Yang Y, Wang J, Rotter S, Pulst S. Keratoconus: non-parametric linkage analysis suggests a gene locus near to the centromere on chromosome 21. Invest Ophthalmol Vis Sci 1999;40(Suppl):2975.
72. Heaven CJ, Lalloo F, McHale E. Keratoconus associated with chromosome 13 ring abnormality. Br J Ophthalmol 2000;84(9):1079.
73. Fullerton J, Paprocki P, Foote S, et al. Identity-by-descent approach to gene localisation in eight individuals affected by keratoconus from north-west Tasmania, Australia. Hum Genet 2002;110(5):462-70.
74. Tyynismaa H, Sistonen P, Tuupanen S, et al. A locus for autosomal dominant keratoconus: linkage to 16q22.3-q23.1 in Finnish families. Invest Ophthalmol Vis Sci 2002;43(10):3160-4.
75. Brancati F, Valente EM, Sarkozy A, et al. A locus for autosomal dominant keratoconus maps to human chromosome 3p14-q13. J Med Genet 2004;41(3):188-92.
76. Hughes AE, Dash DP, Jackson AJ, et al. Familial keratoconus with cataract: linkage to the long arm of chromosome 15 and exclusion of candidate genes. Invest Ophthalmol Vis Sci 2003;44(12):5063-6.

77. Hutchings H, Ginisty H, Le Gallo M, et al. Identification of a new locus for isolated familial keratoconus at 2p24. J Med Genet 2005;42(1):88-94.
78. Udar N, Kenney MC, Chalukya M, et al. Keratoconus—no association with the transforming growth factor beta-induced gene in a cohort of American patients. Cornea 2004;23(1):13-7.
79. Dash DP, Silvestri G, Hughes AE. Fine mapping of the keratoconus with cataract locus on chromosome 15q and candidate gene analysis. Mol Vis 2006;12:499-505.
80. Adachi W, Mitsuishi Y, Terai K, et al. The association of HLA with young-onset keratoconus in Japan. Am J Ophthalmol 2002;133(4):557-9.
81. Udar N, Atilano SR, Brown DJ, et al. SOD1: a candidate gene for keratoconus. Invest Ophthalmol Vis Sci 2006;47(8):3345-51.
82. Bisceglia L, Ciaschetti M, De Bonis P, et al. VSX1 mutational analysis in a series of Italian patients affected by keratoconus: detection of a novel mutation. Invest Ophthalmol Vis Sci 2005;46(1):39-45.
83. Barbaro V, Di Iorio E, Ferrari S, et al. Expression of VSX1 in human corneal keratocytes during differentiation into myofibroblasts in response to wound healing. Invest Ophthalmol Vis Sci 2006;47(12):5243-50.
84. Aldave AJ, Yellore VS, Salem AK, et al. No VSX1 gene mutations associated with keratoconus. Invest Ophthalmol Vis Sci 2006;47(7):2820-2.
85. Kim WJ, Rabinowitz YS, Meisler DM, Wilson SE. Keratocyte apoptosis associated with keratoconus. Exp Eye Res 1999;69(5):475-81.
86. Kaldawy RM, Wagner J, Ching S, Seigel GM. Evidence of apoptotic cell death in keratoconus. Cornea 2002;21(2):206-9.
87. Wilson SE, Kim WJ. Keratocyte apoptosis: implications on corneal wound healing, tissue organization, and disease. Invest Ophthalmol Vis Sci 1998;39(2):220-6.
88. Hollingsworth JG, Efron N, Tullo AB. In vivo corneal confocal microscopy in keratoconus. Ophthalmic Physiol Opt 2005;25(3):254-60.
89. Erie JC, Patel SV, McLaren JW, et al. Keratocyte density in keratoconus. A confocal microscopy study(a). Am J Ophthalmol 2002;134(5):689-95.
90. Kim WJ, Shah S, Wilson SE. Differences in keratocyte apoptosis following transepithelial and laser- scrape photorefractive keratectomy in rabbits. J Refract Surg 1998;14(5):526-33.
91. Wilson SE. Role of apoptosis in wound healing in the cornea. Cornea 2000;19(3 Suppl):S7-12.
92. Chiplunkar S, Chamblis K, Chwa M, et al. Enhanced expression of a transmembrane phosphotyrosine phosphatase (LAR) in keratoconus cultures and corneas. Exp Eye Res 1999;68(3):283-93.
93. Guedez L, Stetler-Stevenson WG, Wolff L, et al. In vitro suppression of programmed cell death of B cells by tissue inhibitor of metalloproteinases-1. J Clin Invest 1998;102(11):2002-10.
94. Matthews FJ, Cook SD, Majid MA, et al. Changes in the balance of the tissue inhibitor of matrix metalloproteinases (TIMPs)-1 and -3 may promote keratocyte apoptosis in keratoconus. Exp Eye Res 2007;84(6):1125-34.
95. Kenney MC, Chwa M, Atilano SR, et al. Increased levels of catalase and cathepsin V/L2 but decreased TIMP-1 in keratoconus corneas: evidence that oxidative stress plays a role in this disorder. Invest Ophthalmol Vis Sci 2005;46(3):823-32.
96. Zhao M, Antunes F, Eaton JW, Brunk UT. Lysosomal enzymes promote mitochondrial oxidant production, cytochrome C release and apoptosis. Eur J Biochem 2003;270(18):3778-86.
97. Roberg K, Kagedal K, Ollinger K. Microinjection of cathepsin d induces caspase-dependent apoptosis in fibroblasts. Am J Pathol 2002;161(1):89-96.
98. Kagedal K, Johansson U, Ollinger K. The lysosomal protease cathepsin D mediates apoptosis induced by oxidative stress. Faseb J 2001;15(9):1592-4.
99. Roberg K, Johansson U, Ollinger K. Lysosomal release of cathepsin D precedes relocation of cytochrome C and loss of mitochondrial transmembrane potential during apoptosis induced by oxidative stress. Free Radic Biol Med 1999;27 (11-12):1228-37.
100. Cirman T, Oresic K, Mazovec GD, et al. Selective disruption of lysosomes in HeLa cells triggers apoptosis mediated by cleavage of Bid by multiple papain-like lysosomal cathepsins. J Biol Chem 2004;279(5):3578-87.
101. Thibodeau MS, Giardina C, Knecht DA, et al. Silica-induced apoptosis in mouse alveolar macrophages is initiated by lysosomal enzyme activity. Toxicol Sci 2004;80(1):34-48.
102. Gondhowiardjo TD, van Haeringen NJ. Corneal aldehyde dehydrogenase, glutathione reductase, and glutathione S-transferase in pathologic corneas. Cornea 1993;12(4):310-4.
103. Gondhowiardjo TD, van Haeringen NJ, Volker-Dieben HJ, et al. Analysis of corneal aldehyde dehydrogenase patterns in pathologic corneas. Cornea 1993;12(2):146-54.
104. Behndig A, Karlsson K, Johansson BO, et al. Superoxide dismutase isoenzymes in the normal and diseased human cornea. Invest Ophthalmol Vis Sci 2001;42(10):2293-6.
105. Buddi R, Lin B, Atilano SR, et al. Evidence of oxidative stress in human corneal diseases. J Histochem Cytochem 2002;50(3):341-51.
106. Atilano SR, Coskun P, Chwa M, et al. Accumulation of mitochondrial DNA damage in keratoconus corneas. Invest Ophthalmol Vis Sci 2005;46(4):1256-63.

107. Wallace DC. Mitochondrial defects in neurodegenerative disease. Ment Retard Dev Disabil Res Rev 2001;7(3):158-66.
108. Brown MD, Wallace DC. Molecular basis of mitochondrial DNA disease. J Bioenerg Biomembr 1994;26(3):273-89.
109. Johns DR. Seminars in medicine of the Beth Israel Hospital, Boston. Mitochondrial DNA and disease. N Engl J Med 1995;333(10):638-44.
110. Green DR, Reed JC. Mitochondria and apoptosis. Science 1998;281(5381):1309-12.
111. Petit PX, Susin SA, Zamzami N, et al. Mitochondria and programmed cell death: back to the future. FEBS Lett 1996;396(1):7-13.
112. Richter C. Oxidative stress, mitochondria, and apoptosis. Restor Neurol Neurosci 1998;12(2,3):59-62.
113. Kenney MC, Brown DJ, Rajeev B. Everett Kinsey lecture. The elusive causes of keratoconus: a working hypothesis. Clao J 2000;26(1):10-3.
114. Chwa M, Atilano SR, Reddy V, et al. Increased stress-induced generation of reactive oxygen species and apoptosis in human keratoconus fibroblasts. Invest Ophthalmol Vis Sci 2006;47(5):1902-10.

***J Bradley Randleman**, MD, **R Doyle Stulting**, MD, PhD*

3 *Keratoconus after Refractive Surgery (Keratoectasia)*

Introduction

Corneal ectasia after laser in situ keratomileusis (LASIK) or photorefractive keratectomy (PRK) is a progressive steepening and thinning of the cornea (keratoectasia) that results in increasing myopia and astigmatism, and in its mild forms, it reduces uncorrected vision with slight loss of best spectacle-corrected visual acuity, In its worst forms, it requires corneal transplantation for visual rehabilitation.[1] Since the first reports in 1998,[2,3] there have been more than 170 reported cases of ectasia after PRK or LASIK.[4] Most of these have appeared as case reports, and very few larger series have been reported.[1, 4-9] From these reports, a variety of risk factors have been identified; however, patients have also developed ectasia without any of these proposed risk factors.[5-7,10-12]

Although less common now,[4] ectasia still occurs too often, and the onset of symptoms may be delayed for years after surgery. As postoperative corneal ectasia has both medical and medicolegal implications,[13] there has been much discussion[14-17] and research into potential mechanisms for this complication.[18-20]

Biomechanics of Postoperative Corneal Ectasia

Corneal refractive surgery alters the shape, thickness, curvature, and tensile strength of the normal cornea. Keratocyte density is greatest in the anterior 10% of the stroma and lowest in the posterior 40% of the stroma;[21,22] it decreases more significantly in the anterior stroma after PRK and in the posterior corneal stroma after LASIK.[23] Preliminary studies indicate that tensile strength is greatest in the anterior one-third and lowest in the posterior two-thirds of the corneal stroma.[18] The corneal flap does not contribute to the tensile strength of the cornea after LASIK.[2, 24]

Routine surgery on normal corneas decreases tensile strength by 13% after PRK and 27% after LASIK.[18] The elastic modulus of the keratoconic cornea was found to be 1.6 to 2.5 (average 2.1) times less than that of a normal cornea.[25] Postoperative ectasia may mimic this altered corneal elastic modulus. Biomechanical modeling approaches addressing corneal plasticity and viscoelasticity[19] and utilizing corneal parameters such as Young's modulus, Poisson's ratio, and curvature radius[20] may provide further insight into the ectatic process. In the future, preoperative corneal interferometry,[26] hysteresis measurements,[27] and dynamic corneal imaging[28] may serve to identify patients at risk for ectasia after LASIK if they are proven in the future to have acceptable sensitivity and specificity in evaluating patients for PRK and LASIK.

Incidence of Postoperative Keratoectasia

The reported incidence of ectasia after LASIK ranges from 0.04 to 0.6%.[1,8,9] These are rough estimations at best, as the incidence of ectasia varies significantly by surgery type and stringency of exclusion criteria used by the operating surgeon. Some feel that these reported incidences are overestimates for the total population of patients undergoing corneal refractive surgery;[29] however, approximately 50% of ophthalmologists who responded to the International Society of Refractive Surgery of the American Academy of Ophthalmology's (ISRS/AAO) practice patterns survey in 2004 had at least one case of keratoectasia in their practice.[30] Thus, the real incidence may actually be higher than has been previously reported.[31] In addition, eyes that eventually develop ectasia may not yet have been followed long enough for this to occur. The vast majority of cases have been reported after myopic LASIK,[4] and very few cases have been reported after hyperopic LASIK[32] or PRK.[33-36]

Diagnosis of Postoperative Corneal Ectasia

Chapter 5 discusses in detail the topographic analysis of ectasia. Of note, initially ectasia leads to increasing myopia and astigmatism and subtle topographic changes that may be misinterpreted as regression of effect **(Figure 3-1)**. Because enhancement of these eyes accelerates ectasia, they should be identified and enhancements should not be performed. Early indicators of ectasia include both reducing corneal thickness and inferior steepening over time. Although Orbscan II and Pentacam posterior float values are less reliable postoperatively, increasing posterior float values may be an early indication of ectasia. In more advanced cases, clinical and topographic changes become obvious **(Figure 3-2)**, including significant inferior steepening, increased anterior and posterior float values, and decreased corneal thickness.

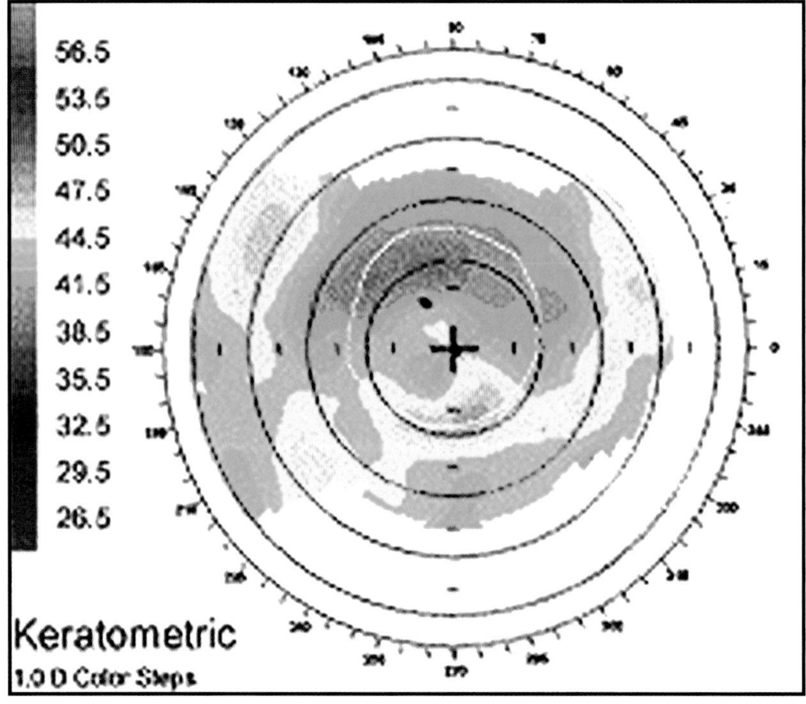

A

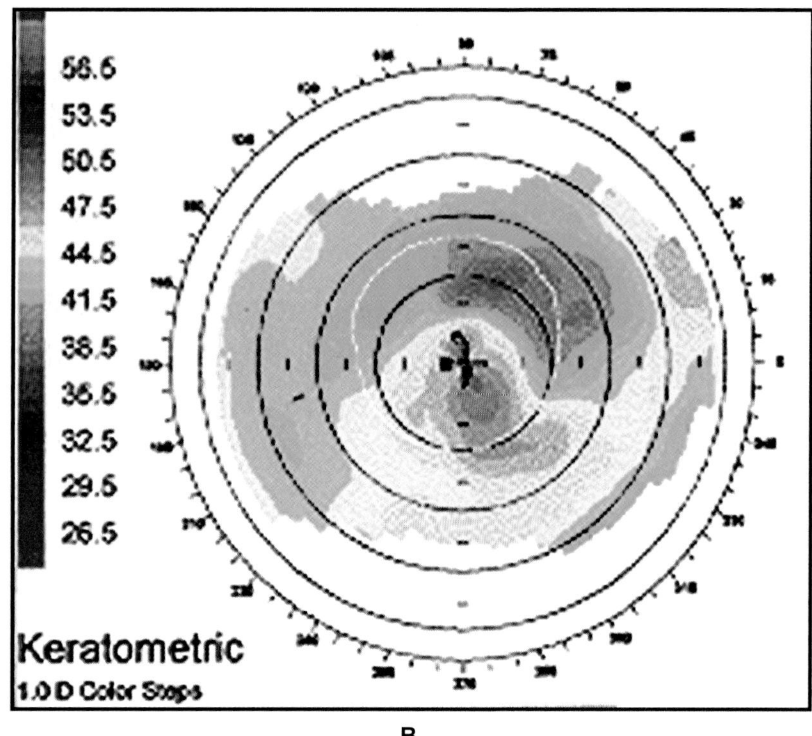

B

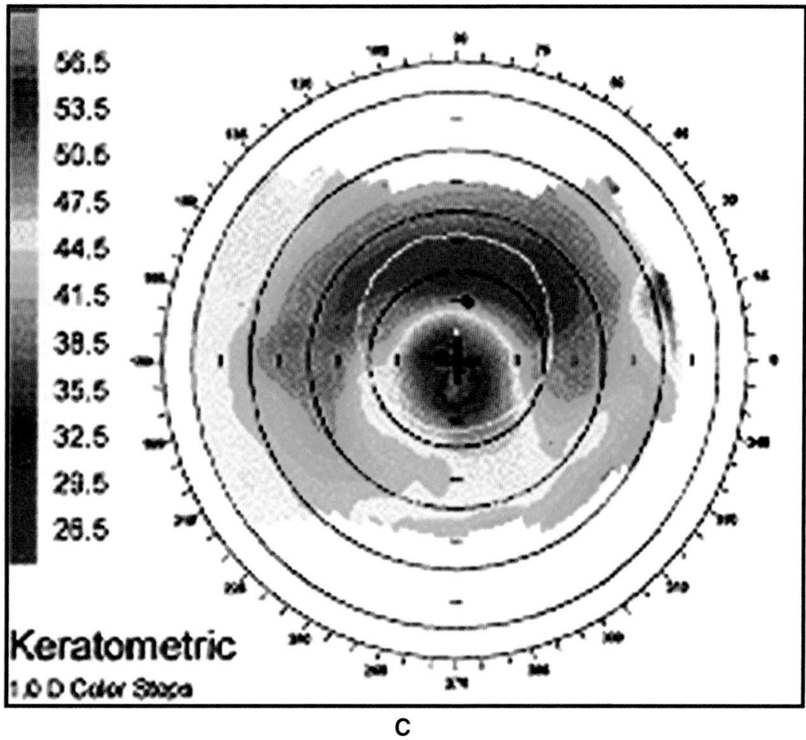

C

FIGURE 3-1: Serial topographies of a patient developing postoperative ectasia after LASIK: (A) 18 months postoperatively there is central irregular astigmatism with mild inferior steepening; (B) 27 months postoperatively there is increased inferior steepening; (C) 30 months postoperatively there is severe central and inferior steepening, with central K greater than 55 D.

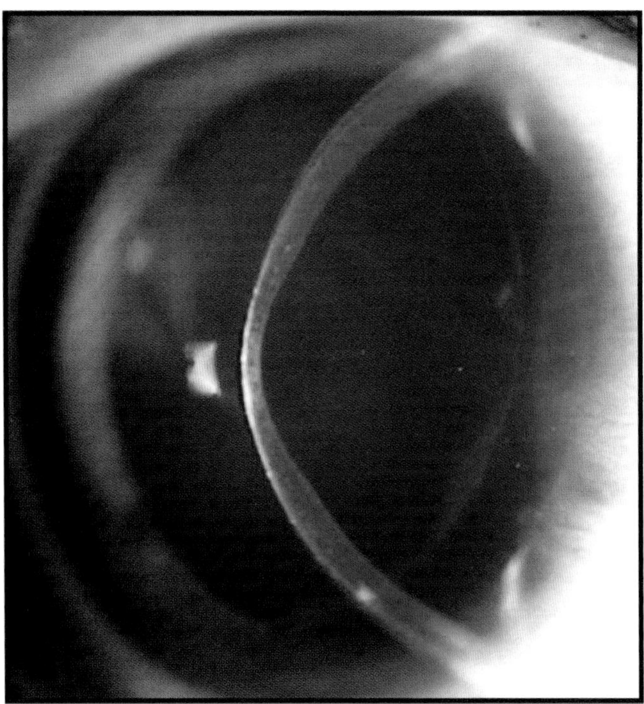

FIGURE 3-2: Keratoectasia after LASIK. Clinical photo demonstrating significant corneal thinning and an iron line circumferentially around the ectatic region.

Risk Factors for Postoperative Ectasia

Risk factors for ectasia include keratoconus and pellucid marginal corneal degeneration, forme fruste keratoconus, low residual stromal bed (RSB) thickness, young age, low preoperative corneal thickness, and high myopia.[4] Among these, abnormal preoperative topography, RSB thickness, and age appear to be the most significant factors, while preoperative corneal thickness and myopia are the least significant independent factors.[4] Abnormal preoperative topography is associated with the greatest relative risk for ectasia.

High Myopia

High myopia (>–12 D) has been reported to be a risk factor for ectasia;[1,4,8,9,33,37,38] however, ectasia can also occur in eyes with low preoperative myopia, and myopia is a poor predictor of ectasia in multivariate analysis.[4]

Thin Corneas

In comparative studies,[1,4] ectasia cases had significantly thinner corneas preoperatively than did controls. There are two potential explanations for these findings:

1. Keratoconic corneas are generally thinner than normal corneas,[39,40] therefore, low preoperative corneal thickness could be indicative of an abnormal cornea that is destined to develop keratoconus.
2. Thinner corneas could be at higher risk for ectasia because there is a higher probability that a thicker than expected corneal flap will result in an extremely low RSB that does not provide sufficient structural integrity to prevent ectasia.

Nevertheless, in multivariate analyses, preoperative corneal thickness was significantly less significant than RSB, age, or preoperative topography.[4]

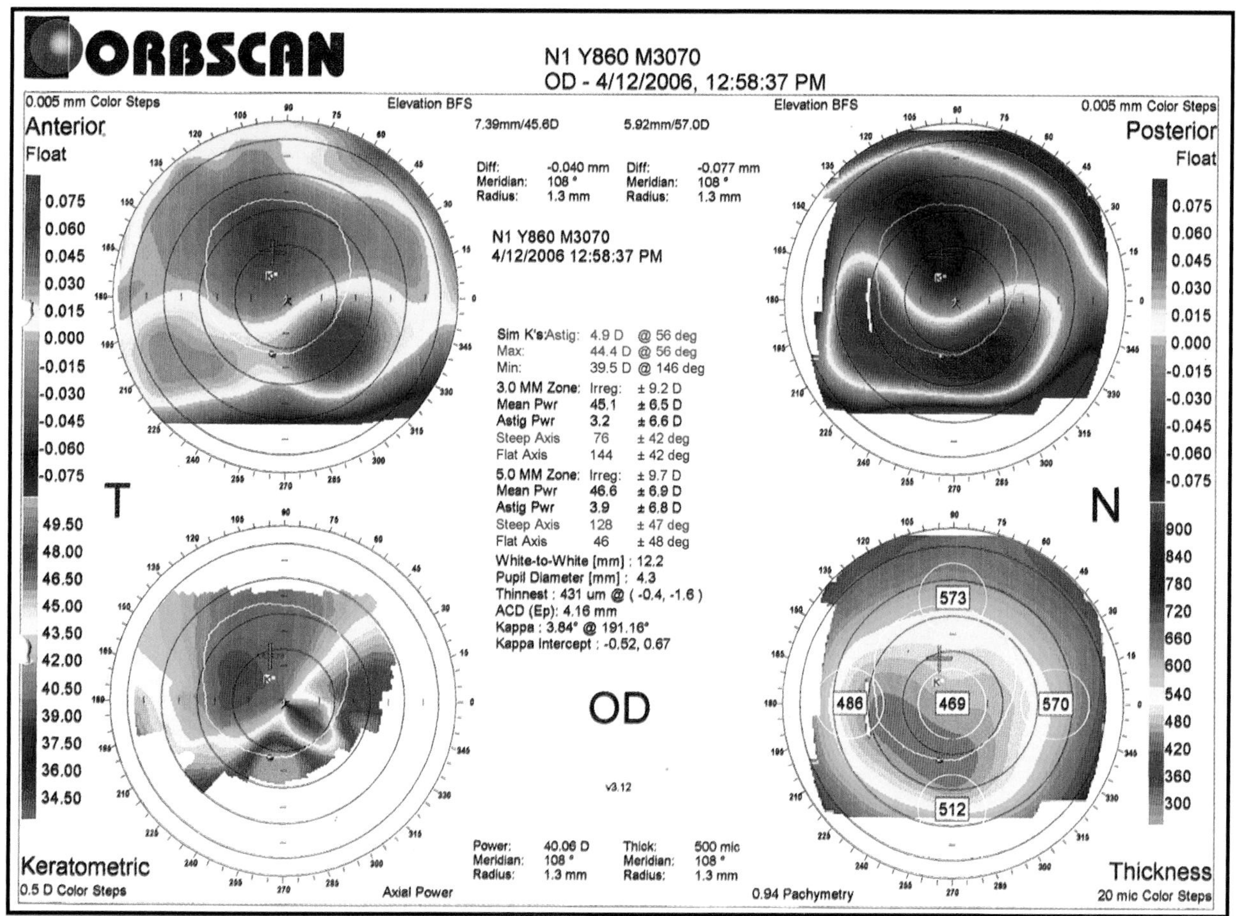

FIGURE 3-3: Representative Orbscan II topography demonstrating classical features of postoperative keratoectasia after LASIK, including significant inferior steepening on the keratometric map (lower left), increased anterior and posterior float elevations (upper right and left, respectively), and inferior thinning (lower right).

Low Residual Stromal Bed Thickness

Ectasia cases have had a significantly lower RSB than controls in comparative studies.[1, 4] Low RSB has always been thought to be one of the most significant risk factors for postoperative ectasia, and a generally accepted minimum RSB of 250 µm has been established.[41]

Factors contributing to low RSB include treatment of high refractive errors, thin preoperative corneas, excessively thick flaps, and deeper than expected stromal ablations. There can be significant variability in the thickness of corneal flaps[42-49] depending on microkeratome technology. While most of the microkeratome plate markings overestimate average actual flap thickness, flap thickness can vary widely with both mechanical microkeratomes and femtosecond lasers.[50, 51] Previous studies have also demonstrated that actual ablation depth is usually greater than estimated ablation depth.[43, 44]

While a 250 µm RSB is commonly accepted as a safe cut-off for LASIK, ectasia has occurred after LASIK in numerous eyes with calculated RSB greater than 250, including eyes with RSB greater than 300 µm confirmed by intraoperative pachymetry and after PRK in eyes with RSB greater than 350 µm.[35, 36, 52] Conversely, many eyes have undergone successful LASIK with RSB less than 225 µm.[1] Thus, decreasing RSB likely represents a continuum of postoperative ectasia risk rather than a definitive safety cut-off.

Only 31% of respondents to the ISRS/AAO survey routinely measure flap or RSB thickness intraoperatively.[30] Using a probability model that accounts for imprecision in corneal thickness, flap thickness, and laser ablation

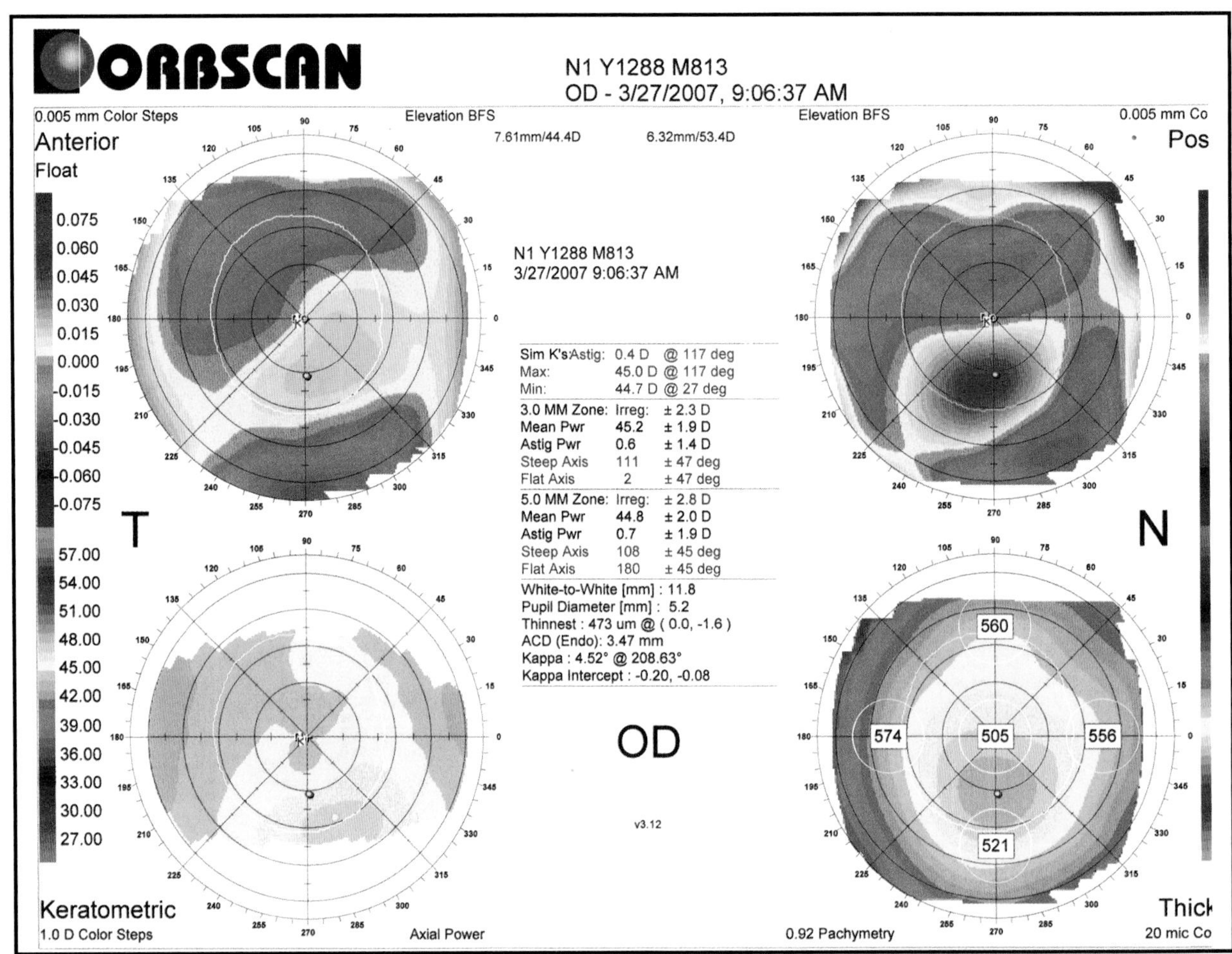

FIGURE 3-4: Preoperative Orbscan II topography demonstrating subtle changes of forme fruste keratoconus (FFKC). Keratometric map of anterior curvature (lower left) exhibits 3 diopters of inferior steepening. There are mild changes in the anterior float map (upper left) and there is significant posterior float elevation inferiorly (upper right) that correlates. Corneal thickness measurement (lower right) shows that the thinnest portion of the cornea is displaced inferiorly, corresponding to the posterior float elevation.

depth measurements, Reinstein and colleagues[53] determined that, depending on the microkeratome used, up to 33% of eyes with calculated RSB thickness of 250 μ could have actual RSB less than 200 μ. Therefore, we recommend that surgeons initially perform intraoperative pachymetry to become familiar with the performance of their microkeratomes and at least for those patients at risk for low RSB, if not for all LASIK cases. It is not necessary to perform intraoperative pachymetry on a routine basis once initial microkeratome evaluation has been performed.

Multiple enhancements further reduce RSB. Corneal thickness measurements taken months after initial LASIK usually overestimate RSB thickness.[54-56] If preoperative information is not available, accurate assessment of actual RSB prior to retreatment is critical to avoid excessive ablation of the posterior stroma. This can be accomplished by utilizing intraoperative pachymetry measurements prior to laser ablation at the time of retreatment, or by utilizing confocal microscopy[57] or high-speed optical coherence tomography (OCT)[58-60] prior to retreatment, as these instruments can accurately measure RSB thickness without ever lifting the flap.

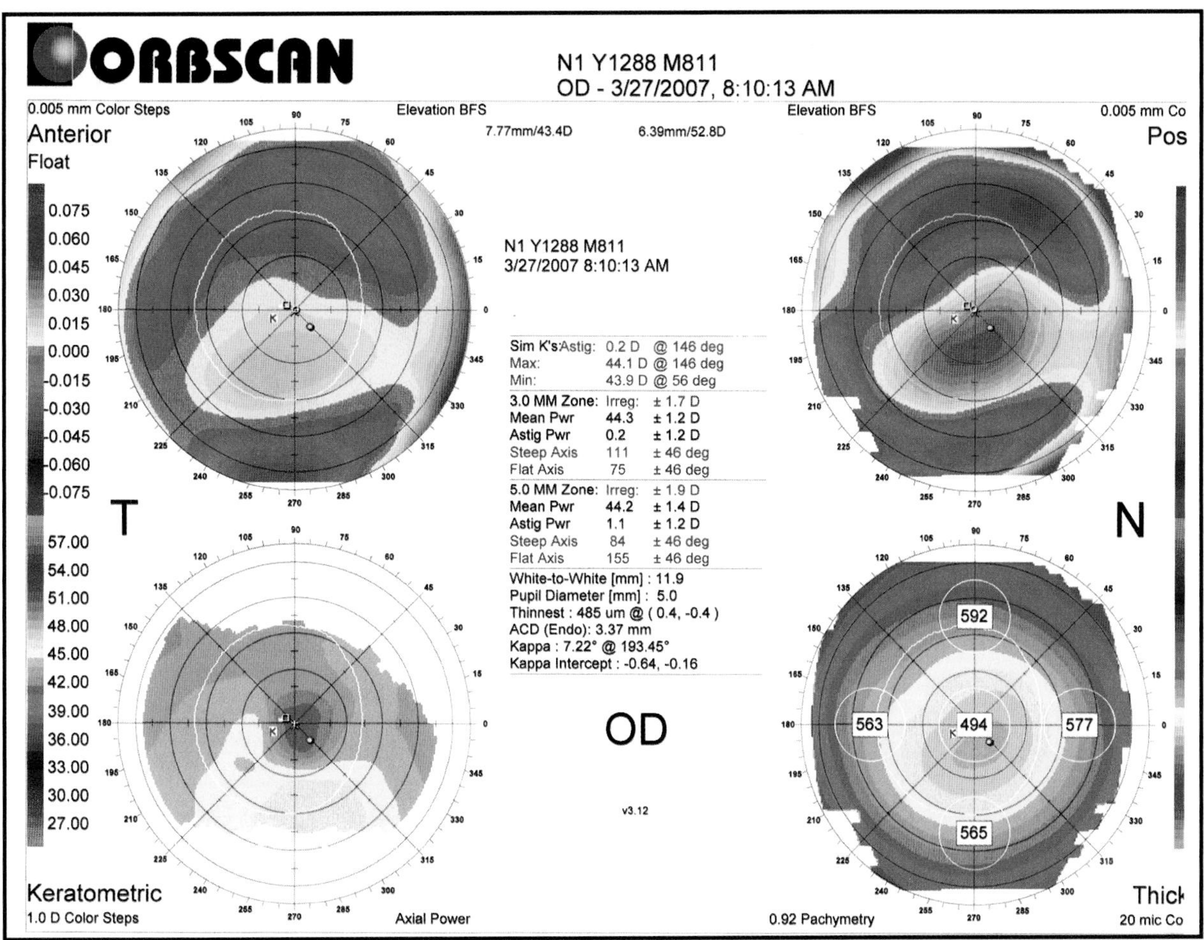

FIGURE 3-5: Preoperative Orbscan II topographies of FFKC in another patient. More pronounced topographic changes indicating FFKC. Keratometric map of anterior curvature (lower left) exhibits 5 diopters of inferior steepening. There are corresponding elevations in the anterior float map (upper left) and posterior float map (upper right). Corneal thickness measurement (lower right) shows that the thinnest portion of the cornea is displaced inferiorly, corresponding to the anterior and posterior float elevation. Patients in Figures 3-4 and 3-5 had more pronounced topographic changes in their contralateral eye.

Young Age

Patients who develop ectasia, especially those without classical, recognized risk factors, tend to be younger than average patients undergoing LASIK.[4, 77, 10-12] This observation may be explained by the fact that younger corneas are more susceptible to structural deformation due to decreased collagen crosslinking that naturally increases with age, or the fact that some younger patients are destined to develop clinical keratoconus in their 4th to 6th decades of life, but have not yet manifested any of the clinical or topographic findings of the disease process.[61, 62]

Ectatic Corneal Disorders and Forme Fruste Keratoconus

Ectatic disorders, including keratoconus, pellucid marginal corneal degeneration, and defined abnormal topographic patterns, such as forme fruste keratoconus (FFKC),[63] are the most significant risk factors for postoperative ectasia. Corneal topography should be carefully evaluated preoperatively in every case before deciding to proceed with surgery **(Figures 3.4 and 3.5)**. Many surgeons rely heavily on topographic software programs designed to identify keratoconus suspects,[29] however, recent evidence suggests that other more subtle topographic abnormalities place patients at increased risk for ectasia after LASIK[4, 64] such as inferior steepening that does not meet FFKC criteria. Additionally, preoperative topographies suggestive of pellucid marginal corneal degeneration may be read as normal with current topographic software.[65] Chapter 5 discusses this topography assessment in more detail.

Other factors, such as contact lens warpage and keratoconjunctivitis sicca, can create topographic changes that resemble those of forme fruste keratoconus.[66] These factors may make it more challenging to differentiate normal from abnormal topographies. We therefore recommend repeating topographic examinations at a later time in questionable cases, and if available, utilizing multiple technologies, since a variety of imaging systems can provide unique information and decrease the odds of artifactual readings.[67]

Other Potential Risk Factors

In addition to the aforementioned risk factors, other factors should be considered, including more subtle topographic abnormalities and higher order aberrations (coma), multiple enhancements, chronic trauma (eye rubbing), family history of keratoconus, and refractive instability (increasing refractive cylinder) with preoperative best spectacle-corrected visual acuity worse than 20/20.

Recommendations from the Joint AAO/ISRS/ASCRS Committee on Corneal Ectasia after LASIK

Recently, a joint committee was formed from members of the American Academy of Ophthalmology (AAO) and the American Society for Cataract and Refractive Surgery (ASCRS) to summarize current knowledge on keratoectasia after LASIK and make recommendations to avoid this complication.[13] This committee emphasized that no single test or evaluation can ultimately determine risk for postoperative ectasia, that ectasia can occur in individuals without any identifiable risk factors, and that the occurrence of postoperative ectasia does not in itself constitute a breach from the standard of care.

They further recommend that preoperative topographies be evaluated in all cases and that intraoperative pachymetry be measured in all cases where the patient may be at risk for low RSB. In addition to forme fruste keratoconus, the members of the AAO/ASCRS joint committee further recommend avoiding LASIK in patients with asymmetric inferior corneal steepening or asymmetric bowtie patterns with skewed steep radial axes.[13]

Conclusion

Postoperative corneal ectasia after LASIK or PRK is a relatively rare, but very serious complication of modern refractive surgery. New insights into the biomechanical mechanisms underlying the development of ectasia, combined with the detection of previously unrecognized risk factors have resulted in improved preoperative screening techniques and should further reduce the incidence of this complication. To date, there is no single characteristic that identifies all at-risk patients; therefore, screening strategies that weigh all of the known potential risk factors should be more effective than considering any of the factors in isolation. In spite of extensive screening efforts, some patients will still develop postoperative ectasia without any of the aforementioned risk factors. Further research may allow the identification of underlying biomechanical abnormalities that may explain some cases of ectasia that occur without currently identified risk factors.

Acknowledgments and Grant Support: Supported in part by Research to Prevent Blindness, Inc. New York, and the National Institutes of Health Core Grant P30 EYO6360, Bethesda, Maryland.

References

1. Randleman JB, Russell B, Ward MA, et al. Risk factors and prognosis for corneal ectasia after LASIK. Ophthalmology 2003;110(2):267-75.
2. Seiler T, Koufala K, Richter G. Iatrogenic keratectasia after laser in situ keratomileusis. J Refract Surg 1998;14(3):312-7.
3. Seiler T, Quurke AW. Iatrogenic keratectasia after LASIK in a case of forme fruste keratoconus. J Cataract Refract Surg 1998;24(7):1007-9.
4. Randleman JB, Woodward M, Lynn MJ, Stulting RD. Risk assesment for ectasia after corneal refractive surgery. Ophthalmology (in press).
5. Amoils SP, Deist MB, Gous P, Amoils PM. Iatrogenic keratectasia after laser in situ keratomileusis for less than –4.0 to –7.0 diopters of myopia. J Cataract Refract Surg 2000;26(7):967-77.
6. Argento C, Cosentino MJ, Tytiun A, et al. Corneal ectasia after laser in situ keratomileusis. J Cataract Refract Surg 2001;27(9):1440-8.
7. Klein SR, Epstein RJ, Randleman JB, Stulting RD. Corneal ectasia after laser in situ keratomileusis in patients without apparent preoperative risk factors. Cornea 2006;25(4):388-403.
8. Pallikaris IG, Kymionis GD, Astyrakakis NI. Corneal ectasia induced by laser in situ keratomileusis. J Cataract Refract Surg 2001;27(11):1796-802.
9. Rad AS, Jabbarvand M, Saifi N. Progressive keratectasia after laser in situ keratomileusis. J Refract Surg 2004;20(5 Suppl):S718-22.
10. Lifshitz T, Levy J, Klemperer I, Levinger S. Late bilateral keratectasia after LASIK in a low myopic patient. J Refract Surg 2005;21(5):494-6.
11. Piccoli PM, Gomes AA, Piccoli FV. Corneal ectasia detected 32 months after LASIK for correction of myopia and asymmetric astigmatism. J Cataract Refract Surg 2003;29(6):1222-5.
12. Wang JC, Hufnagel TJ, Buxton DF. Bilateral keratectasia after unilateral laser in situ keratomileusis: a retrospective diagnosis of ectatic corneal disorder. J Cataract Refract Surg 2003;29(10):2015-8.
13. Binder PS, Lindstrom RL, Stulting RD, et al. Keratoconus and corneal ectasia after LASIK. J Cataract Refract Surg 2005;31(11):2035-8.
14. Comaish IF, Lawless MA. Progressive post-LASIK keratectasia: biomechanical instability or chronic disease process? J Cataract Refract Surg 2002;28(12):2206-13.
15. Koch DD. The riddle of iatrogenic keratectasia. J Cataract Refract Surg 1999;25(4):453-4.
16. Kohnen T. Iatrogenic keratectasia: current knowledge, current measurements. J Cataract Refract Surg 2002;28(12):2065-6.
17. Seiler T. Iatrogenic keratectasia: academic anxiety or serious risk? J Cataract Refract Surg 1999;25(10):1307-8.
18. Dawson DG, O'Brien TP, Dubovy SR, et al. Post-LASIK Ectasia: Histopathology, Ultrastructure, and Corneal Physiology from Human Corneal Buttons and Eye Bank Donors Presented at the AAO Annual Meeting, Las Vegas NV 2006.
19. Dupps WJ, Jr. Biomechanical modeling of corneal ectasia. J Refract Surg 2005;21(2):186-90.
20. Guirao A. Theoretical elastic response of the cornea to refractive surgery: risk factors for keratectasia. J Refract Surg 2005;21(2):176-85.
21. Moller-Pedersen T, Ledet T, Ehlers N. The keratocyte density of human donor corneas. Curr Eye Res 1994;13(2):163-9.
22. Patel S, McLaren J, Hodge D, Bourne W. Normal human keratocyte density and corneal thickness measurement by using confocal microscopy in vivo. Invest Ophthalmol Vis Sci 2001;42(2):333-9.
23. Erie JC, Patel SV, McLaren JW, et al. Corneal keratocyte deficits after photorefractive keratectomy and laser in situ keratomileusis. Am J Ophthalmol 2006;141(5):799-809.
24. Chang DH, Stulting RD. Change in intraocular pressure measurements after LASIK the effect of the refractive correction and the lamellar flap. Ophthalmology 2005;112(6):1009-16.
25. Andreassen TT, Simonsen AH, Oxlund H. Biomechanical properties of keratoconus and normal corneas. Exp Eye Res 1980;31(4):435-41.
26. Jaycock PD, Lobo L, Ibrahim J, et al. Interferometric technique to measure biomechanical changes in the cornea induced by refractive surgery. J Cataract Refract Surg 2005;31(1):175-84.
27. Luce DA. Determining in vivo biomechanical properties of the cornea with an ocular response analyzer. J Cataract Refract Surg 2005;31(1):156-62.
28. Grabner G, Eilmsteiner R, Steindl C, et al. Dynamic corneal imaging. J Cataract Refract Surg 2005;31(1):163-74.
29. Condon PI. 2005 ESCRS Ridley Medal Lecture: will keratectasia be a major complication for LASIK in the long-term? J Cataract Refract Surg 2006;32(12):2124-32.
30. Duffey RJ, Leaming D. US trends in refractive surgery: 2004 ISRS/AAO Survey. J Refract Surg 2005;21(6):742-8.
31. Randleman JB. Post-laser in-situ keratomileusis ectasia: current understanding and future directions. Curr Opin Ophthalmol 2006;17(4):406-12.
32. Randleman JB, Banning CS, Stulting RD. Corneal ectasia after hyperopic LASIK. J Refract Surg 2006;22 (in press).

33. Holland SP, Srivannaboon S, Reinstein DZ. Avoiding serious corneal complications of laser assisted in situ keratomileusis and photorefractive keratectomy. Ophthalmology 2000;107(4):640-52.
34. Lovisolo CF, Fleming JF. Intracorneal ring segments for iatrogenic keratectasia after laser in situ keratomileusis or photorefractive keratectomy. J Refract Surg 2002;18(5):535-41.
35. Malecaze F, Coullet J, Calvas P, et al. Corneal ectasia after photorefractive keratectomy for low myopia. Ophthalmology 2006;113(5):742-6.
36. Randleman JB, Caster AI, Banning CS, Stulting RD. Corneal ectasia after photorefractive keratectomy. J Cataract Refract Surg 2006;32(8):1395-8.
37. Alio J, Salem T, Artola A, Osman A. Intracorneal rings to correct corneal ectasia after laser in situ keratomileusis. J Cataract Refract Surg 2002;28(9):1568-74.
38. Spadea L, Palmieri G, Mosca L, et al. Iatrogenic keratectasia following laser in situ keratomileusis. J Refract Surg 2002;18(4):475-80.
39. Haque S, Simpson T, Jones L. Corneal and epithelial thickness in keratoconus: a comparison of ultrasonic pachymetry, Orbscan II, and optical coherence tomography. J Refract Surg 2006;22(5):486-93.
40. Ucakhan OO, Kanpolat A, Ylmaz N, Ozkan M. In vivo confocal microscopy findings in keratoconus. Eye Contact Lens 2006;32(4):183-91.
41. Checklist of information usually submitted in an investigational device exemption (IDE) application for refractive surgery lasers. Ophthalmic Devices Advisory Panel, Food and Drug Administration. J Refract Surg 1997;13(6):579-88.
42. Dougherty PJ, Wellish KL, Maloney RK. Excimer laser ablation rate and corneal hydration. Am J Ophthalmol 1994;118(2):169-76.
43. Durairaj VD, Balentine J, Kouyoumdjian G, et al. The predictability of corneal flap thickness and tissue laser ablation in laser in situ keratomileusis. Ophthalmology 2000;107(12):2140-3.
44. Chang AW, Tsang AC, Contreras JE, et al. Corneal tissue ablation depth and the Munnerlyn formula. J Cataract Refract Surg 2003;29(6):1204-10.
45. Iskander NG, Anderson Penno E, Peters NT, et al. Accuracy of Orbscan pachymetry measurements and DHG ultrasound pachymetry in primary laser in situ keratomileusis and LASIK enhancement procedures. J Cataract Refract Surg 2001;27(5):681-5.
46. Prisant O, Calderon N, Chastang P, et al. Reliability of pachymetric measurements using orbscan after excimer refractive surgery. Ophthalmology 2003;110(3):511-5.
47. Salz JJ, Azen SP, Berstein J, et al. Evaluation and comparison of sources of variability in the measurement of corneal thickness with ultrasonic and optical pachymeters. Ophthalmic Surg 1983;14(9):750-4.
48. Yildirim R, Aras C, Ozdamar A, et al. Reproducibility of corneal flap thickness in laser in situ keratomileusis using the Hansatome microkeratome. J Cataract Refract Surg 2000;26(12):1729-32.
49. Jacobs BJ, Deutsch TA, Rubenstein JB. Reproducibility of corneal flap thickness in LASIK. Ophthalmic Surg Lasers 1999;30(5):350-3.
50. Binder PS. One thousand consecutive IntraLase laser in situ keratomileusis flaps. J Cataract Refract Surg 2006;32(6):962-9.
51. Talamo JH, Meltzer J, Gardner J. Reproducibility of flap thickness with IntraLase FS and Moria LSK-1 and M2 microkeratomes. J Refract Surg 2006;22(6):556-61.
52. Kim H, Choi JS, Joo CK. Corneal ectasia after PRK: clinicopathologic case report. Cornea 2006;25(7):845-8.
53. Reinstein DZ, Srivannaboon S, Archer TJ, et al. Probability model of the inaccuracy of residual stromal thickness prediction to reduce the risk of ectasia after LASIK part I: quantifying individual risk. J Refract Surg 2006;22(9):851-60.
54. Flanagan GW, Binder PS. Precision of flap measurements for laser in situ keratomileusis in 4428 eyes. J Refract Surg 2003;19(2):113-23.
55. Randleman JB, Hewitt SM, Lynn MJ, Stulting RD. A comparison of 2 methods for estimating residual stromal bed thickness before repeat LASIK. Ophthalmology 2005;112(1):98-103.
56. Das S, Sullivan LJ. Comparison of residual stromal bed and flap thickness in primary and repeat laser in situ keratomileusis in myopic patients. J Cataract Refract Surg 2006;32(12):2080-4.
57. Vinciguerra P, Torres I, Camesasca FI. Applications of confocal microscopy in refractive surgery. J Refract Surg 2002;18(3 Suppl):S378-81.
58. Avila M, Li Y, Song JC, Huang D. High-speed optical coherence tomography for management after laser in situ keratomileusis. J Cataract Refract Surg 2006;32(11):1836-42.
59. Maldonado MJ, Ruiz-Oblitas L, Munuera JM, et al. Optical coherence tomography evaluation of the corneal cap and stromal bed features after laser in situ keratomileusis for high myopia and astigmatism. Ophthalmology 2000;107(1):81-7; discussion 8.
60. Li Y, Netto MV, Shekhar R, et al. A longitudinal study of LASIK flap and stromal thickness with high-speed optical coherence tomography. Ophthalmology 2007.
61. Owens H, Gamble G. A profile of keratoconus in New Zealand. Cornea 2003;22(2):122-5.

62. Zadnik K, Barr JT, Gordon MO, Edrington TB. Biomicroscopic signs and disease severity in keratoconus. Collaborative longitudinal evaluation of keratoconus (CLEK) study group. Cornea 1996;15(2):139-46.
63. Rabinowitz YS, McDonnell PJ. Computer-assisted corneal topography in keratoconus. Refract Corneal Surg 1989;5(6):400-8.
64. Abad JC, Rubinfeld RS, Valle MD, et al. Vertical D A Novel topographic pattern in some keratoconus suspects. Ophthalmology 2007.
65. Klein SR, Muller LT, Uwaydat S, et al. Poor visual outcomes following corneal surgery refractive surgery in patients with clinically unsuspected pellucid marginal degeneration. AAO Annual Meeting, Anaheim CA 2003.
66. De Paiva CS, Harris LD, Pflugfelder SC. Keratoconus-like topographic changes in keratoconjunctivitis sicca. Cornea 2003;22(1):22-4.
67. Quisling S, Sjoberg S, Zimmerman B, et al. Comparison of Pentacam and Orbscan IIz on posterior curvature topography measurements in keratoconus eyes. Ophthalmology 2006;113(9):1629-32.

Section 2

Diagnosing Keratoconus and Keratoectasia

Michael K Smolek, *PhD*

4 Clinical Signs

External Signs

There are relatively few external signs for keratoconus. The most well-known is Munson's sign. The patient is asked to look downward towards the floor and the examiner views the lower eyelid margin from a slightly superior vantage point. Slight adjustments of the patient's direction of gaze may be necessary to obtain the best view of the eyelid profile. A lower, peripheral cone (the most common form of keratoconus) will deform the inferior eyelid margin in a mild V-shaped profile as the margin conforms to the rather pointed cornea which differs than the contour of the eyelid with a normal cornea **(Figure 4-1)**. Rare, superiorly located cones are less likely to have a visible effect on the profile of the lower eyelid. Moderate to severe keratoconus tends

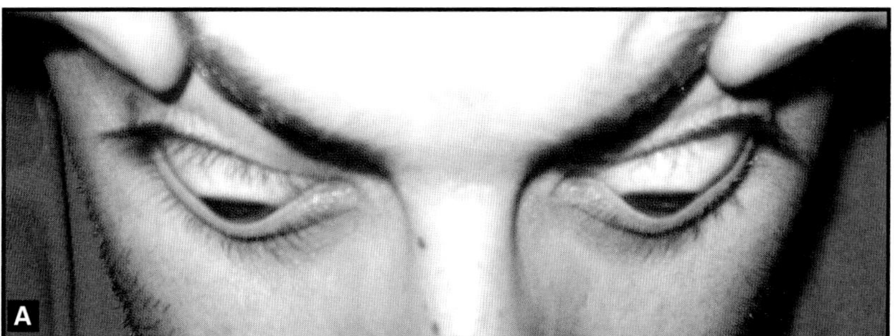

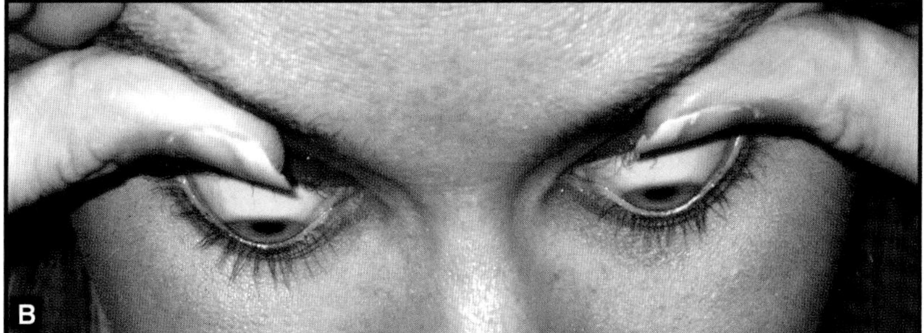

FIGURE 4-1: Eyelid contours. There is a V-shaped protrusion of the eyelid with keratoconus (A) compared to lid contour from normal cornea (B) (Courtesy: Brian S Boxer Wachler, MD).

to produce Munson's sign, while mild cases of keratoconus will not produce this sign since corneal bulging is more subtle.

Rizzuti's sign is another external sign for keratoconus. This sign is observed by focusing a light on the nasal anterior sclera where the light is directed into the cornea from the temporal direction. The optics of the cone refracts the incoming light back onto the nasal sclera, whereas in the normal cornea, this focusing effect is not seen. As with Munson's sign, this Rizzuti's sign is more reliable for screening moderate to severe cones and is less sensitive for mild keratoconus.

Retinoscopy Signs

The scissoring effect of the retinal reflex seen with manual retinoscopy is largely diagnostic of keratoconus. Because the optical pathlength through the eye is longer along the direction that light travels through the cone apex compared to the surrounding region, the retinoscopic reflex will tend to appear distorted and flash unevenly as the light streak from the retinoscope is passed across the pupil of the patient. This distortion is commonly referred to as a scissoring effect. Retinoscopy is best performed with dilated pupils which allows exposure of the corneal periphery, the location of most cones. Unlike Munson's sign, the scissoring effect is considered to be sensitive to even mild forms of keratoconus.

Slit Lamp Biomicroscopy Signs

The slit lamp examination has been the traditional workhorse in the diagnosis of keratoconus, but as with many tests, the signs are often based on subjective observations rather than objective measurements. This does not mean that such tests are invalid, but rather that the subtle nature of the signs need to be learned. The experienced clinician who has observed many examples of the disease at different stages of development will be far more skilled than the less experienced clinician who has seen only a handful of cases.

One of the most useful slit lamp signs is focal thinning at the cone apex, which is often in the lower cornea. This is considered a sensitive test because assessing corneal thinning is a "hyperacuity" task for a clinician. Hyperacuity is the ability to recognize spatial displacement, such as a curve or bend in an otherwise straight edge.[1] The clinician views an optical cross-section produced by a thin slit beam under high magnification. Localized thinning in the patient's cornea will be seen as a change in the width (anterior to posterior distance) of the optical section caused by a deviation in the curvature along one or both of the edges of the illuminated section that demarcate the front and back surfaces of the patient's cornea. A potential limitation of visually assessing corneal thickness with the slit lamp is the inability to recognize thinning in regions that are not typical for keratoconus. A cone may occasionally be located in the superior, nasal, or temporal quadrants as well as centrally. In particular, when mild thinning occurs centrally, it may be difficult to detect this as a sign of pathology because this region is naturally thinner relative to the peripheral cornea.

Fleischer's iron ring is sign of keratoconus and it partially or completely encircles the base of the cone **(Figure 4-2)**. Fleischer's ring is due to accumulations of ferritin particles in corneal basal epithelial cells. In normal corneas, ferritin particles are randomly and diffusely scattered throughout the corneal epithelium and basal cells of the conjunctiva, but are not found in corneal stroma or endothelium.[2]

As the cornea continues to thin and bulge out, "stretch marks" may develop in the form of anterior stromal scars, which may be small or large **(Figure 4-3)**. The size and location of scar determines its impact on visual function. Vogt's striae are a sign of corneal stretching and protrusion. These thin, brightly vertical lines appear to be located deep in the stroma adjacent to Descemets' layer **(Figure 4-4)**. Vogt's striae may be explained by an increase in the light reflectivity that occurs from changes in the relative index of refraction in stromal

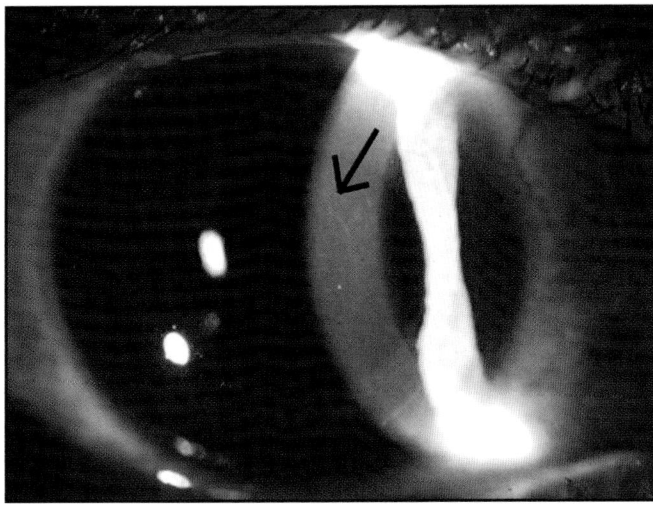

FIGURE 4-2: Fleischer's ring. Note the brown circular ring (arrow) that surrounds the cone (Courtesy: Brian S Boxer Wachler, MD).

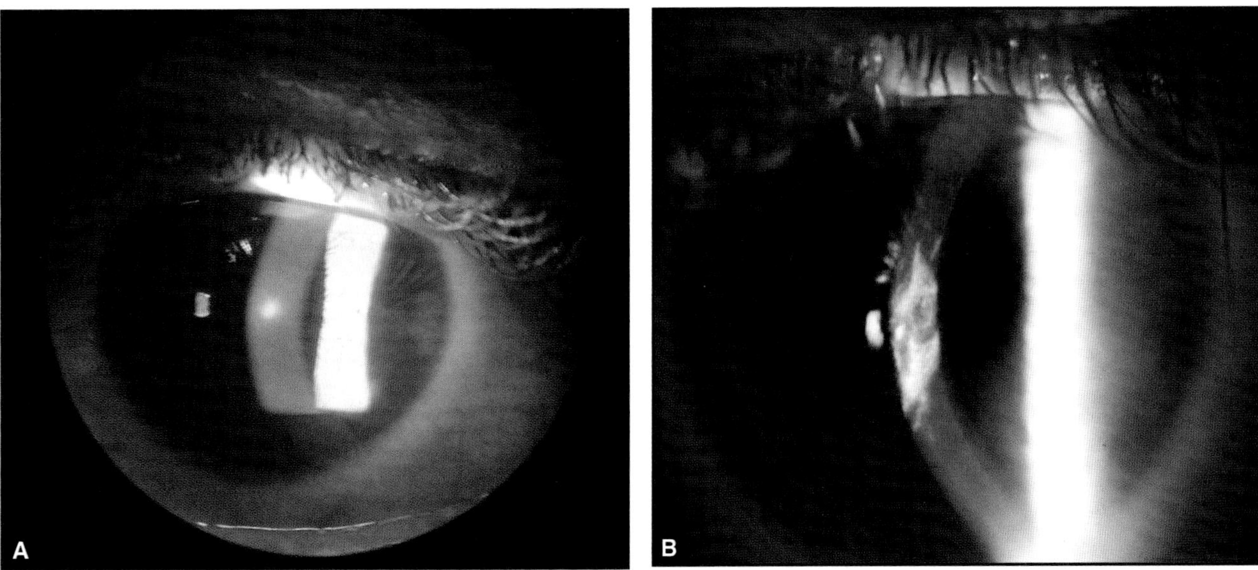

FIGURE 4-3: Corneal scarring. Note the small, non-significant scar (A) compared to the large, reticular scar (B) (Courtesy: Brian S Boxer Wachler, MD).

collagen that is under shearing tension from increased strain. Such forces may be a combination of eyelid shearing forces and tension, the weight of corneal acting upon its own weakened structure, and forces of intraocular pressure within the eye. When the cornea is depressed, Vogt's striae often disappear, only to return once the externally applied tension is released.

If stretching becomes excessive, the cornea may eventually tear in the posteriorly located Descemets' layer. This tear allows aqueous fluid to enter the otherwise protected corneal stroma. Normal corneal stroma is compact like a dry sponge. With a Descemet's tear, fluid has immediate access to the stroma and it swells like a sponge. This intense stromal edema often results in acute blurred vision since the tears often occur centrally. When the endothelium migrates to cover the tear, edema resolves and a posterior scar forms **(Figure 4-5)**. Tears can occur in the corneal periphery which may have minimal impact on vision **(Figure 4-6)**.

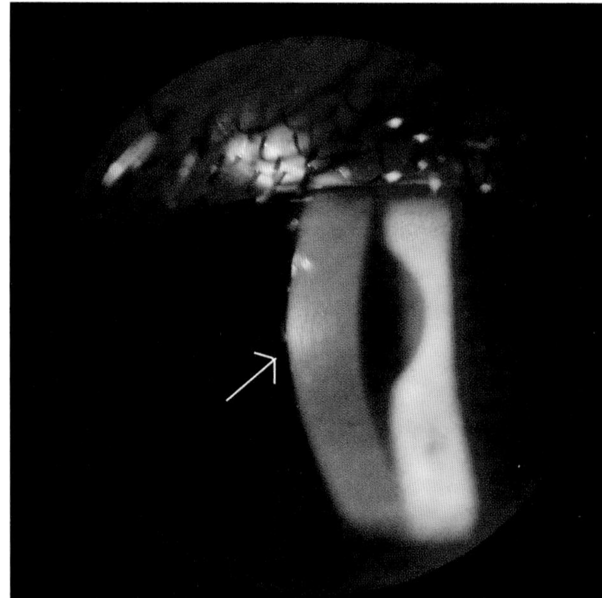

FIGURE 4-4: Vogt's striae. There are posterior vertical stress lines (arrow) result from focal outward stretching of the cornea (Courtesy: Brian S Boxer Wachler, MD).

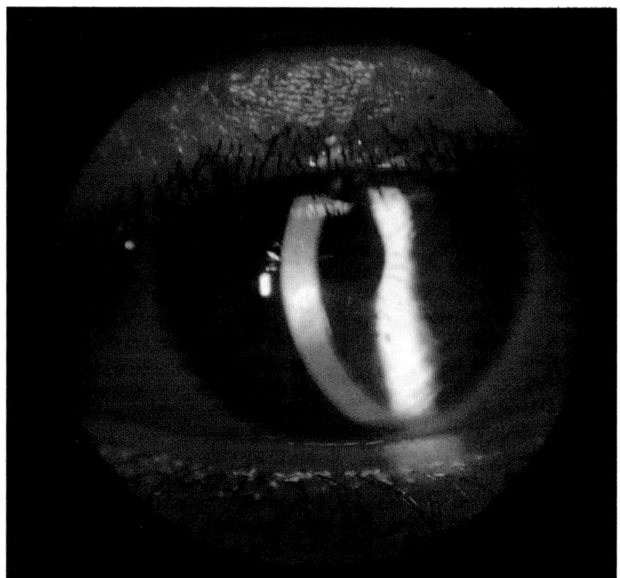

FIGURE 4-5: Central scar after hydrops episode had healed (Courtesy: Brian S Boxer Wachler, MD).

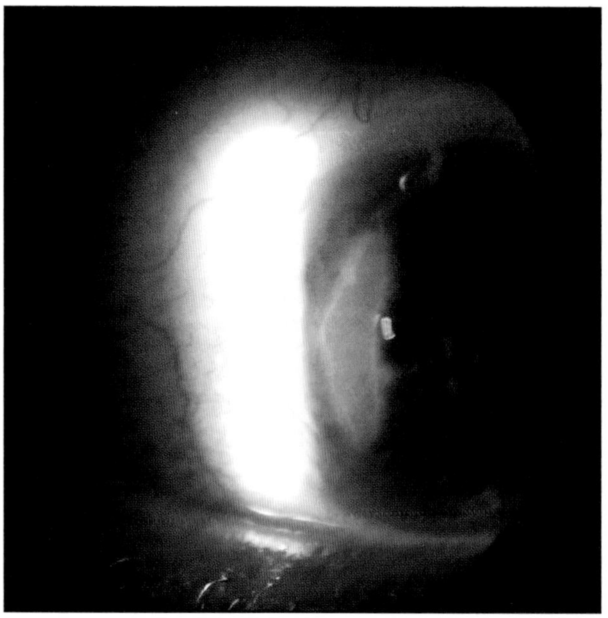

FIGURE 4-6: Active temporal hydrops (white area), an uncommon location for hydrops (Courtesy: Brian S Boxer Wachler, MD).

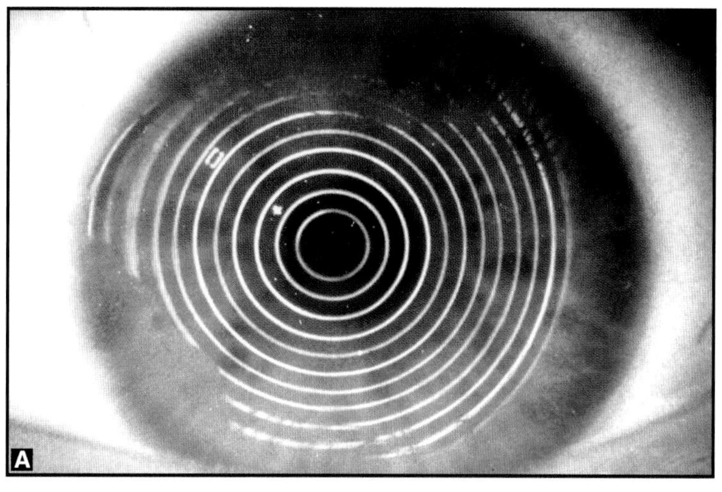

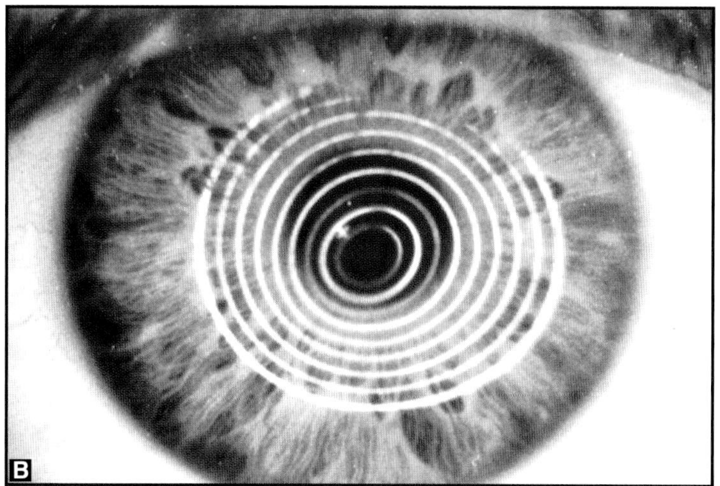

FIGURE 4-7: Photokeratoscopy: (A) Normal cornea. Note the round, concentric rings. (B) Keratoconic cornea. Note the asymmetric, concentric rings (Courtesy: Brian S Boxer Wachler, MD and Daniel S. Durrie, MD).

Keratoscopy and Photokeratoscopy Signs

Keratoscopy is the precursor to modern corneal topography, which still relies on keratoscopy principles. Keratoscopy uses a pattern of concentric rings (mires) called a Placido disk with approximately 9 alternating bright and dark rings.[3] The rings are reflected off the anterior cornea surface via Purkinje image number one and viewed directly by the clinician. The Placido disk is nothing more than a simple, inexpensive hand-held device with a central peep-hole for the clinician through which to look. The clinician subjectively analyzes the pattern of the rings to assess if irregular astigmatism or keratoconus exists. Photokeratoscopy is the same basic device as the keratoscope except that the Placido disk is back-illuminated with a strobe flash and a camera replaces the clinician's eye at the viewing port that takes a picture of the reflected mire pattern.

When the curved surface of the cornea is viewed with the keratoscope or photokeratoscope, the rings appear to be thin and tightly squeezed together in those regions where the curvature was steep and broadly dispersed wherever the curvature was flat. The clinician needs to be familiar with these patterns in order to interpret them. At the time, computers were not linked and did not interpret the ring patterns as occurs with corneal topography.

For a normal spherical cornea the rings appeared to be circular **(Figure 4-7)**. With corneal astigmatism, the rings appeared to be oval with the short axis corresponding to the steep meridian. In keratoconus, the rings were distorted and grouped more closely in the region of the cone (steep curvature) **(Figure 4-7)**. Moderate and severe forms of keratoconus were easy to distinguish using these mires, but subtly compressed rings were difficult to appreciate in mild keratoconus. Central keratoconus detection was also a challenge for keratoscopy as the mires tended to be uniformly tight, which was not as obvious as the asymmetry which was found in peripheral keratoconus. Keratoscopy and photokeratoscopy were replaced by corneal topography, which incorporates their principles. Modern topography uses computer processing of the mires to yield accurate color maps with numerical indices.

Conclusion

In the past, clinical diagnosis of keratoconus allowed identification of moderate to severe forms of keratoconus. As technology developed, use of a circular pattern of lighted rings (Placido disk) that reflected off the cornea allowed more accurate assessment of corneal shape. The Placido disk is the foundation for modern corneal topography, which presently uses this disk.

References

1. Watt RJ, Andrews DP. Contour curvature analysis: hyperacuities in the discrimination of detailed shape Vision Res. 1982; 22:449-60.
2. Iwamoto T, DeVoe AG. Electron microscopical study of the Fleisher ring. Archives of Ophthalmology 1975;94:1579-84.
3. Knoll HA. Corneal contours in the general population as revealed by the photokeratoscope. American Journal of Optometry & Archives of American Academy of Optometry 1961;38:389-97.

Michael K Smolek, PhD, **Brian S Boxer Wachler,** MD

5 Corneal Topography

Introduction

Corneal topography (formerly known as videokeratography) is the current gold standard for keratoconus screening and is based upon prior technology used for keratoconus assessment.[1,2] There are confounding conditions such as corneal scarring, hyperopic refractive surgery, and contact lens-induced corneal warpage that can produce topography maps similar to keratoconus. Patient history, corneal pachymetry, and slit lamp evaluation for prior corneal surgery can rule out these other conditions.

Axial and Instantaneous Maps

Most corneal topographers use a Placido disk **(Figure 5-1)** while others use slit scanning methods or a combination of both. It is not possible here to describe in detail the advantages and disadvantages of each system, but

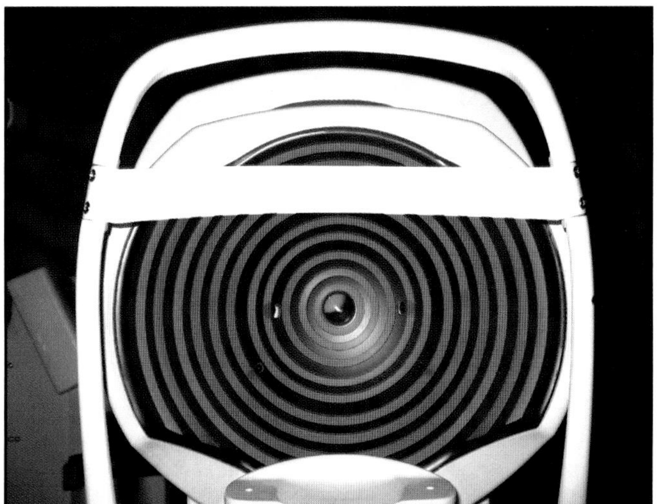

FIGURE 5-1: Placido disk. The concentric red circles of the Nidek device are projected on to the cornea. A camera captures the reflected image and analyzes the pattern for the topography display map that is used by the clinician.

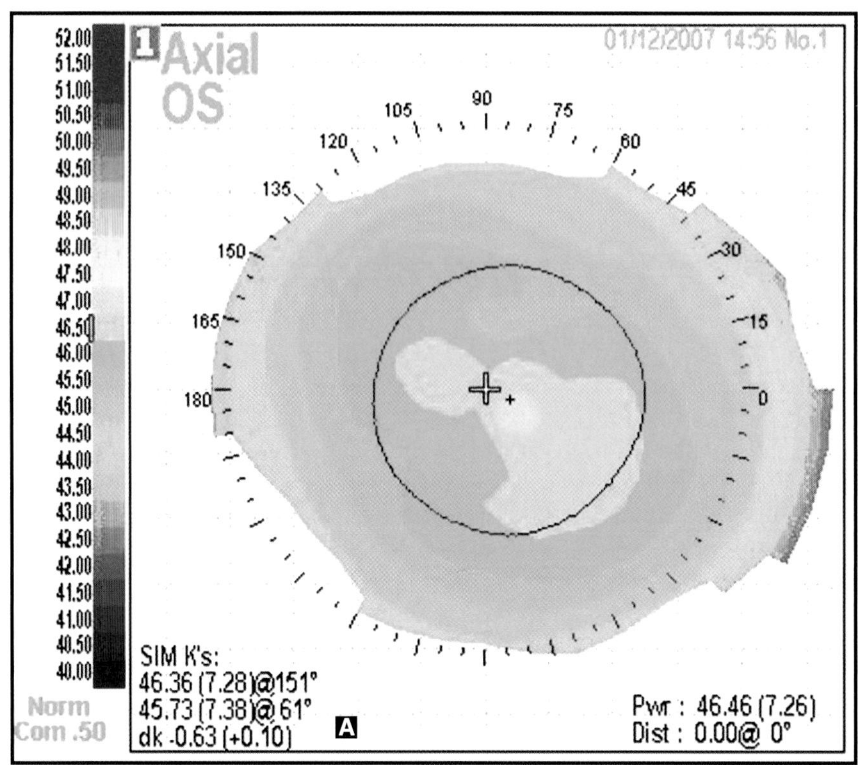

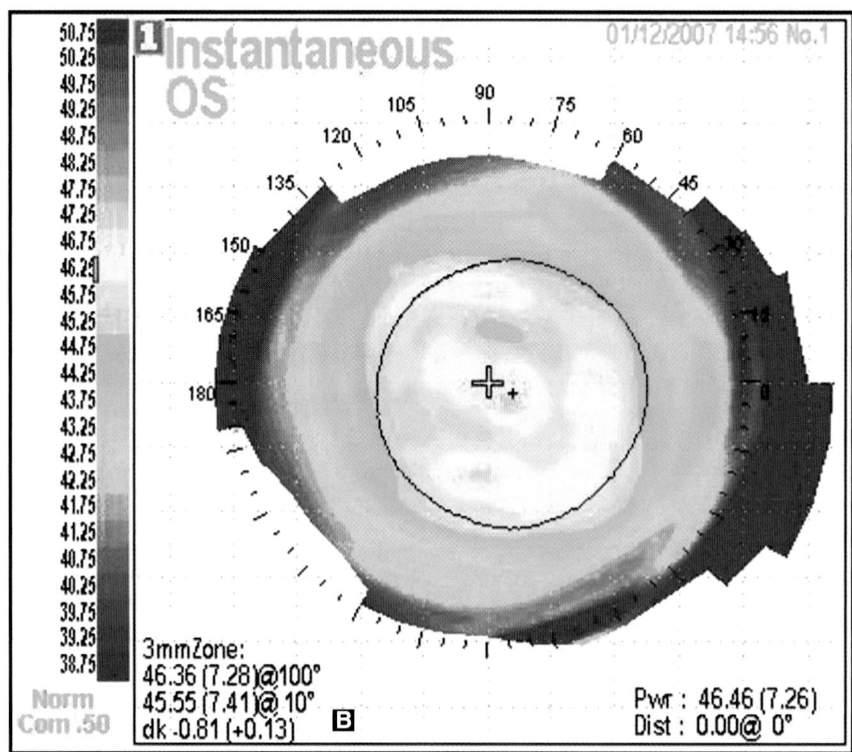

FIGURE 5-2: Axial and instantaneous maps. Axial map (A) compared to an instantaneous map (B) shows the latter is too sensitive and displays "noise" that is irrelevant. In this example, the center of the cornea appears significantly steeper than the periphery.

review articles exist that provide an overview of those that are commercially available. The most popular method of mapping corneal curvature is *axial curvature* display. Other methods include *tangential (instantaneous) curvature* as well as *mean curvature*. In some cases, the user can select the method to be used. Some users suggest that tangential curvature maps provide a better view of keratoconus, because the cone apex corresponds more accurately to the point of highest curvature power on the map. Axial maps do not have the extraneous data in the map that occurs with instantaneous maps **(Figure 5-2)**. There are more keratoconus numerical indices designed for axial curvature maps than for instantaneous maps. Some topographers provide refraction and elevation height maps. Refraction maps do not appear to provide an advantage over curvature maps. Elevation maps will be discussed below.

Keratometry Values

Keratometry provides information on corneal astigmatism by imaging two pairs of mire reflection points located approximately 3 mm apart from the central portion of the cornea. Corneal astigmatism (i.e. corneal cylinder) is expressed as curvature in diopters (D) and is determined along the steepest and flattest meridians. In a normal cornea, the steep and flat meridians are orthogonal (90 degrees perpendicular) to each other. Any loss of orthogonality is a sign of irregular astigmatism, which in turn suggests keratoconus.

Smolek reported that normal corneas had a steep simulated keratometry (SimK) value of 43.9 +/– 1.12 D while keratoconus suspect corneas had a higher value of 45.1 +/– 1.64 D and mild keratoconus corneas was higher with 47.8 +/– 1.93 D.[3] To evaluate usefulness of SimK values, Smolek compared SimK values to the Tomey TMS-2 modified I-S index and to a keratoconus classification neural network with respect to screening for inferior midperipheral keratoconus. Sensitivity for the neural network and I-S index was 100%, but SimK only achieved 76%. Specificity for the neural network approached 100%, I-S was just under 89% and SimK was just over 80%. In summary, keratometry does not perform as well as methods designed specifically for keratoconus screening.[3]

Selecting and Using Corneal Topographers

Not all corneal topographers are created equal. Some systems have higher resolutions or encompass larger areas of the cornea. Some systems have more informative graphical interfaces, provide better numerical analysis of the cornea, and have tools to specifically screen for keratoconus. Therefore, choosing a topography system is an important step in being able to screen for keratoconus. It is not a matter of choosing the most popular device or the latest system on the market, but involves choosing a device that has been experimentally verified as being repeatable and accurate. A system that provides sufficient information will allow the user to accomplish more than visual screening alone.

Understanding Absolute and Normalized Scales

A common question about topography screening is: What scale should I use — *normalized scale* or *absolute scale*? There are advantages and disadvantages for each scale. When using an absolute scale, colors are permanently assigned to K values and this relationship never changes from map to map or from patient to patient. The maximum is 67.5 D and minimum is 30 D **(Figure 5-3A)**. This can be easier for clinicians to see more extremes in abnormal patterns and significant increases in steepness based simply on the color. With a normalized scale, colors representing K values can vary from map to map. There is a smaller difference between maximum and minimum values in the normalized scale: maximum is 49.5 D and minimum is 40.5 D **(Figure 5-3B)**. The upper and lower limits can change from eye to eye. Using a normalized scale, the clinician

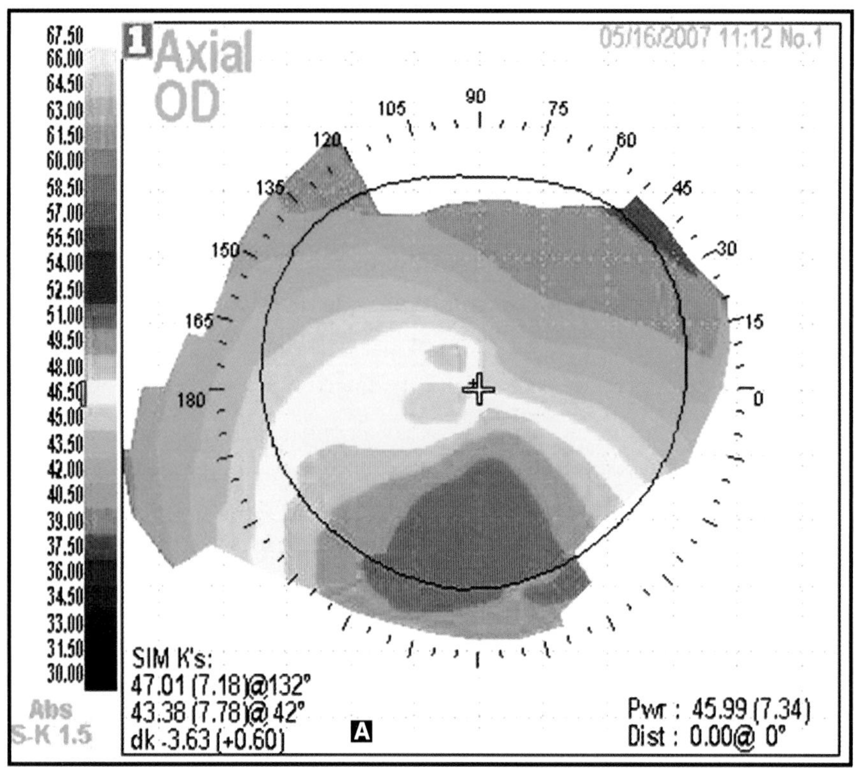

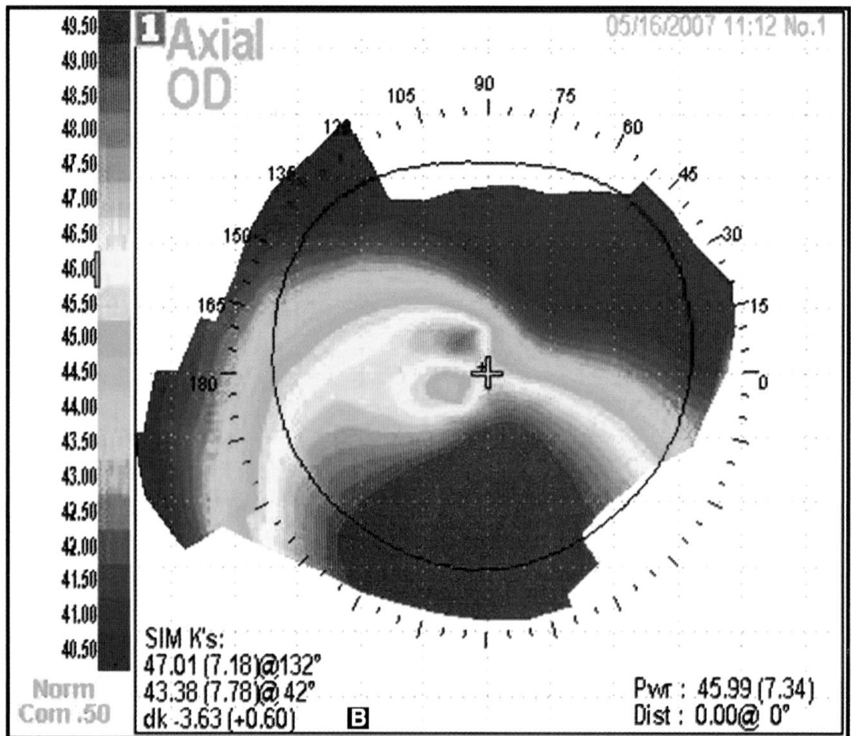

FIGURE 5-3: Same cornea with two different displays. Absolute scale (A) always has maximum value of 67.5 D and minimum value of 30 D in 1.5 D steps between colors. The same eye with normalized scale (B) has a maximum of 50.0 D and minimum of 41.0 D (which can vary among eyes). The display is manually set for 0.5 D steps.

should manually set the topography program for 0.5 D steps to allow maximum sensitivity in the displays. Setting 1.0 D or 1.5 D steps with a normalized scale will mask potentially important information. With a normalized scale, the clinician needs to examine the color assignments and note which color signifies a normal 43 D curvature and which color signifies a steeper 48 D curvature and so on.

The Smolek-Klyce (S-K) color scale is a well-researched and published absolute scale that was designed so that each 1.5 D color contour step corresponds to approximately 1 standard deviation for normal corneas.[4] Because of their largely spherical surfaces, normal corneas have the lowest curvature variance of any type of corneal category and this becomes the criterion by which all topographies are measured and compared. The 1.5 D contour step allows the user to easily determine for a mapped cornea how many standard deviations below or above it is from the normal mean cornea curvature **(Figure 5-3A)**. In contrast with a normalized scale, 0.5 D contour steps should be used **(Figure 5-3B)** since range of minimum and maximum values is not as large as with the S-K scale.

It is possible to use 1 D absolute scale successfully in clinical screening, although there are tradeoffs. First, there will be a slight increase in the noise in the map. Second, more color steps must be used in order to make the scale effective over a large enough range of corneal powers. Finally, the association is lost between a single color difference on the scale being equivalent to a 1 standard deviation change in curvature.

It has been stated that using 1.5 D steps with an absolute scale will cause useful information to be hidden "between the steps" compared to a 0.5 D steps in normalized scale. This is not typically observed, since biomechanical tissue coupling means that a change in curvature in one location causes another curvature change elsewhere on the corneal surface through surface slope. For frank keratoconus, it is difficult to "hide" a significant change in curvature "between the steps" of the absolute scale map **(Figure 5-4)**. Masking subtle changes could occur in corneas after LASIK or other types of surgery.

Each clinician can use both absolute and normalized scales and decide which is preferred. Dr Smolek prefers to use the absolute scale, while Dr Boxer Wachler prefers to use the normalized scale. Either way, the clinician should ultimately choose one scale type and use it to maintain consistency.

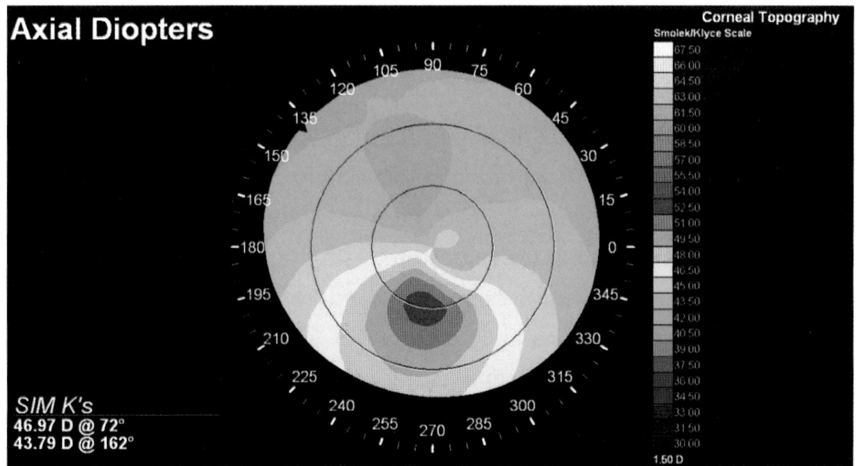

FIGURE 5-4: Frank keratoconus topography. With an absolute scale using 1.5 diopter steps, the increased curvature in lower cornea is obvious.

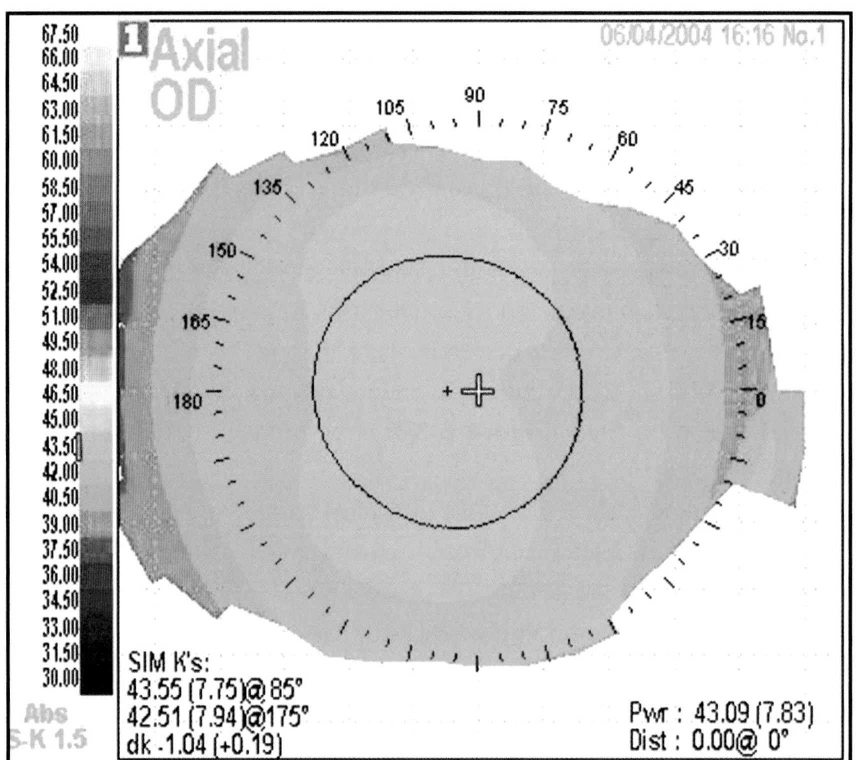

FIGURE 5-5: Normal topography, absolute scale. Green color corresponds to average curvature of approximately 43 D. All green colors represent curvatures within 2 standard deviations from average population curvature using absolute scale.

Visual Screening of Topography Maps

It is important for the clinician to become proficient at visual analysis of corneal topography when screening for keratoconus as well as when evaluating patients for LASIK. Even the best automated screening systems are not reliable all of the time, so the clinician should know signs that are clinically meaningful. Comparing maps in fellow eyes of the same patient is an important technique.

Absolute Scale

Using an absolute scale, the first step in visual analysis of a map is to determine if steepening exists by looking for warm colors in the map. As an overview, all green colors signify curvature values that are within 2 standard deviations from normal **(Figure 5-5)**. As each 1.5 D interval represents 1 standard deviation from the average (green), yellow and blue colors signify curvature values are 3 standard deviations above and below the mean, respectively. Specifically, yellow indicates mild steepening and orange corresponds to moderate steepening **(Figure 5-6A)**. Red represents advanced steepening **(Figure 5-6B)** and pink hues indicate severe steepening. Cool hues (light blue and dark blue) are indicative of flatter curvature. It can be useful to simply count the number of visible steps which represent 1.5 D intervals. If there are more than 4 or 5 intervals, the cornea is likely abnormal.

Normalized Scale

With a normalized scale, green often represents normal curvature (43 to 45 D) **(Figure 5-7)**. The clinician should also inspect which curvature on the scale corresponds to the green color since there can be occasions

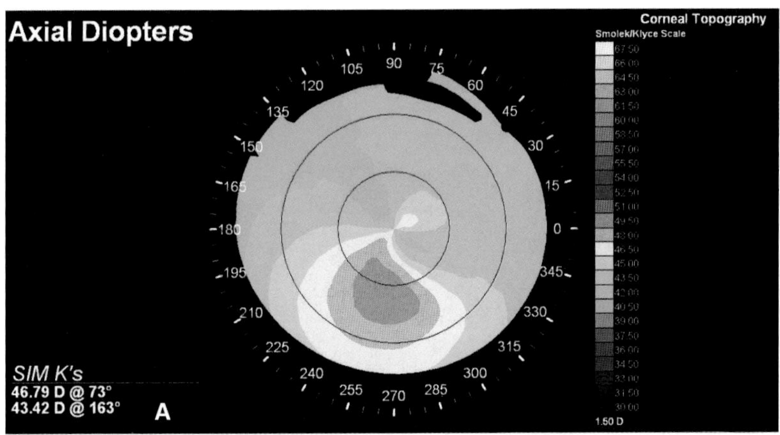

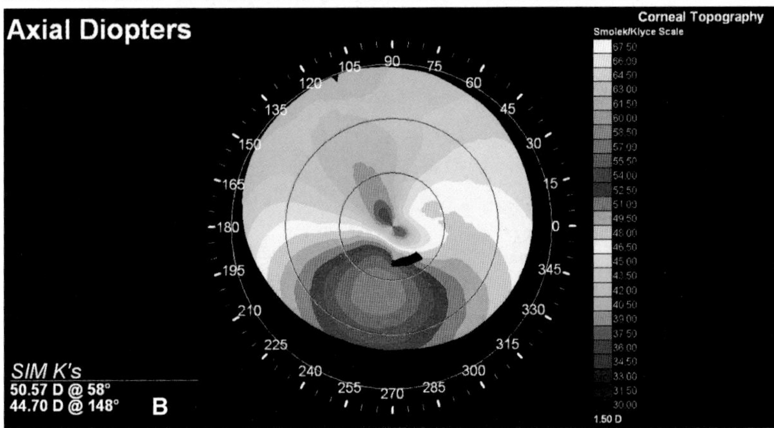

FIGURE 5-6: Moderate and advanced keratoconus, absolute scale. Moderate keratoconus (A) is signified by orange color of lower steepening while another eye with advanced keratoconus (B) is identified with a red inferiorly located cone.

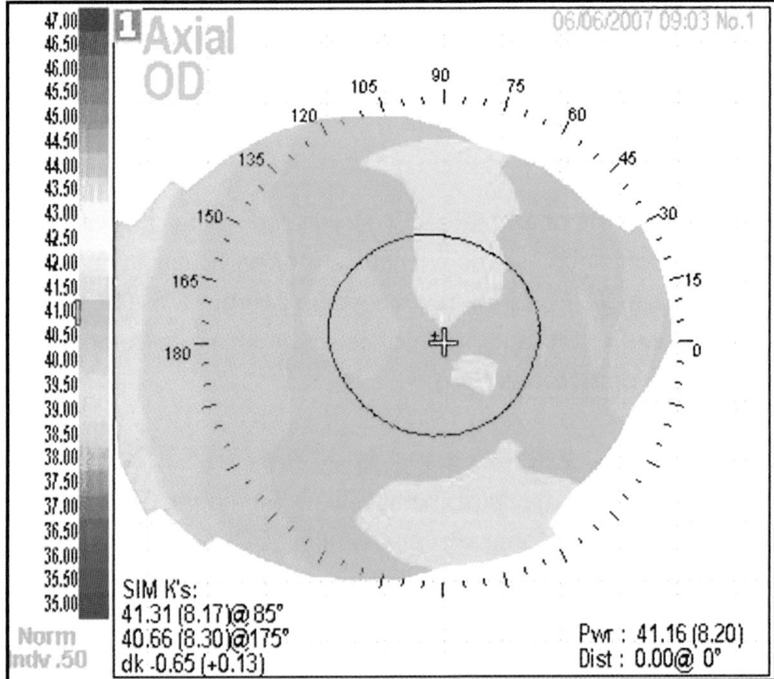

FIGURE 5-7: Normal eye topography, normalized scale. Green color corresponds to an average curvature of 41.16 D.

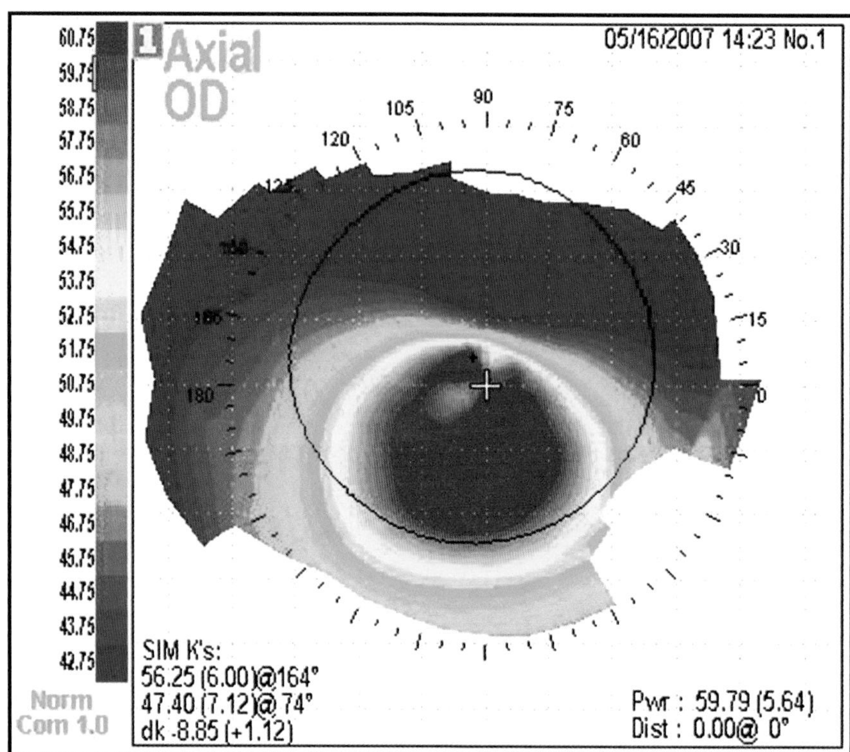

FIGURE 5-8: Advanced keratoconus, normalized scale. Topography shows the yellow, orange, and red colors that indicate the degree of steepening.

where green could represent a normally shaped cornea that is a little steeper at 46 D or 47 D. Irregular shaped patterns can be easy to recognize with a normalized scale since the 0.5 D steps in the context of a more narrow range of maximum and minimum values that yield more variety in colors. As with an absolute scale, warmer colors such as yellow, orange, and red in the normalized scale signify greater amounts of steepening **(Figure 5-8)**.

Comparison of Absolute and Normalized Maps

Single Axial Maps

For most cases, using either an absolute or normalized scale will enable the clinician to detect abnormal corneal shapes. For LASIK screening, more subtle shape changes are of particular interest and should be identified. Forme fruste keratoconus **(Figure 5-9)** and inferior steepening **(Figure 5-10)** may be easier to appreciate with a normalized scale compared to absolute scale since there are more colors displayed in the map with the normalized scale which aids pattern detection.

Difference Maps

After LASIK is performed, some patients may postoperatively present to the office with a decline in uncorrected visual acuity (UCVA) and/or best spectacle-corrected visual acuity (BSCVA). If the cause of decline is keratoectasia, it becomes critical that this condition is identified as unknowingly performing a LASIK retreatment on an ectatic cornea will likely exacerbate the keratoectasia and lead to worse vision (see Chapter 3 for more information on keratoectasia). Postoperatively, difference maps allow easy detection of keratoectasia. A difference map is a display of two different topographies of the same eye that were taken at different time intervals accompanied by the mathematical subtraction map of the topographies, known as the difference map.

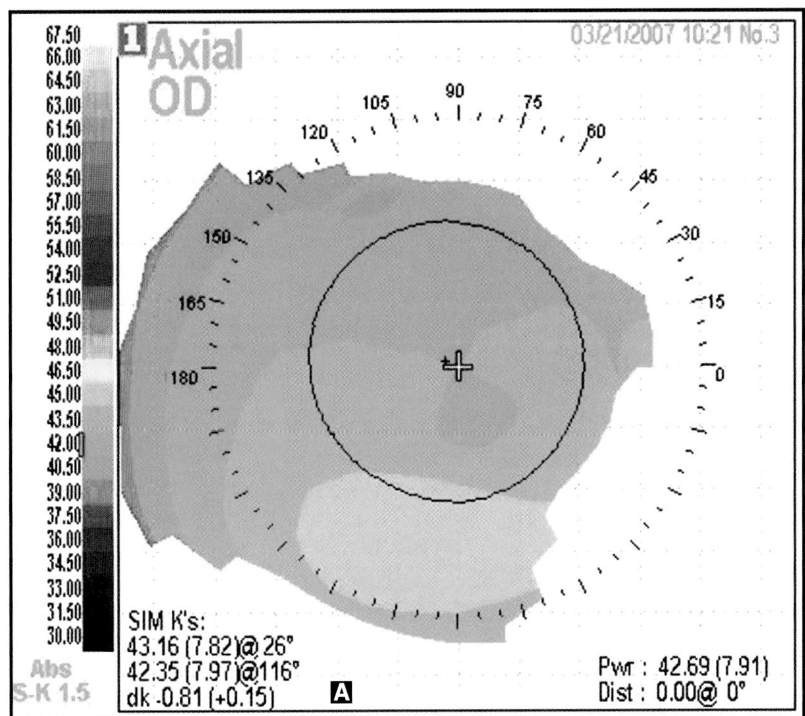

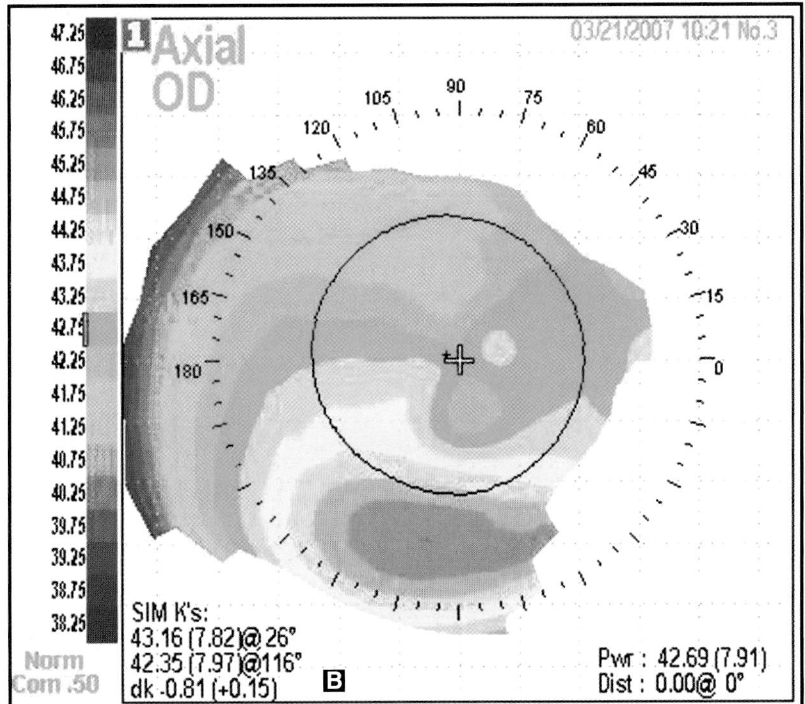

FIGURE 5-9: Forme fruste keratoconus. Absolute scale (A) and normalized scale (B) for the same eye are compared. The normalized scale enables easier identification of an abnormality.

The difference map is sensitive for displaying both obvious and subtle changes in shape that occur over time versus two single topography maps without the difference map. **Figure 5-11A** shows the difference map using an absolute scale for an eye that developed new onset of keratoectasia and **Figure 5-11B** shows the same eye with a normalized scale. For both types of scales, the difference map clearly shows red color which

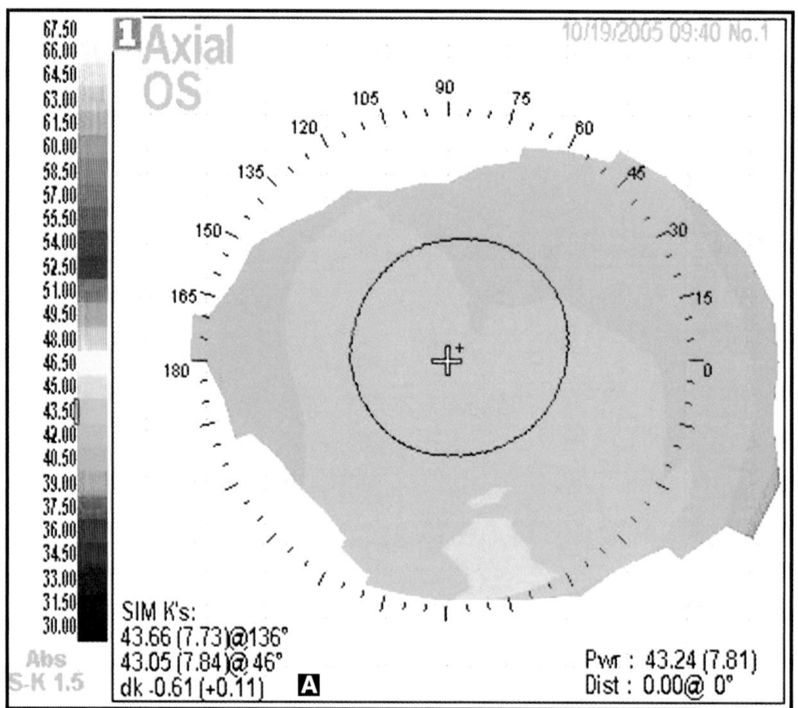

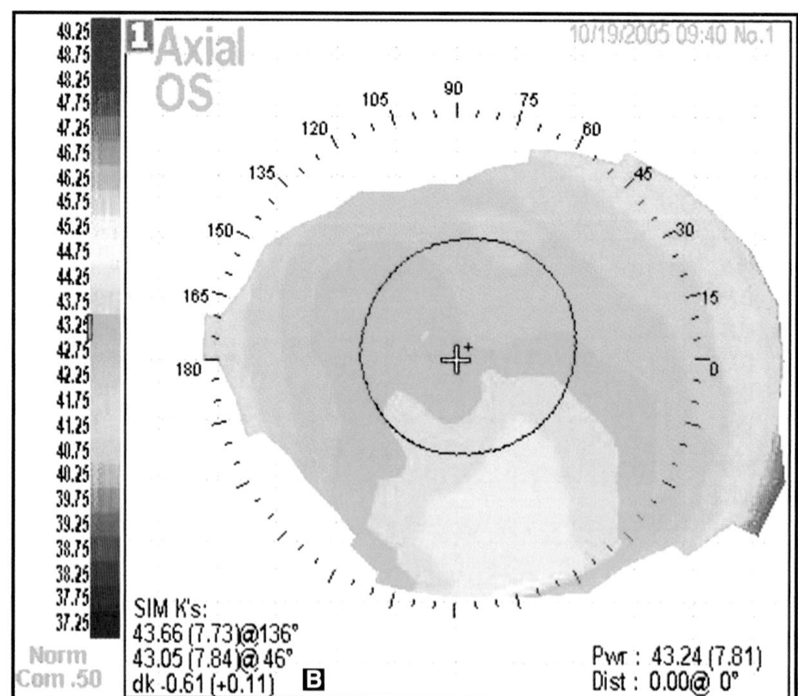

FIGURE 5-10: Inferior steepening. Absolute scale (A) could be considered normal, but normalized scale (B) of same eye provides more of a clue that this cornea requires further evaluation regarding being a candidate for LASIK.

indicates steepening that developed after LASIK. For less obvious keratoectasia after LASIK, the difference maps using either absolute or normalized scales make the condition easy to identify **(Figures 5-12A and B)**. If one was relying only on single maps (only upper and lower topographies on left side of display), it would be hard to recognize that new onset of inferior steepening has occurred after LASIK in this case.

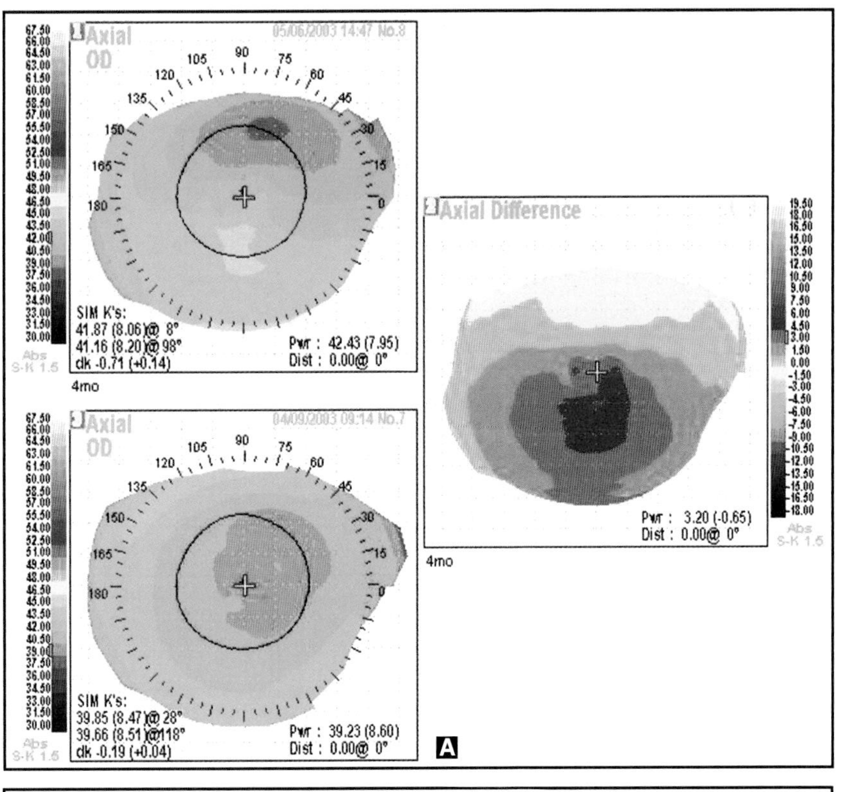

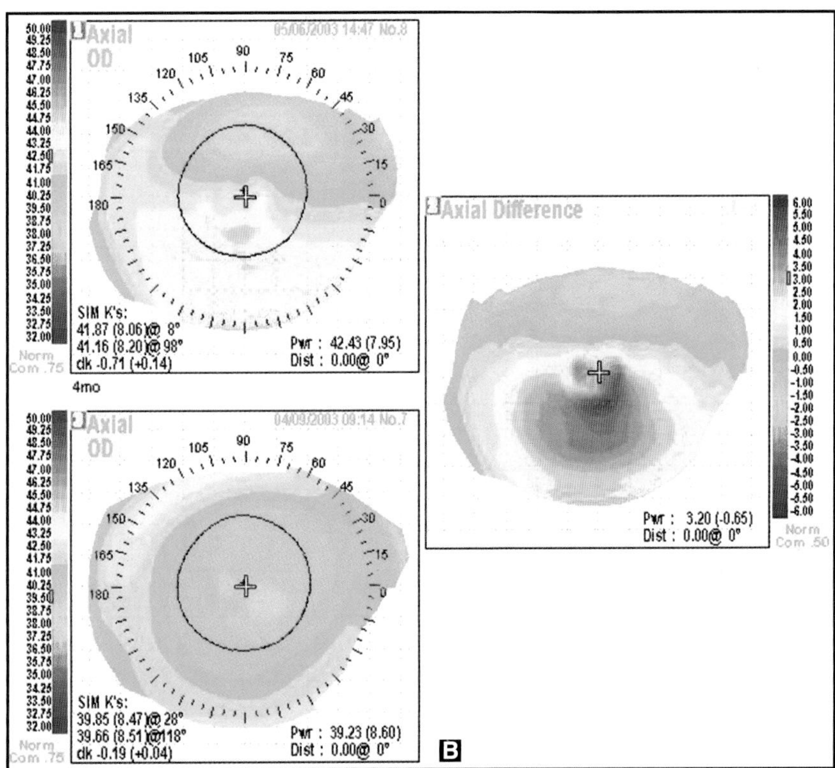

FIGURE 5-11: New keratoectasia after LASIK shown with difference maps. Absolute scale (A) and normalized scale (B) for same eye are shown. Lower left shows prior map and upper left shows recent map. The obvious red color in the difference map on right of (A) and (B) makes it obvious the ectasia has occurred. If one was relying only on two single maps for comparison, the lower steepening could go unrecognized by the clinician. Note normalized scale (B) is displayed in 0.75 D steps. Note: even though the computer default is set to 0.50 D, the computer may increase the interval from 0.50 to 0.75 D in difference map displays.

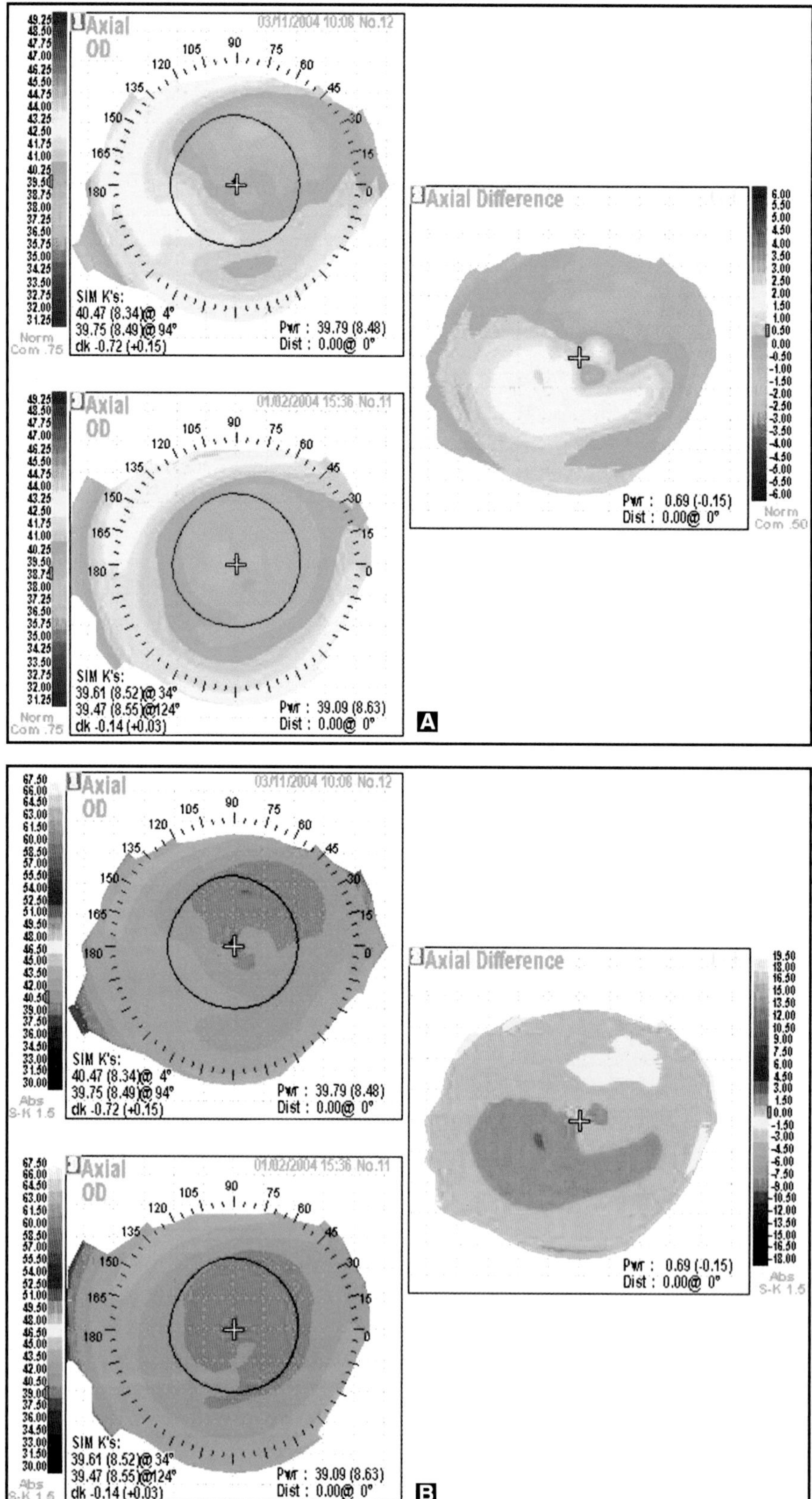

FIGURE 5-12: New subtle keratoectasia after LASIK shown with difference maps. Absolute scale (A) and normalized scale (B) for same eye. As with Figure 5-11, difference maps show the new steepening, which would be very hard to detect without the difference map display.

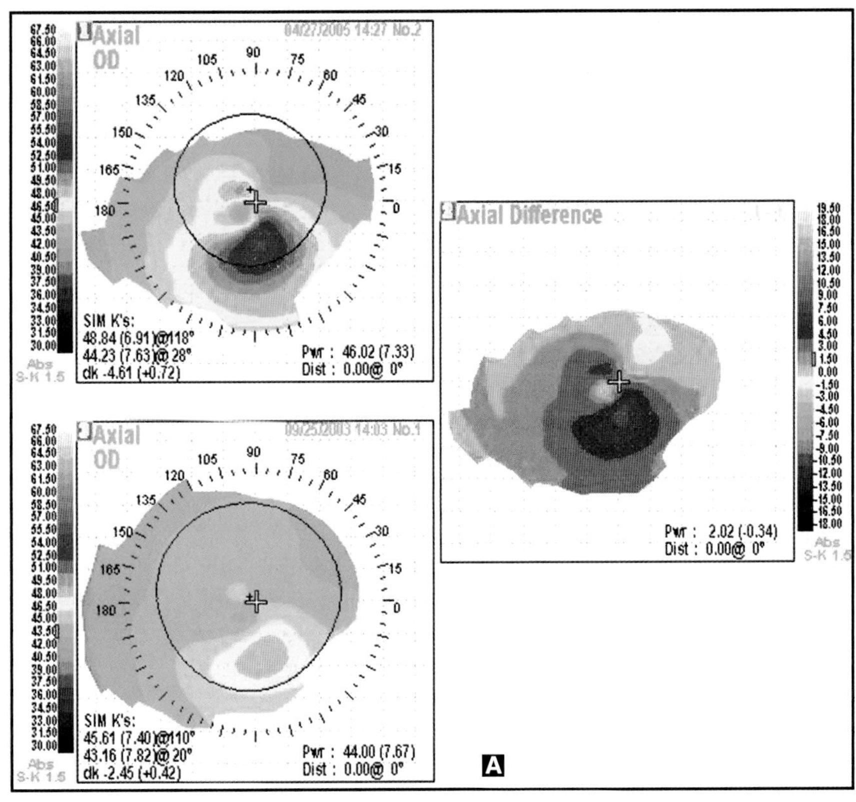

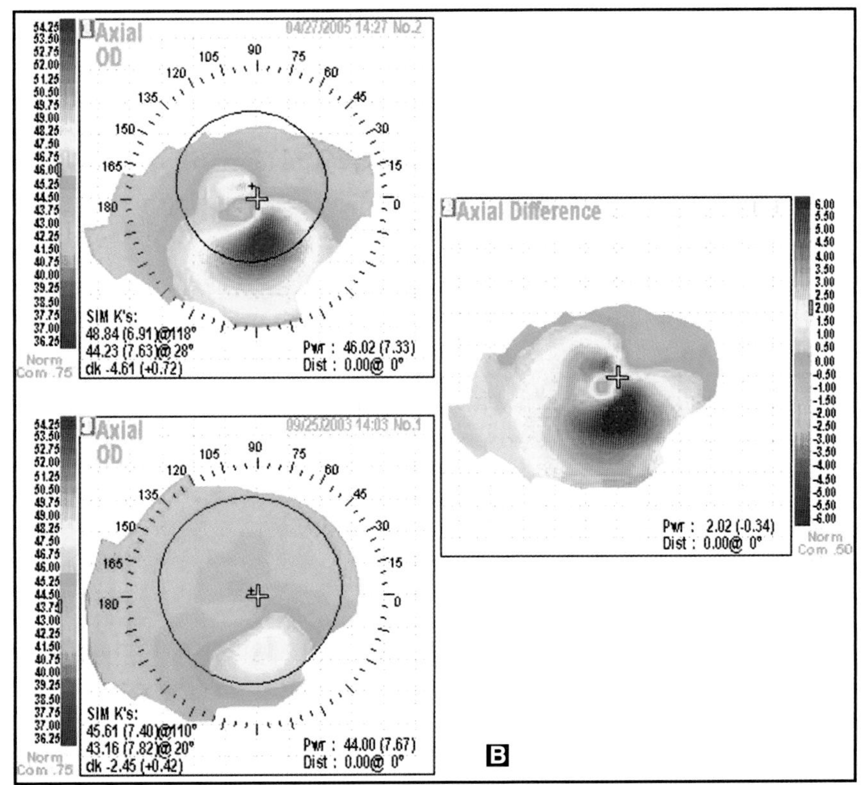

FIGURE 5-13: Progression of keratoconus with difference maps. Absolute scale (A) and normalized scale (B) for same eye clearly shows progression.

Difference maps are also useful for following progression of keratoconus **(Figure 5-13)**. Evaluation of the difference map reveals red which leaves no doubt that this patient experienced progression and may be a candidate for certain procedures such as Intacs® and C3-R.®

Keratoconus and Keratoectasia Topography Patterns

There are two essential factors involved in screening corneal topography:

1. Evaluate the range and magnitude of curvature that is present in the pattern, which is related to the severity of the keratoconus.
2. Evaluate asymmetry or irregularity of the contour pattern.

For the classical form of inferior, mid-peripheral cones, the steepness will tend to arise in the inferior quadrant of the map. For off-center cones, there tends to be a distinct asymmetry to the topographic pattern. As the cone distends over time, the asymmetry will become more noticeable and the bull's eye-like pattern of yellow, orange, and red hued contours will be more obvious. When the cone arises in the direct center of the cornea, asymmetry is less pronounced and the obvious pattern of a peripheral cone is absent, which makes identifying purely central cones more difficult to see. When visually screening topographies, it is prudent that one considers the possibility of a central cone, because it may be easy to overlook.

Peripheral Keratoconus and Keratoectasia: Bow-tie Pattern

Peripheral keratoconus and keratoectasia are characterized by a pattern shaped like a bow-tie (also called an hour-glass, figure-8, or propeller), which is the most common form of keratoconus compared to less common central keratoconus that is discussed below. Each side of the bow-tie is called a lobe. The bow-tie pattern may have symmetrical lobes which indicates corneal astigmatism, a naturally occurring shape that by itself is not indicative of keratoconus **(Figure 5-14)**.

With keratoconus and keratoectasia, there are four main types of patterns. Any of these patterns with localized steepening are strong signs for keratoconus or a keratoconus-like shape being present. Please note there are many variations of the below topography examples.

1. Lobes of the bow-tie may be unequal in area (size), but lobes are not bent **(Figure 5-15)**.
2. Lobes of bow-ties may be equal in area and are not bent (uncommon pattern) **(Figure 5-16)**.
3. Lobes may be equal in size and have the same colors in each lobe, but they may show distortion in the form of a bend along the axis that connects the lobes **(Figure 5-17)**. This effect is called by various names, including a lazy-8 pattern, a bent propeller, or a sagging bow-tie (if horizontally located).
4. Lobes of bow-tie may be unequally sized with a bent axis, and curvature in lobes may be equal to each other or different **(Figure 5-18)**. This is a common pattern.

Central Keratoconus and Keratoectasia: Bull's Eye Pattern

When steepening is localized into a round, central (bull's eye) cone pattern with the steepest curvatures near the center, it is highly indicative of central keratoconus and keratoectasia **(Figure 5-19)**. In most cases, the pattern does not appear this perfect.

Bow-tie Combined with Central Pattern

Both a bow-tie and central cone pattern can occur together because corneas can exhibit astigmatism along with the localized distension of the cone simultaneously, which will produce a distorted bow-tie pattern **(Figure 5-20)**.

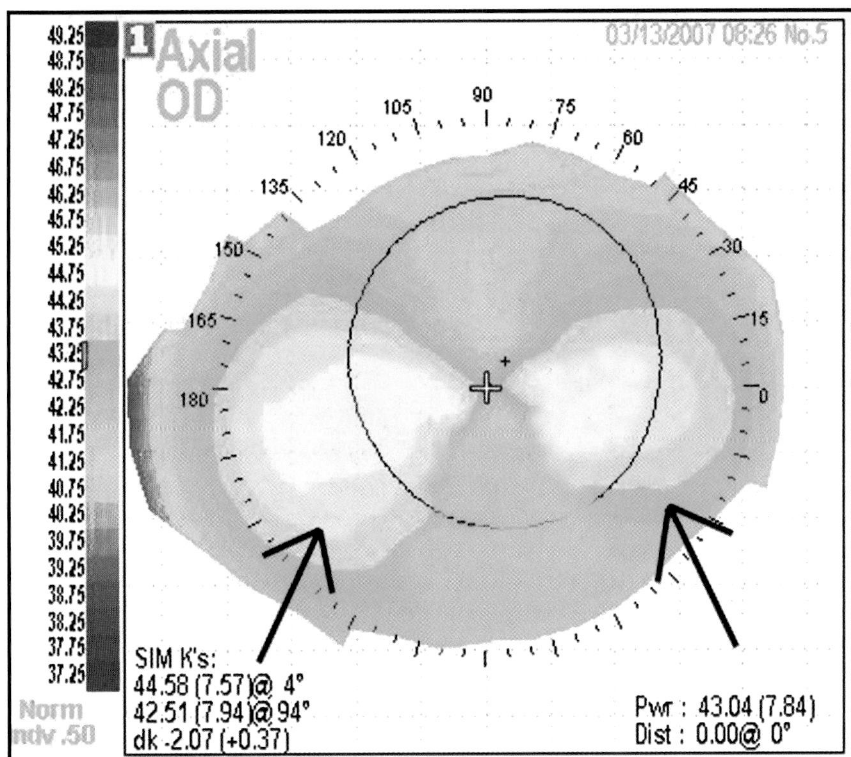

FIGURE 5-14: Normal astigmatism with the bow-tie pattern. The bow-tie is comprised of two fairly symmetrical lobes (arrows) which indicates normal astigmatism, not keratoconus.

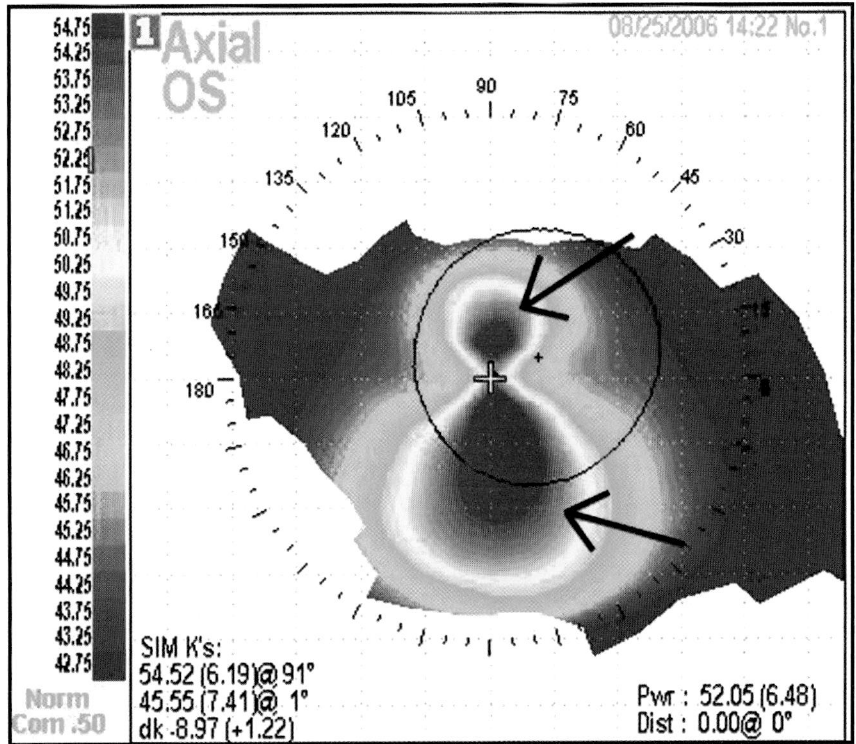

FIGURE 5-15: Keratoconus with asymmetric sized lobes of bow-tie. The lower lobe is larger than the upper lobe. Both lobes (arrows) show similar amount of steepening (red).

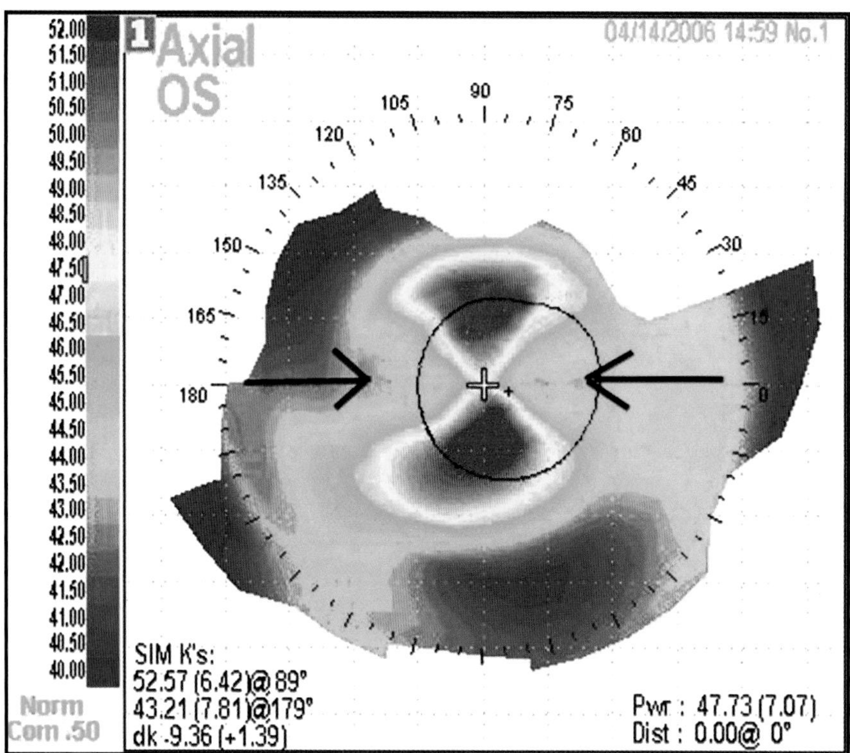

FIGURE 5-16: Keratoconus with similar sized lobes of bow-tie. The lobes are also of similar steepening (red). Note the symmetrically flat (blue) areas (arrows) between the lobes. This is an uncommon pattern of keratoconus.

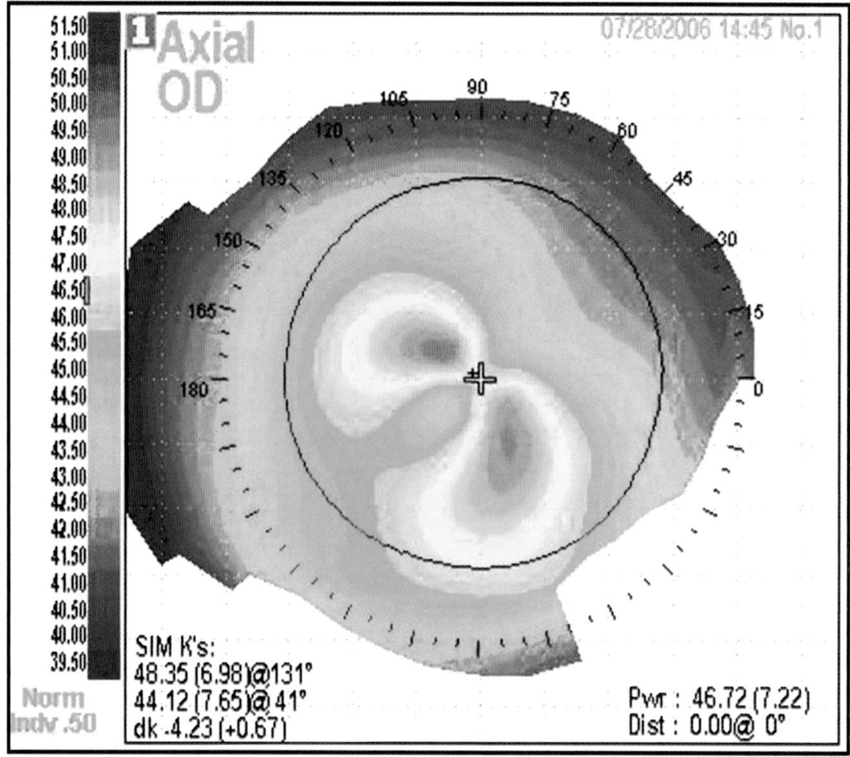

FIGURE 5-17: Keratoconus with bent bow-tie lobes. The lobes are equally sized with same steepening (red), but the bow-tie is mildly bent. Note the asymmetrically flat (blue) areas between the lobes.

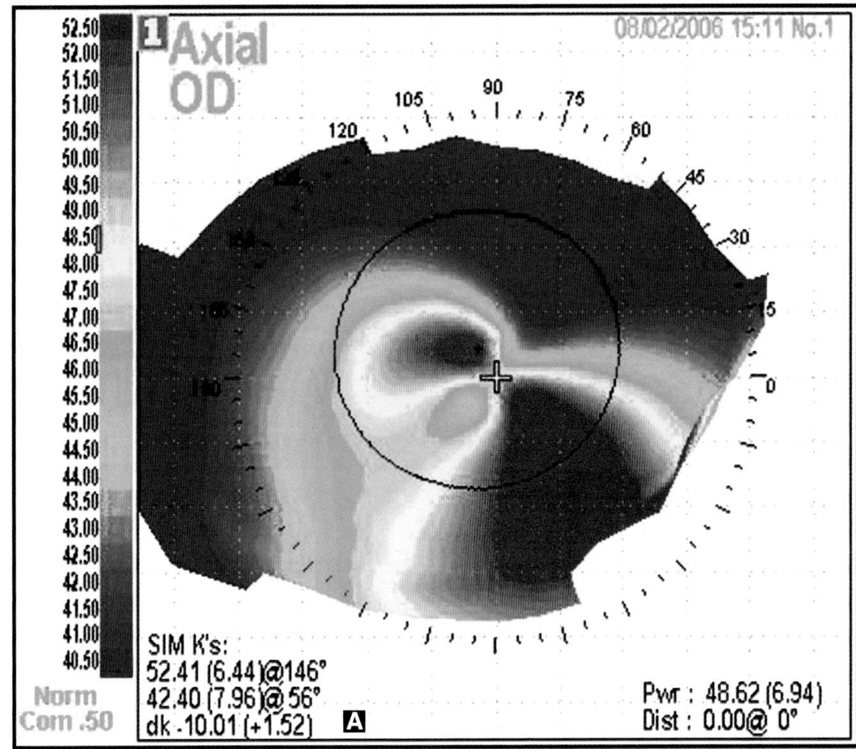

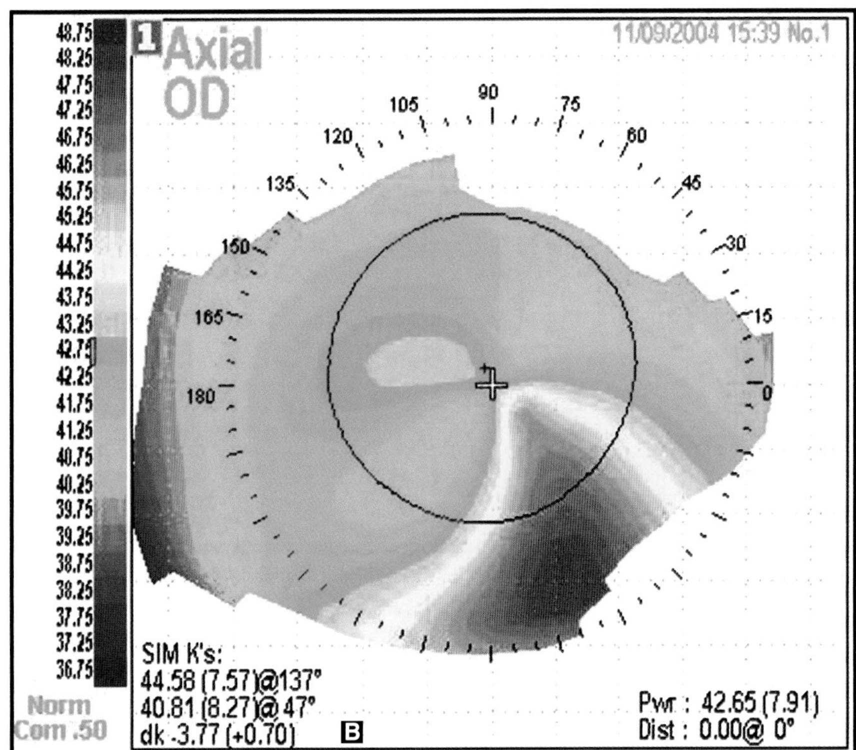

FIGURE 5-18: Keratoconus with bent bow-tie with the different sized lobes. The lobes may have same steepness (A) or different steepness (B). These are the most common forms of keratoconus.

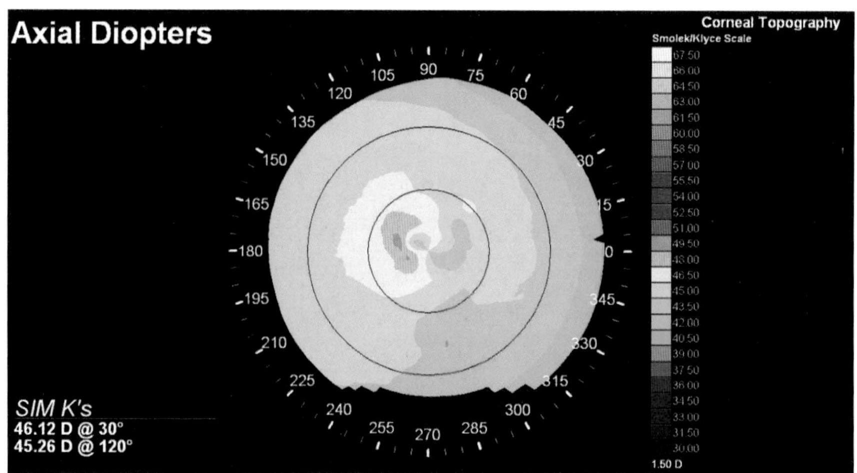

FIGURE 5-19: Central keratoconus. The round, bull's eye of steepening is in the center of the map.

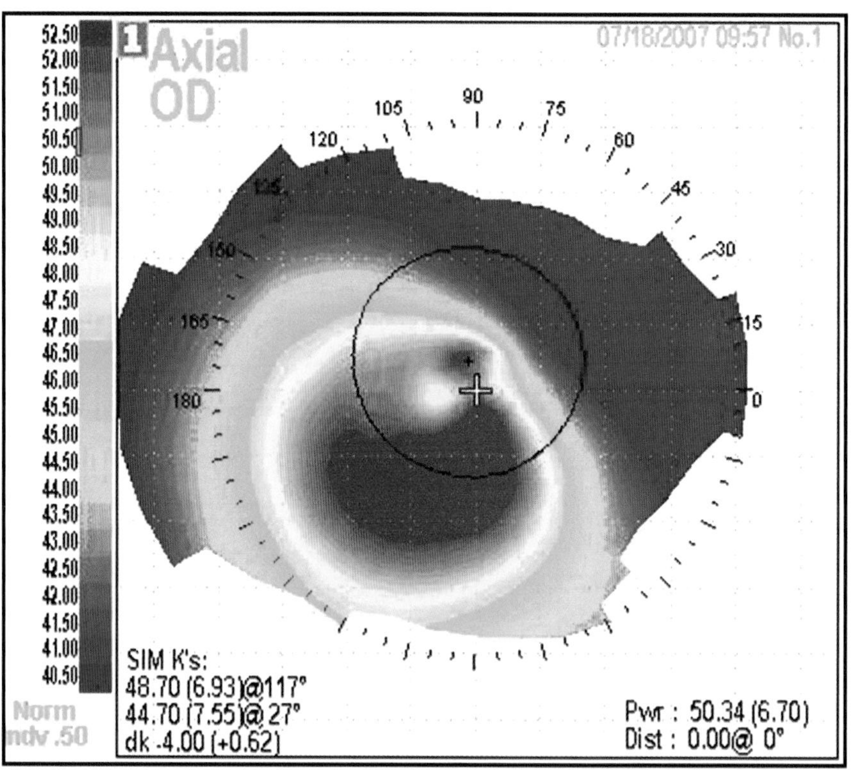

FIGURE 5-20: Combined peripheral and central keratoconus. There can be overlap between keratoconus patterns.

Forme Fruste Keratoconus and "Inferior Steepening"

When screening patients for LASIK, positive identification of a subclinical form of keratoconus known as forme fruste keratoconus (FFKC) is important. Performing LASIK on patients with FFKC significantly increases the risk of developing keratoectasia. Therefore, it is prudent to identify such patients and if appropriate consider alternative corrective procedures such as phakic IOLs (e.g. Staar ICL) or photorefractive keratectomy (PRK). FFKC differs from keratoconus in that the latter can be diagnosed clinically with use of slit lamp examination (as discussed in Chapter 4) and characteristic pattern on corneal topography as discussed above. FFKC has no identifiable slit lamp signs, but corneal topography shows a cone pattern. In other words, FFKC is diagnosed by topography alone **(Figure 5-9)**. FFKC may or may not exhibit astigmatism on manifest refraction and BSCVA may be 20/20 or it may be reduced.

Another finding of interest when evaluating a patient for LASIK is the subtle entity known simply as "inferior steepening" **(Figure 5-10)**. Like FFKC, this entity also is strictly a topography diagnosis. Slit lamp examination is unremarkable. Manifest refraction will usually not have any astigmatism and BSCVA is typically 20/20 (assuming no unrelated pathology is present such as amblyopia or macular scarring, for examples). Performing LASIK on these corneas can evoke a higher keratoectasia risk as well. There can be overlap between FFKC and inferior steepening, so these conditions are not mutually exclusive. FFKC topography maps tend to show marked steeper colors such as red, while inferior steepening may have normal curvatures, but the inferior pattern is the only unusual sign.

Pellucid Marginal Degeneration

Pellucid marginal degeneration is a condition with the same underlying biomechanical etiology as keratoconus, but the corneal thinning is in the far periphery close to the lower limbus. Some clinicians simply consider pellucid as a subtype of keratoconus. Biomechanical strength testing of donor tissue has shown that normal corneas have an inherent weakness in the inferior part of the cornea that tends to correspond with the apex location of the cone in keratoconus.[5] The weakness patterns of individual eyes have been shown to be both in the central cornea and at the limbus, which corresponds to central keratoconus and pellucid marginal degeneration, respectively. The pattern of weakness in the right and left eyes were often mirror images of one another, just as the topography patterns for keratoconus and pellucid are similar in fellow eyes (although one eye is delayed in time of progression). This unusual correspondence of biomechanical and topographical patterns suggests that the inherent structural strength of the cornea mediates the form of the ectasia, its location and magnitude.

The topographic signs of pellucid include a lobster-claw pattern where the steep contours arise all the way from the limbus and appear to pinch the center of the cornea **(Figure 5-21)**. In addition, one will often see a vertical, flattened curvature (blue colored), bow-tie pattern with one blue lobe contained within the claw and the other lobe above the claw **(Figure 5-22)**. This flat bow-tie is sometimes distorted and not perfectly symmetrical. Occasionally it appears to be absent. Use of difference maps is helpful for detecting progression of pellucid marginal degeneration **(Figure 5-23)**.

In some instances, the claw-like pattern does not extend all the way to the limbus, but it looks more like a croissant roll. It therefore has topographic signs of both keratoconus and pellucid—a claw-like pattern, but no steep curvatures at the limbus. In such cases, the condition is probably not true pellucid, because of the lack of involvement of the limbus. It is more likely a very peripheral keratoconus cone. For simplicity purposes, some clinicians simply lump pellucid in to the keratoconus category since distinction seems only to be of academic interest; the clinical implications and treatments for both conditions are often not different.

Sometimes, it is prudent to look at the picture of the Placido disk mires on the cornea. The pellucid pattern may aberrantly result from the Placido disk mires being disrupted by eyelashes, tear film pooling, or totally missing tear film due to interference by the lower eyelid. If the mires were disrupted, extrapolated data may cause a keratoconus condition to appear more like pellucid or vice versa. In such cases, the slit lamp microscope or pachymetry is used to determine the location where the maximum thinning is occurring. Given that pellucid and keratoconus are so closely related, there will be some cases where the signs are vague and point to either condition being present. Assuming no topography artifacts, this is the reason some clinicians just consider pellucid as very peripheral keratoconus.

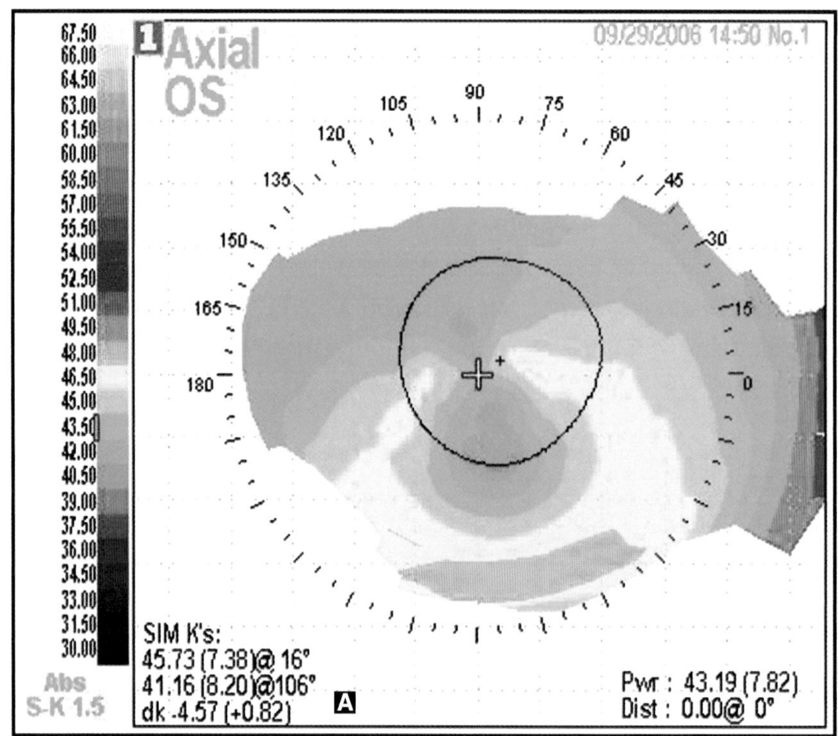

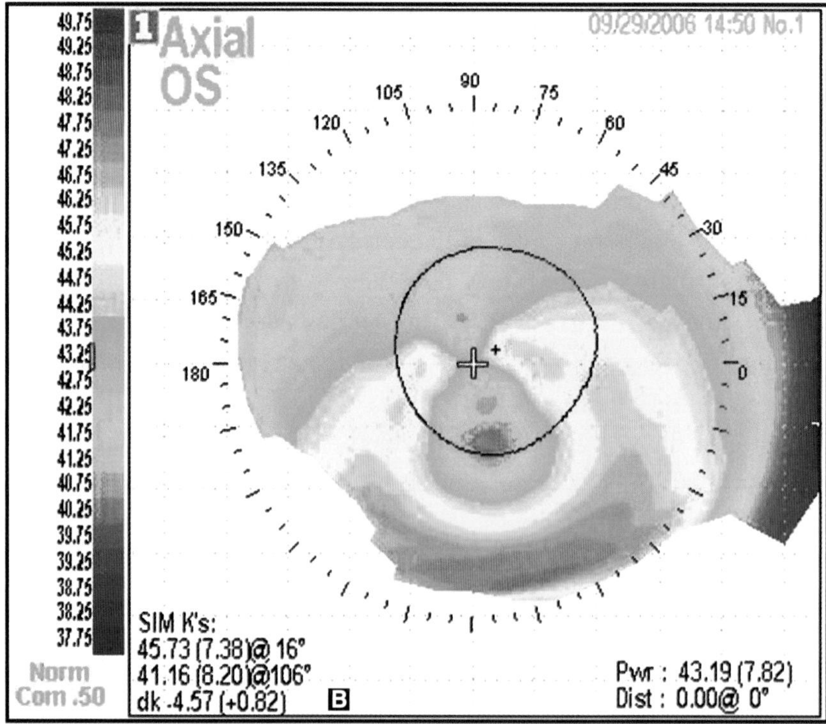

FIGURE 5-21: Pellucid marginal degeneration, The "lobster-claw" pattern is displayed in absolute scale (A) and normalized scale (B).

Topography Pattern Summary

There are many variations of keratoconus patterns depending on the location of the cone and the severity of the condition. It is possible to have more than one clinical condition present on the same cornea. For example, contact lens wear over an existing cone may make keratoconus difficult to diagnose as one would initially

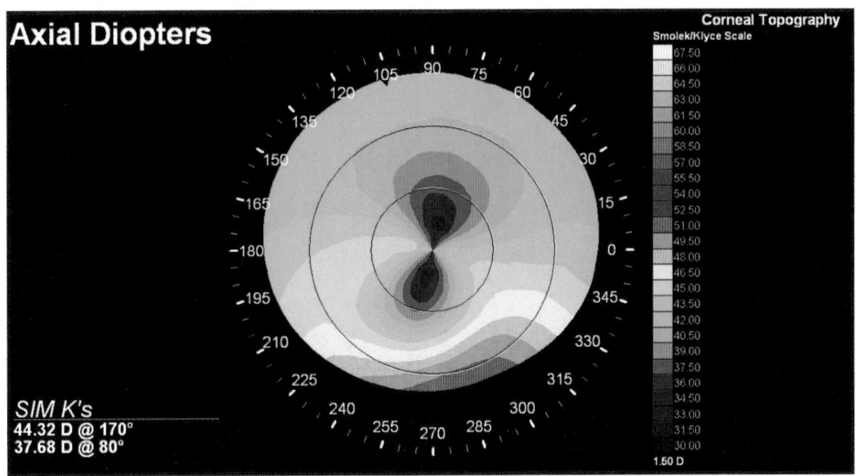

FIGURE 5-22: Pellucid marginal degeneration, absolute scale. There is a vertical blue bow-tie with one blue lobe above the "lobster claw" and the other blue lobe contained within the claw.

presume the steepening is contact lens warpage. It is therefore advisable that the initial goal of screening is to first look for any signs of abnormal topography such as unusual asymmetry and/or steepening. Then the clinician can focus on determining how and why a particular topography map is abnormal. In addition, occasionally a correct diagnosis cannot be made at the first examination, and a follow-up examination can be scheduled. For example, in order to rule out a diagnosis of contact lens-induced corneal warpage, it may be necessary to have the patient out of contact lenses for several weeks to assess if the ectasia-like patterns resolve, or if the contact lens wear was covering up a true cone.

Numerical Indices Derived from Topography Maps

While many keratoconic topography maps are easy to visually identify, some mild cases of keratoconus may be more challenging. Corneal numerical indices were developed as an aid to make screening easier, objective, and repeatable.

One of the oldest indices was the Inferior-Superior or I-S index.[6] Because the most typical form of keratoconus arises in the inferior midperiphery, steep corneal curvatures in this region compared to flatter corneal curvature in the opposite superior quadrant provides a numerical value that is a sign for keratoconus. The I-S keratoconus threshold was originally determined to be 1.67, but was later refined to 1.40 D. This means that a topography with an I-S value above 1.4 is highly suspicious for keratoconus. Unfortunately, the I-S index does generate false-negatives because it is not valid for central keratoconus and for those instances where keratoconus arises in some other quadrant besides the inferior one. It also will generate false-positives because it is not specific for keratoconus alone.[7] It is therefore best applied in combination with visual screening or with other numerical indices and not used alone.

In an effort to make keratoconus screening with the I-S index value more sensitive to central keratoconus, the KISA% method was developed that incorporated keratometry and asymmetry of the corneal astigmatism.[8] Although it was a much-needed improvement over I-S alone, it still was not specific for keratoconus, nor was it widely accepted for routine clinical use.

A further modification of the I-S index came in the form of L-U (Lower-Upper) index.[9] The I-S index uses the horizontal, 180 degrees meridian the reference axis for inferior and superior topography comparison. Many cones are not directly inferiorly located as shown in this chapter for examples, but are inferior obliquely located. The I-S index will not accurate characterize obliquely located cones **(Figure 5-24)**. The L-U index customizes

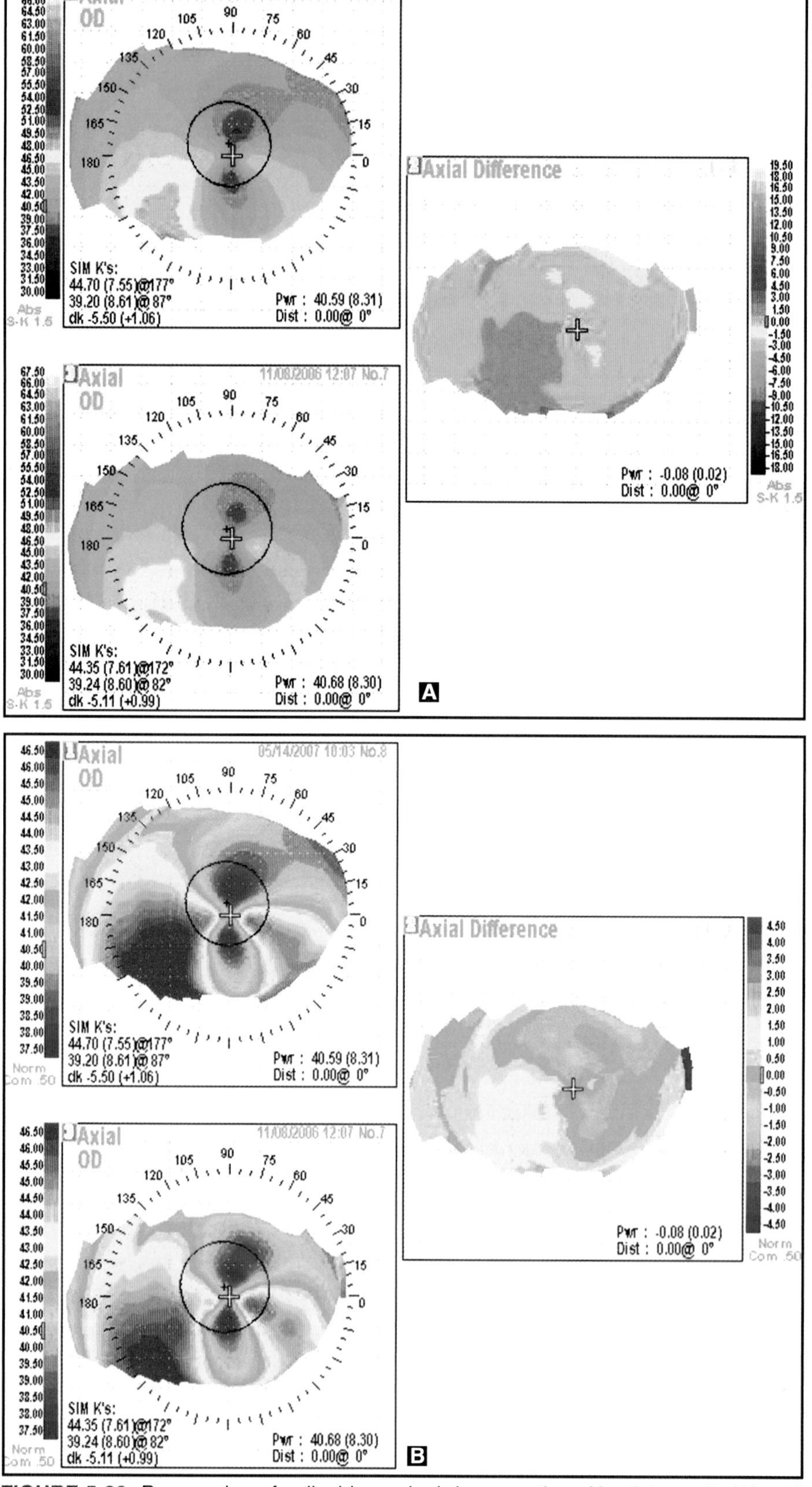

FIGURE 5-23: Progression of pellucid marginal degeneration. Absolute scale (A) and normalized scale (B) for same eye show temporal progression has occurred as signified by red color on difference map.

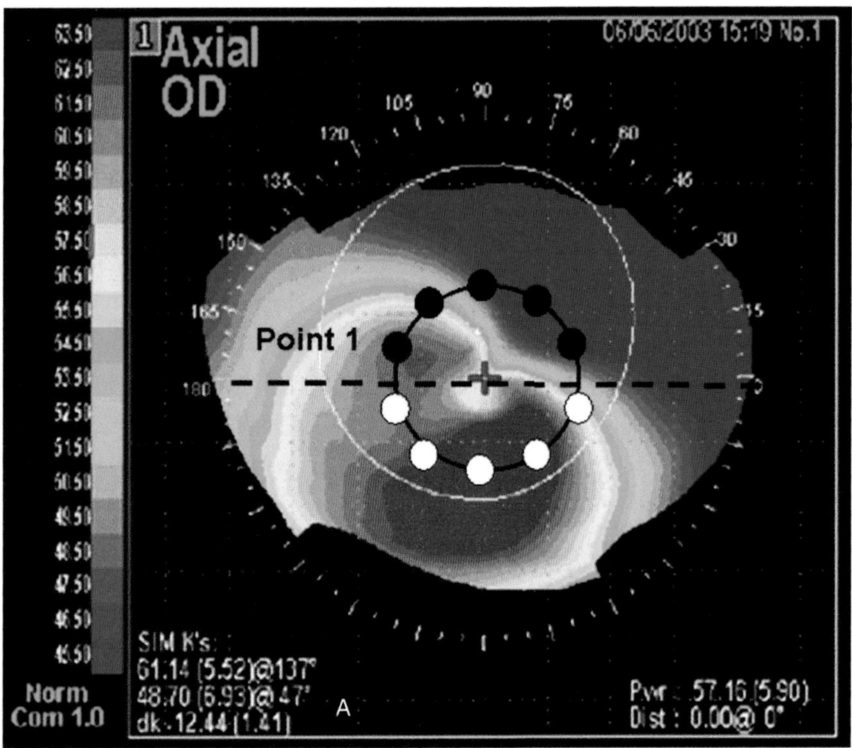

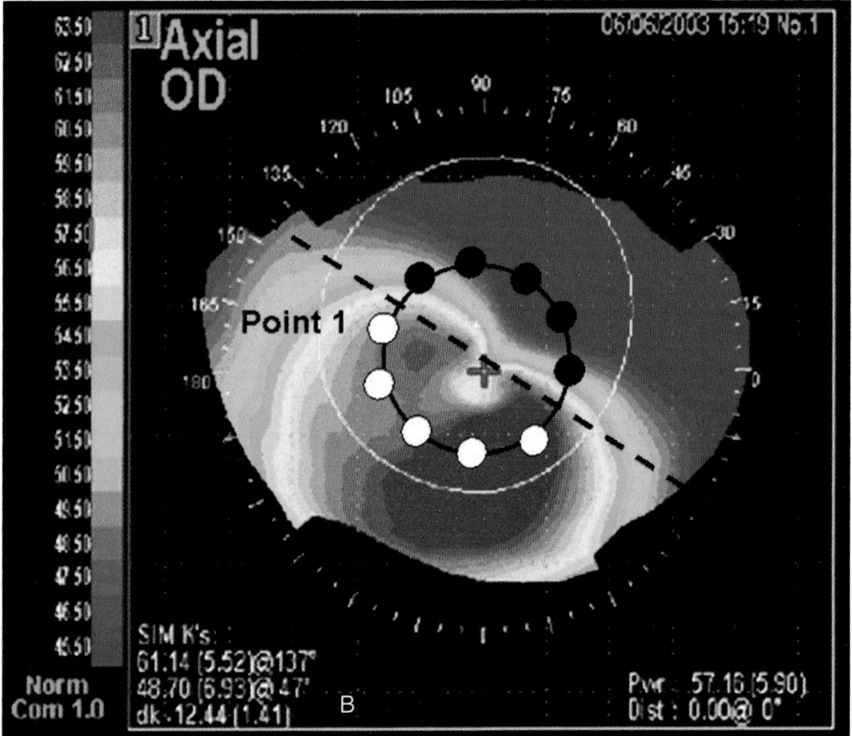

FIGURE 5-24: Comparison of I-S and L-U indices. The I-S index (A) shows the horizontal reference line is not in the axis of the cone, while the reference line for L-U index (B) is appropriately rotated and matched to axis of the cone. With I-S (A), point 1 would inadvertently be considered in the superior (assumed flat part) of the cornea. With the custom reference line rotation, L-U (B) will accurately consider point 1 in the lower, steeper cornea for calculation of this index. This is the reason the L-U index is more accurate than I-S index.

the reference axis for cone displayed on topography and then calculates a similar index as I-S for comparison of lower and upper topography curvatures. L-U has been shown to be more accurate than I-S.

Klyce and his research team developed over a dozen unique corneal indices or statistics for use in topographical analysis, many of which were designed specifically to be sensitive to and specific for keratoconus when used in combination.[10,11] These include indices that are sensitive to corneal irregularity such as the surface regularity index (SRI), the irregular astigmatism index (IAI), and the potential visual acuity (PVA). Other indices were designed to be sensitive to corneal asymmetry which include: the differential sector index (DSI), opposite sector index (OSI), and the center-surround index (CSI). Still other indices described characteristics about the curvature of the cornea that include: simulated keratometry values for the steep and flat axes (SimK1 and SimK2), minimum value of keratometry (MinK), coefficient of variation of power (CVP), and the average corneal power (ACP).

While the Tomey **(Figure 5-25)** and Nidek **(Figure 5-26)** systems make extensive use of the corneal indices developed by Klyce's research group, other systems also have their own sets of corneal indices. The Humphrey Atlas topographer includes simulated keratometry values with cylinder, maximum axial and tangential curvature, the corneal shape factor (CSF), the corneal irregularity measure (CIM), maximum elevation, and the mean reference toric K value (TKM).[12] Unfortunately, the CSF and CIM components are not particularly sensitive to central keratoconus.

In addition, Holladay developed a set of maps and corneal statistics that he called the "Holladay diagnostic summary" for use in screening keratoconus, among other uses.[13] Chastang reported development of a set of corneal statistics for use in keratoconus screening with the EyeSys corneal topographer[14] and others have advocated new and assorted indices designed to measure shape or curvature.[15]

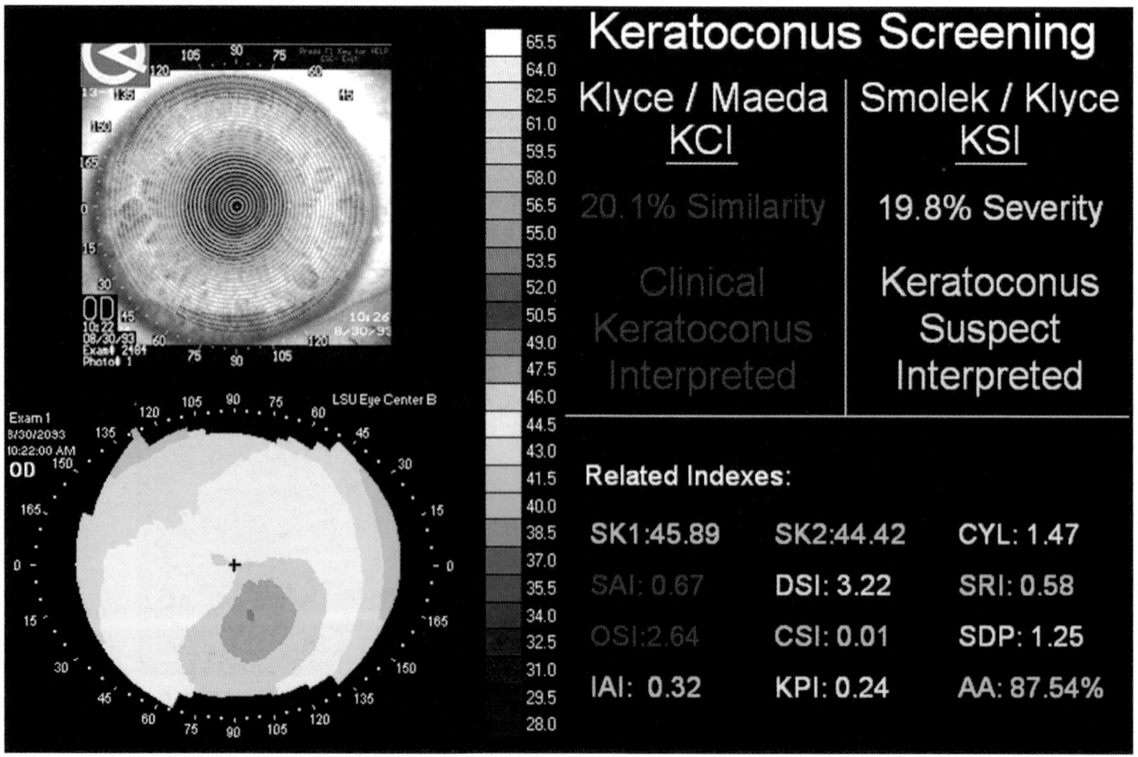

FIGURE 5-25: Tomey display. Screening indices provide helpful automated tools for the clinician.

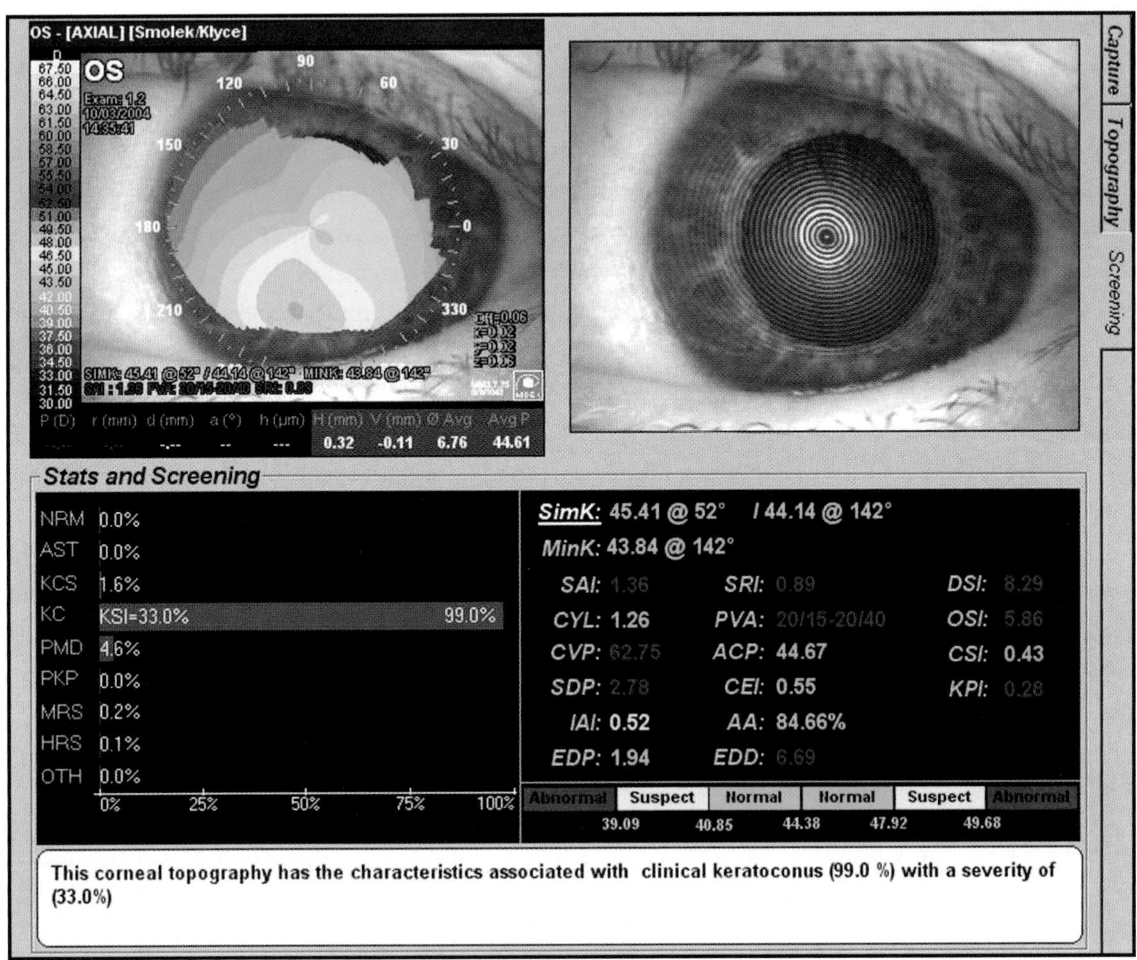

FIGURE 5-26: Nidek display. Screening indices also have proven useful in clinical practice.

A unique two-index graphical approach to keratoconus screening and grading was the "keratomorphic diagram".[16] This method plotted individual corneas in two axes with the X-axis signifying the steepness of the cornea and the Y-axis signifying the irregularity of the surface. Normal corneas are clustered in the lower left-hand part of the graph, with keratoconus corneas running along a diagonal trail toward the upper right-hand quadrant from mild to moderate to severe cases. Contact lens-induced corneal warpage cases exhibit signs of irregularity, but no significant increase in steepness, so they tend to lie in the upper left hand quadrant. The lower right hand quadrant contains atypically steep normal corneas. This same methodology could be used today with data that more readily available, such as plotting higher order aberrations (3rd order and above) versus the 2nd order (spherocylinder) components, then establishing cutoff thresholds, and testing for sensitivity.

Artificial Intelligence Methods of Keratoconus Screening

Maeda et al used the Klyce corneal indices numerical signs to derive a discriminant analysis routine (combined with an expert system) to screen for keratoconus using the Tomey TMS topographer. The discriminate analysis method was termed the keratoconus prediction index (KPI) and the overall result from the expert system was termed KCI for keratoconus index.[17] The method is noteworthy not only because it was the first true artificial intelligence method applied to the problem of keratoconus screening, but also because it was designed to ignore corneal topographies from confounding conditions. Consequently, it has both good specificity as well as good sensitivity to keratoconus. This method is still in use in the TMS system approximately 13 years after it was first developed.

Maeda et al,[11] and Smolek et al,[18] later applied the corneal indices to train a neural network to grade the severity of keratoconus and assess keratoconus suspects (FFKC). This method was called the keratoconus severity index (KSI). It too was trained to ignore confounding topographies and was subsequently added to the Tomey TMS system to replace the I-S index which has poor specificity.

Smolek and Klyce went on to develop an even more sophisticated approach to keratoconus screening by developing a series of individual neural networks using corneal indices as inputs.[19] These neural networks were individually sensitive and specific to different types of corneal conditions including both pellucid and keratoconus as well as keratoconus suspects and grading the severity of keratoconus. This method is currently available with both the Nidek-Magellan topographer and the Nidek OPD-scan aberrometer via the navigator software.[20]

Even though the Magellan and OPD-scan devices have different Placido disks with different resolutions, a Fourier filter was devised to resample the data at a standard resolution, regenerate new statistics, and provide these data to the same neural network software for analysis.[21] The ability to use an independent screening approach across different topography devices has long been a goal of those working in the field.

Conclusion

Corneal topography is a valuable tool for evaluating keratoconus, FFKC, and inferior steepening. The clinician can use either absolute or normalized scales to identify patterns of irregular corneal contour. Corneal topographer also offers objective numerical indices that can aid the clinician in assessment.

References

1. Knoll HA. Corneal contours in the general population as revealed by the photokeratoscope. American Journal of Optometry & Archives of American Academy of Optometry 1961;38:389-97.
2. Wilson SE, Klyce SD. Screening for corneal topographic abnormalities before refractive surgery. Ophthalmology 1994;101:147-52.
3. Rabinowitz YS, Rasheed K. KISA% index: a quantitative videokeratography algorithm embodying minimal topographic criteria for diagnosing keratoconus. J Cataract Refract Surg 1999; 25:1327-35.
4. Smolek MK, Klyce SD, Hovis JK. The universal standard scale: proposed improvements to the ANSI standard scale for corneal topography. Ophthalmology 2002;109:361-9.
5. Smolek MK. Interlamellar cohesive strength in the vertical meridian of human eyebank corneas. Invest Ophthalmol Vis Sci 1993; 34:2962-9.
6. Rabinowitz YS. McDonnell PJ. Computer-assisted corneal topography in keratoconus. Refractive & Corneal Surgery 1989;5:400-8.
7. Klyce SD, Smolek MK, Maeda N. Keratoconus detection with the KISA% method-another view. Journal of Cataract & Refractive Surgery 2000;26:472-4.
8. Rabinowitz YS, Rasheed K. KISA% index: a quantitative videokeratography algorithm embodying minimal topographic criteria for diagnosing keratoconus. Journal of Cataract & Refractive Surgery 1999;25:1327-35.
9. Chan CC, Sharma M, Boxer Wachler BS. Effect of inferior-segment Intacs with and without C3-R on keratoconus. J Cataract Refract Surg 2007;33:75-80.
10. Klyce SD, Wilson SE. Methods of analysis of corneal topography. Refractive & Corneal Surgery 1989;5:368-71.
11. Maeda N, Klyce SD, Smolek MK. Neural network classification of corneal topography. Preliminary demonstration. Investigative Ophthalmology & Visual Science 1995;36:1327-35.
12. Lebow KA, Grohe RM. Differentiating contact lens induced warpage from true keratoconus using corneal topography. CLAO Journal 1999;25:114-22.
13. Holladay J T. Corneal topography using the Holladay diagnostic summary. Journal of Cataract & Refractive Surgery 1997; 23:209-21.

14. Chastang P J, Borderie V M, Carvajal-Gonzalez S, Rostene W, Laroche L. Automated keratoconus detection using the EyeSys videokeratoscope. Journal of Cataract & Refractive Surgery 2000;26:675-83.
15. Szczotka LB, Roberts C, Herderick EE, Mahmoud A. Quantitative descriptors of corneal topography that influence soft toric contact lens fitting. Cornea 2002;21:249-55.
16. Smolek MK, Klyce SD, Maeda N. Keratoconus and contact lens-induced warpage analysis using the keratomorphic diagram. Invest Ophthalmol Vis Sci 1994; 35:4192-204.
17. Maeda N, Klyce SD, Smolek MK, Thompson HW. Automated keratoconus screening with corneal topography analysis. Investigative Ophthalmology & Visual Science 1994;35:2749-57.
18. Smolek MK, Klyce SD. Current keratoconus detection methods compared with a neural network approach. Invest Ophthalmol Vis Sci 1997; 38:2290-9.
19. Smolek MK, Klyce SD, Karon MD. Device-Independent Corneal Topography Classification and Keratoconus Grading by Neural Networks [abstract 2867]. Association for Research in Vision & Ophthalmology (ARVO), Ft. Lauderdale, Florida, April 27, 2004.
20. Klyce SD, Karon MD, Smolek MK. Screening patients with the corneal navigator. J Refract Surgery 2005; 21:S617-22.
21. Karon MD, Klyce SD, Smolek MK. Device-Independent Statistical Indexes in Corneal Topography [abstract 2874]. Association for Research in Vision & Ophthalmology (ARVO). Ft. Lauderdale, Florida, April 27, 2004.

Michael K Smolek, *PhD*

6 Non-Topography Diagnostic Devices

Corneal Elevation Maps

Corneal measurement systems, such as the Orbscan, the PAR, and the Pentacam, provide elevation maps for the anterior and/or posterior corneal surfaces. These maps are often referred to as elevation float maps or simply as floats **(Figure 6-1)**. Some believe that elevation mapping can provide better information than

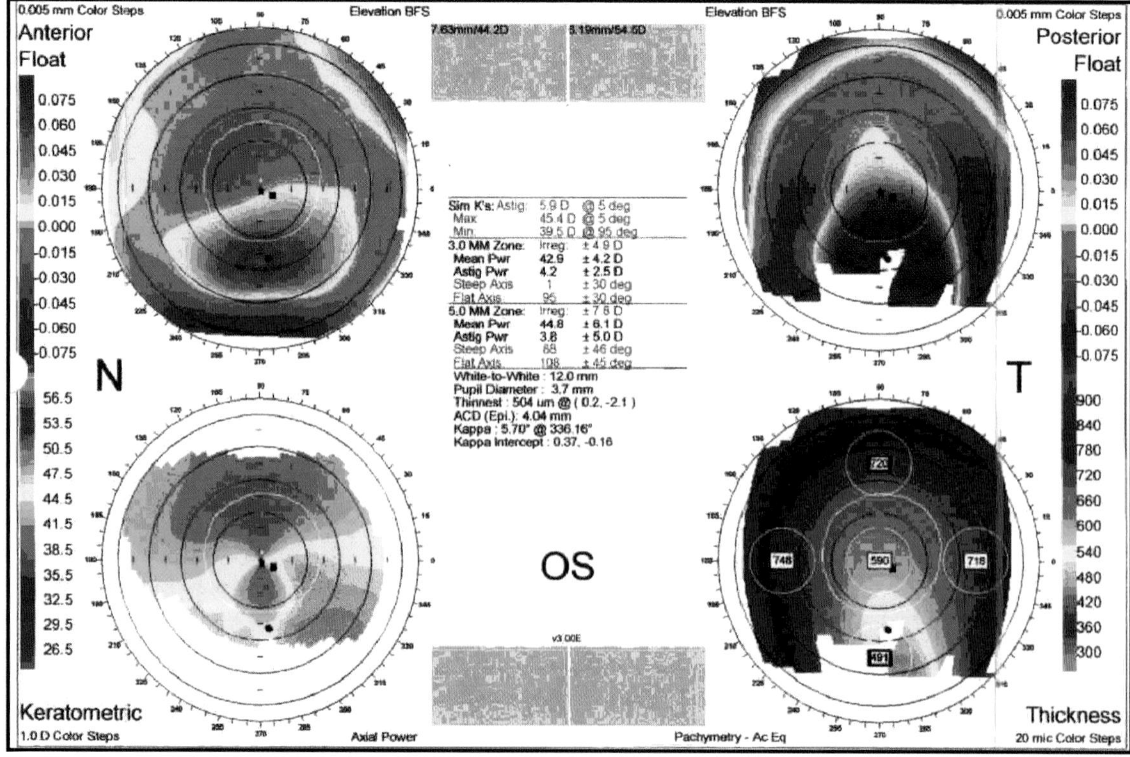

FIGURE 6-1: Orbscan map of peripheral keratoconus. The anterior elevation (upper left) and posterior elevation (upper right) display results in reference to a best fit sphere to the corneal shape. Keratometric (topography) map (lower left) and pachymetry map (lower right) are also shown. This map could also be called pellucid marginal degeneration as well (Courtesy: Brian S Boxer Wachler, MD).

axial curvature maps for screening purposes.[1] It is asserted that posterior surface maps show earlier signs of ectasia than can be seen on the anterior surface via Placido disk topography, but studies have yet to prove this claim due to a wide range of confounding corneal variables.[2] It is unclear which are the ideal base curves that need to be used for elevation-based systems in order to achieve optimum sensitivity.[3]

Elevation maps do have shortcomings that make them difficult to use and in some cases fail to show signs of keratoconus which may include severe forms of keratoconus. By necessity, elevation maps use a floating (normalized) color scale due to the extreme range of heights that may be present on the anterior or posterior surface. Floating scales do not link the numerical height values to specific color contours of the map, so the clinician needs to inspect the microns of the float as well as the pattern of the float

Users of the elevation mapping systems need to appreciate that when elevation height is mapped, a reference surface (typically a base sphere) is subtracted from the shape. Removing the base sphere also removes critical information about central keratoconus **(Figures 6-2 and 6-3)**. In these examples, the elevation map fails to show the presence of a central cone because it was subtracted off with the reference sphere. The central elevation is given as values close to zero even though a prominent cone exists in that location.

While elevation maps do show peripheral keratoconus **(Figure 6-1)**, subtraction of the base sphere removes height information about a central cone. It has occurred where a surgeon exclusively relied on the elevation

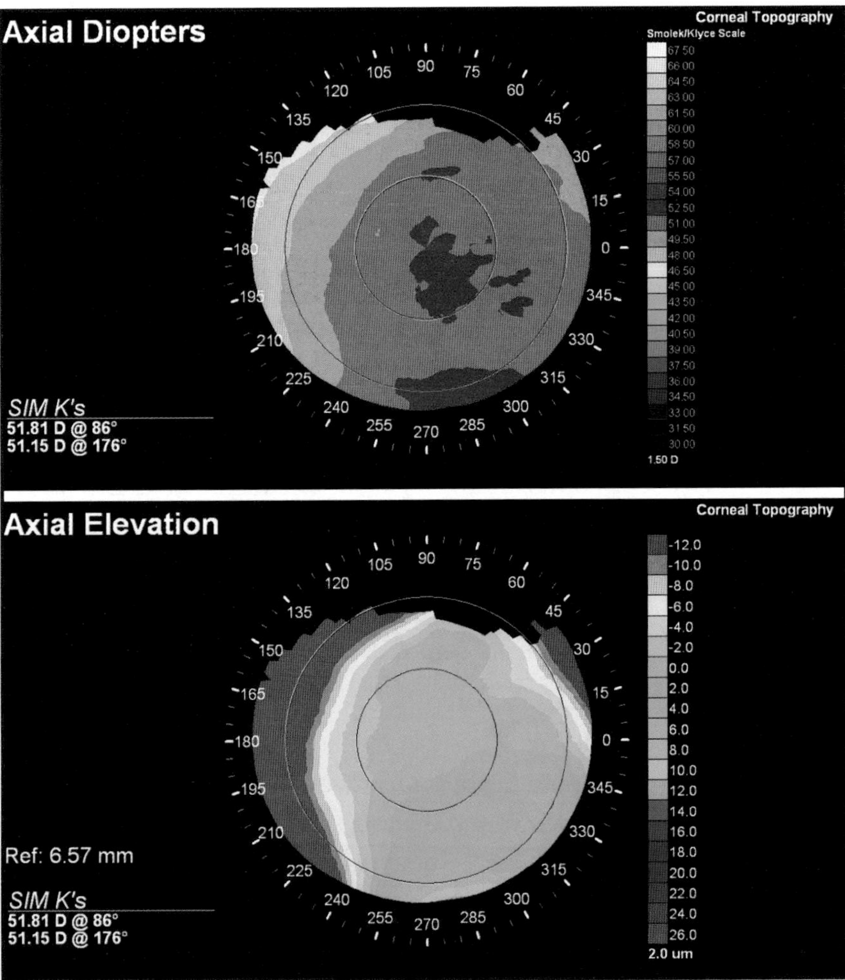

FIGURE 6-2: Comparison of axial topography map (top) and elevation map (bottom) of central keratoconus. Despite the presence of a significant central cone with curvature over 51 D, the elevation map appears normal.

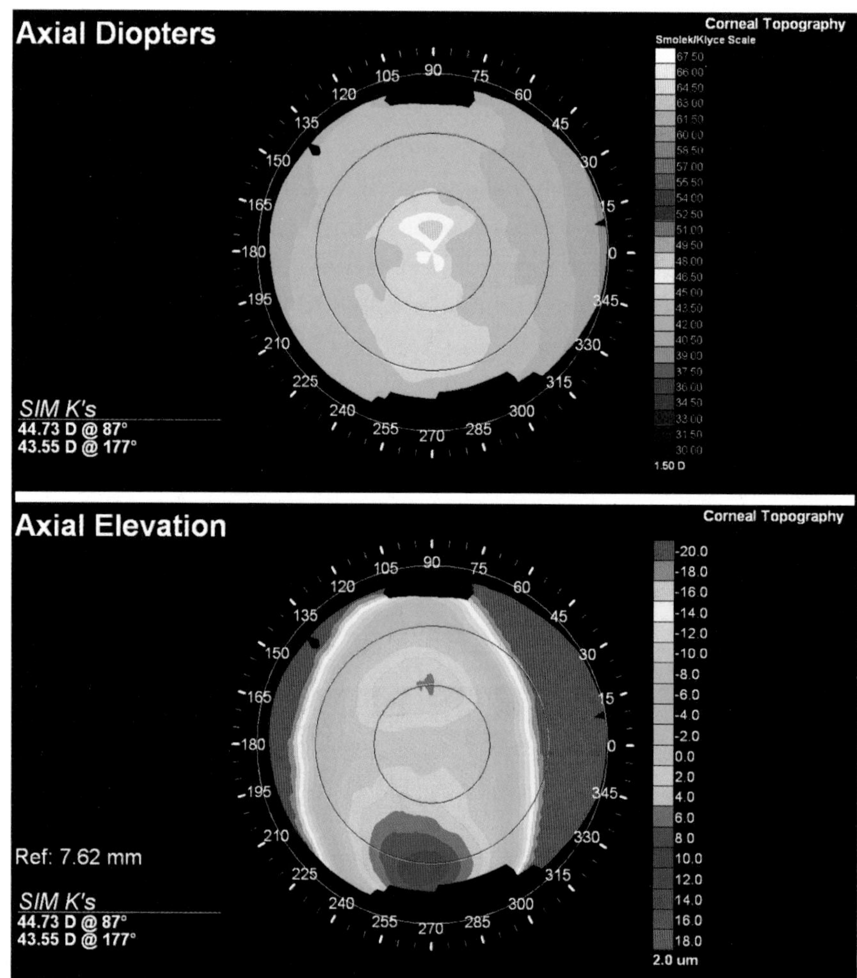

FIGURE 6-3: Comparison of axial topography map (top) and elevation map (bottom) of central keratoconus. The axial map shows a small, central cone, but the elevation map shows no hint of it.

map and inadvertently interpreted it as normal during a patient evaluation for LASIK. LASIK was subsequently performed and the patient unfortunately experienced keratoectasia. In this instance, central keratoconus was preoperatively visible on the axial curvature map. It seems prudent that users of elevation-based systems continue to also use axial curvature maps to be certain that keratoconus in all forms is being properly screened.

Wavefront Aberrometry Maps

Wavefront aberrometry has been suggested as a possible means of screening for keratoconus. In aberrometry, the deviation of a plano standard wavefront of light is recorded after passing through the optics of the whole eye. The wavefront error is then typically decomposed into a series of Zernike coefficients whose terms reflect radial and angular frequency harmonics of shape.[4] Comparisons can then be made between each aberration term of the keratoconus condition to the coefficient values for a typical normal cornea.[5]

It is also possible to convert corneal topography elevation information into wavefront error maps, thus allowing only the shape of the anterior corneal surface to be examined for aberrations.[6] Corneal wavefronts therefore will not be confounded by the aberrations of the lens, but on the other hand, they also will not provide information about the posterior surface of the cornea.

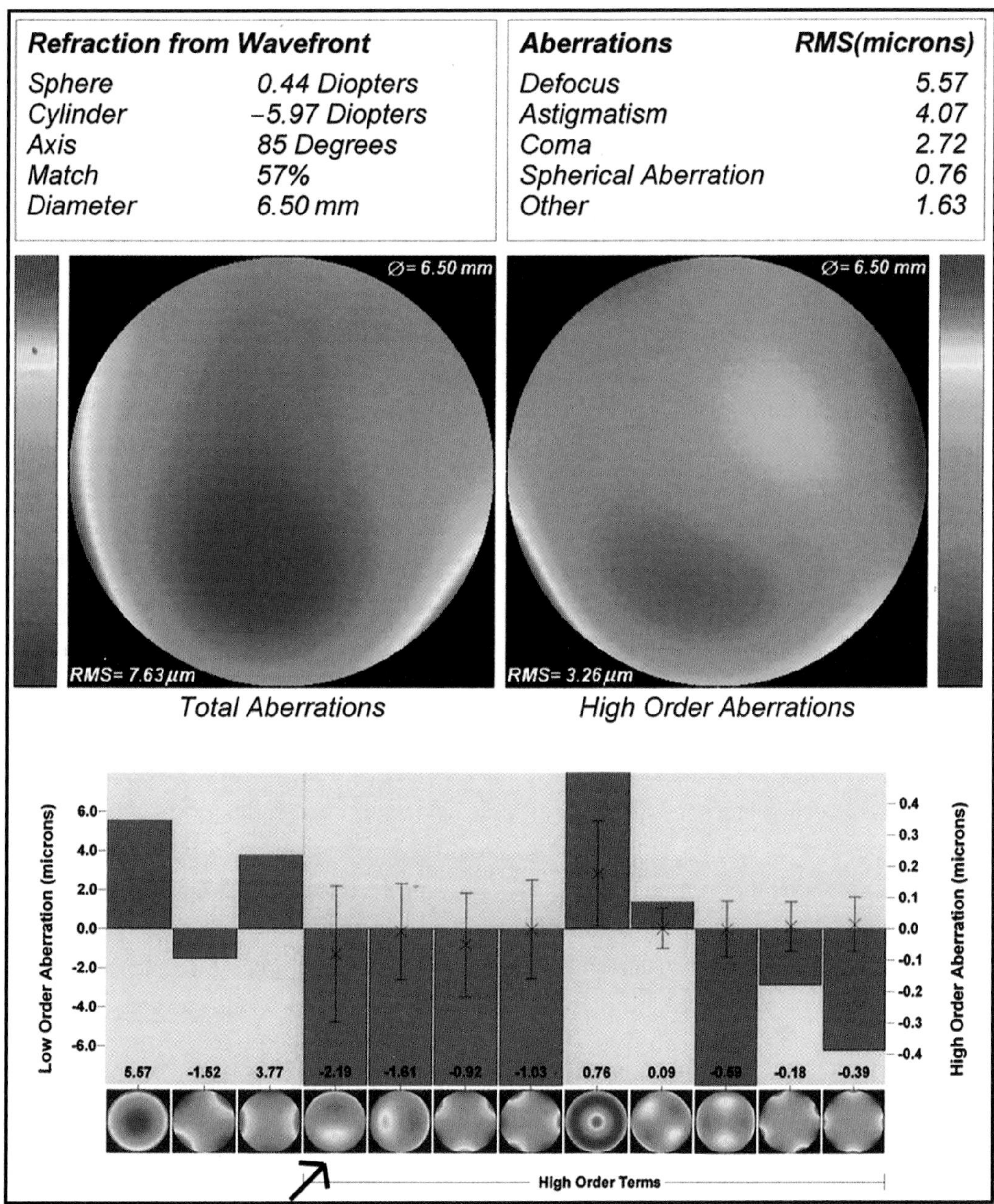

FIGURE 6-4: Wavefront map of keratoconus. Vertical coma (arrow) is typically high in keratoconus as shown here which measures 2.19 microns. Coma in the normal population is typically under 0.20 microns (Courtesy: Brian S Boxer Wachler, MD).

One of the earliest reports on aberrometry applied to keratoconus screening was use of the trefoil term as a sign for keratoconus.[7] Subsequent analysis has shown that vertical coma is a more sensitive Zernike term **(Figure 6-4)**. Prism is the most sensitive term because it picks up the asymmetry of the wavefront shape induced by the cone.[8] However, prism is not normally present on many aberrometry displays because the afocal tip and tilt prism terms are often discarded.

Unfortunately, there is a high likelihood that central keratoconus will not be readily detected with aberrometry. Central keratoconus, particularly the milder form, will tend to have little or no prism, coma, or trefoil, making it difficult to distinguish from the normal condition. Central keratoconus will have higher amounts of radially symmetric aberrations such as defocus and spherical aberration, but unfortunately, neither of these terms is unique to keratoconus alone.

Another challenge with aberrometry is that the mapped patterns of wavefront error are not particularly specific for keratoconus. If the wavefront error map for keratoconus was placed beside a wavefront map from a hyperopic LASIK procedure, most clinicians would be unable to distinguish any appreciable difference in the maps or in the underlying numerical microns of aberrations. Use of axial topography maps allows the clinician to distinguish the two procedures since each entity has distinctly different topography patterns.

Using Zernike coefficients as keratoconus screening indices have met with only limited success. While they are very sensitive indicators for keratoconus, their specificity for keratoconus is low which makes wavefront analysis vulnerable to many false-positives during screening.[9] Large amounts of coma or trefoil can occur in a variety of conditions including post-surgical corneas and contact-lens wearing corneas. By contrast, corneal topography axial curvature maps typically have both high sensitivity and high specificity for keratoconus. In general, wavefront analysis of keratoconus may be best performed when there is a need to either determine the severity of keratoconus or when there is a need to determine a threshold value of an aberration term between the normal and keratoconus conditions.[10] This becomes more complicated as Zernike coefficient values are dependent on the number of terms that are decomposed in the Zernike equation and can change based on diameter of the pupil.

Pachymetric Maps

As previously discussed, corneal thickness is an important sign for the correct diagnosis of keratoconus.[11] Using a slit lamp microscope, relative changes in thickness across the cornea can often be quickly judged by visual inspection. However, methods that provide numerical values of thickness with a high degree of accuracy and precision are preferred. There are at least 9 different methods for measuring corneal pachymetry including: traditional ultrasound, very high frequency ultrasound, confocal microscopy, optical slit-lamp, specular microscopy, slit scanning systems, optical coherence tomography (OCT), low coherence reflectometry, and laser Doppler interferometry.

Traditional ultrasound and optical slit lamp measurements have historically been popular methods. Their limitation is that they provide only point-based measurements. Slit scanning systems such as the Orbscan (Bausch and Lomb), Pentacam (Oculus) **(Figure 6-5)**, and Visante OCT (Zeiss) devices provide three-dimentional maps of pachymetry across the entire cornea, which is very useful for keratoconus screening.

While mean pachymetry values vary from system to system and from study to study, the typical mean normal central corneal thickness using traditional ultrasound is approximately 550 +/– 40 μm. Using two standard deviations from the mean as an indication of the normal range, the lower limit for normal corneas is approximately 470 μm. Clinicians should keep this number in mind as a cutoff criterion that can help distinguish keratoconus from normal corneas.

The Pentacam device uses pachymetry mapping of the cornea to produce unique tomography indices for keratoconus.[12] **Figure 6-6** shows a graph for corneal thickness over a 10 mm diameter as well as a graph for progression of corneal thickness. The patient's pachymetry curve is plotted against the population curves and if the patient's curve follows a pattern divergent from that of the population, it is of concern for keratoconus. This analysis may complement other devices for keratoconus analysis and screening.

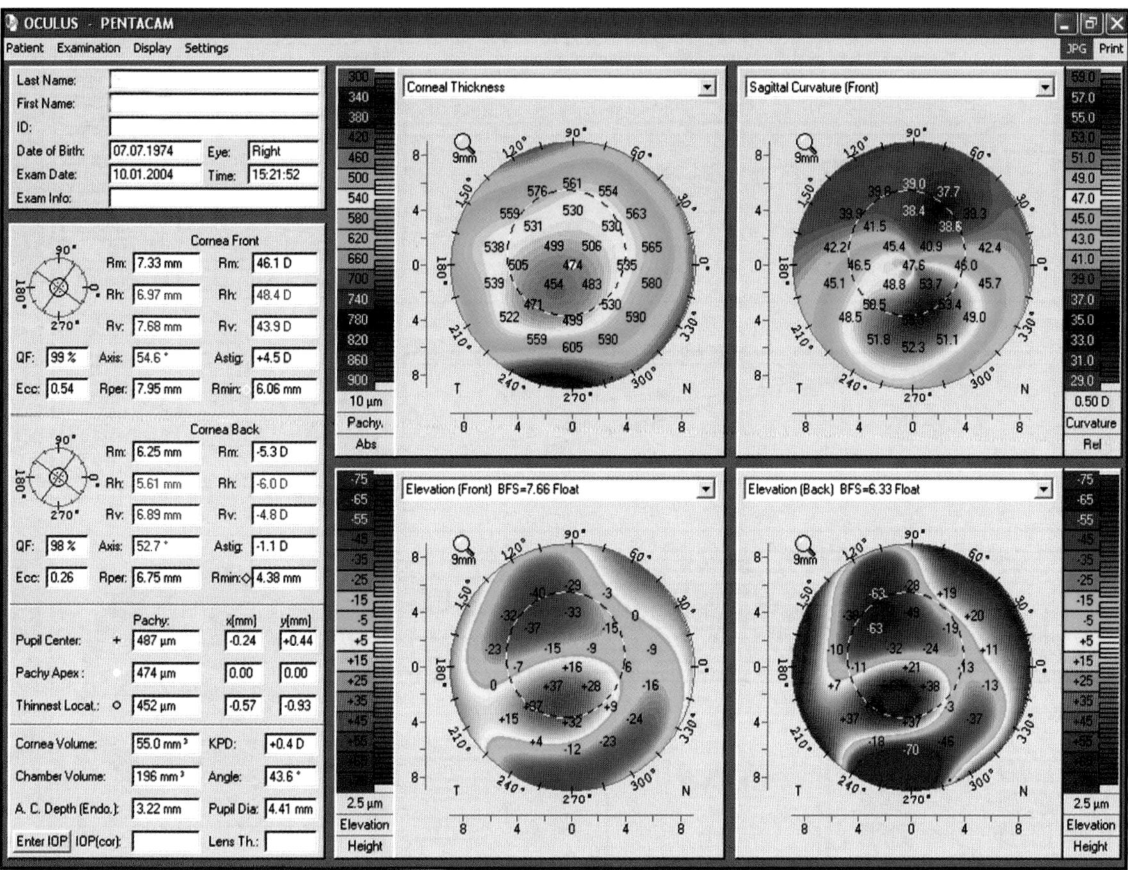

FIGURE 6-5: Pentacam map of keratoconus. Corneal thickness (upper left) shows thinning down to 454 microns, topography (upper right) shows inferior cones, and anterior elevation (lower left) and back or posterior elevation (lower right) both show protrusion (Courtesy: Michael Belin, MD).

Corneal Hysteresis

A relatively new approach to keratoconus screening is the use of in vivo biomechanical measurements of the corneal tissue properties.[13] The Ocular Response Analyzer (Reichert) utilizes a rapid pulse of air to move the cornea inward and outward under the force through a "dynamic bi-directional applanation process." An electro-optical optical system monitors the shape change of the cornea. Applanation pressure is recorded at two points: when the cornea is bending inward and when the cornea is returning to its normal state. Due to bending resistance of the tissue, there are delays in the expected times when the cornea bends and returns to a normal state and the difference in the applanation pressure at these two points is termed corneal hysteresis. Depending on the properties of the cornea for different conditions, one would expect to see different hysteresis values. For example, normal corneas have significantly higher hysteresis values (on average) than do keratoconic corneas **(Figure 6-7)**. At the time of this publication, only one peer-reviewed paper has been published related to hystersis in keratoconus and normal eyes.

While the technology looks promising, there is a question as to how well the method can distinguish between normal and mildly keratoconic tissue. Data plots of normal and keratoconus corneas show there is significant overlap in hysteresis values in the two groups. This implies that hysteresis is neither very sensitive nor specific for keratoconus. At this time, the technology does not appear to have any advantage over current screening methods that are more sensitive to the disease. Further modifications may make it more useful.

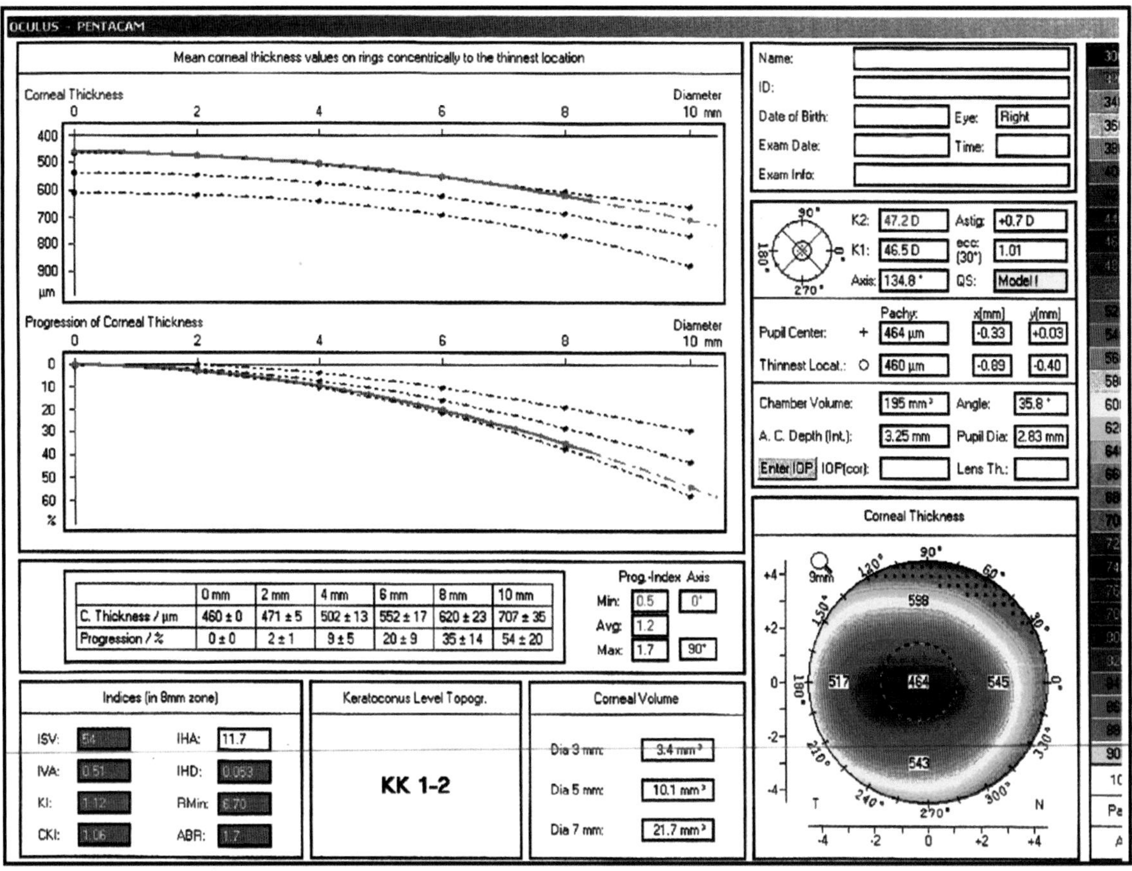

FIGURE 6-6: Pentacam OCT pachymetry graphs and map. Corneal thickness graph in microns (upper left) shows patient's pachymetry distribution (red line) compared to non-keratoconus population (upper and lower black lines represent two standard deviations, middle black line is mean). This patient's cornea is very thin and outside standard deviation curve, but proportionally thin as the red line is parallel to black lines across the corneal diameter. Progression of corneal thickness graph in percentage (lower left) shows that the patient's thickness progression across the cornea (red line) is parallel to and within the border of the population curves (black lines). Corneal thickness map is displayed as well (lower right). (Courtesy: Brian S Boxer Wachler, MD).

Confocal Microscopy Signs

The use of confocal microscopy for keratoconus is still a fairly recent addition to the clinician's choice of screening tools. This device has added considerable information about the morphology of keratoconus at the microscopic level. As the magnification is higher and the optical imaging/sectioning methods are different from slit lamp biomicroscopy, confocal findings are distinctly different from those seen with the slit lamp examination.

The list of confocal microscopy signs associated with keratoconus is fairly extensive and includes thinning of the stroma; elongated, exfoliating superficial epithelial cells; enlarged wing and basal epithelial cells; bright reflective material deposited within basal epithelial cells; prominent, thickened subbasal nerves with additional structural changes seen along nerve fibers; increased stromal haze; pronounced reflectivity and an irregular arrangement of the stromal keratocytes; structurally abnormal anterior stromal keratocyte nuclei; lower densities of anterior and posterior stromal keratocytes; Z-shaped folds in the anterior, mid, and posterior stroma; folds in Descemet's membrane; pleomorphism and enlargement of endothelial cells; increased endothelial cell density; and endothelial guttata.[14-16] **Figure 6-8** shows a confocal image of an eye with keratoconus.

While these signs may occur with keratoconus, most are not specific to keratoconus, but may be also seen with other corneal disorders. Nevertheless, efforts are underway to automatically recognize many of these findings

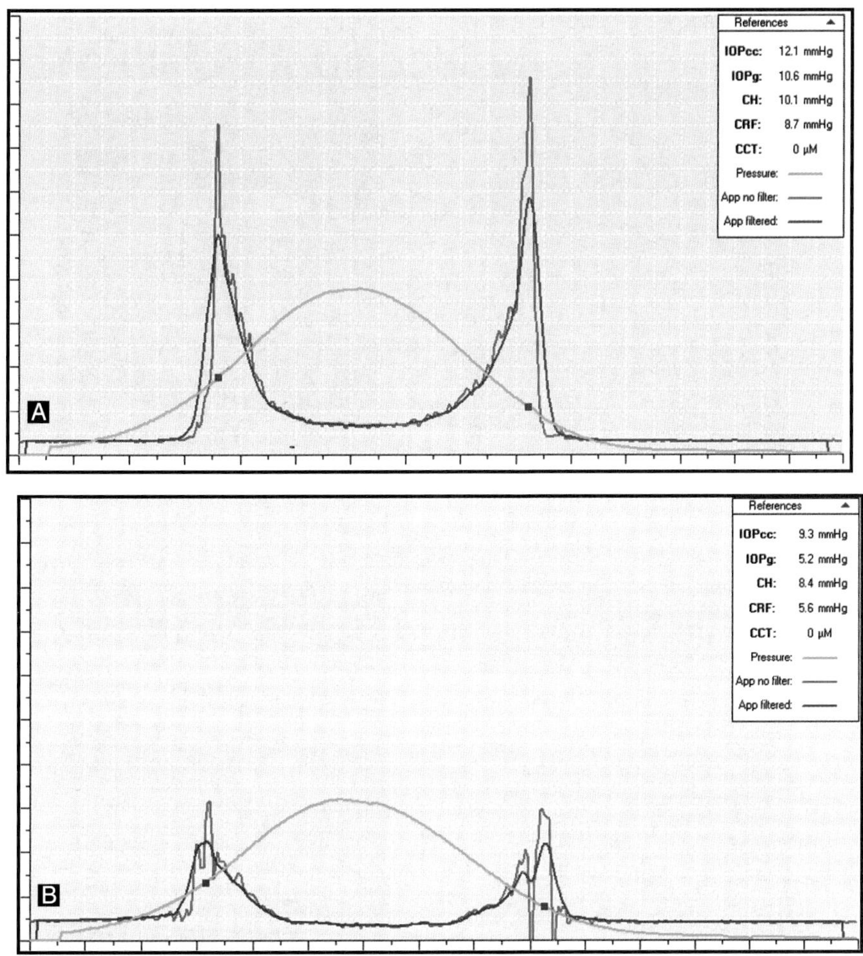

FIGURE 6-7: Corneal hysteresis graphs. A normal hysteresis graph (A) and keratoconus hysteresis graph (B) which shows lower values than normal cornea (A). (Illustration copyright © 2007 Reichert, Inc, all rights reserved).

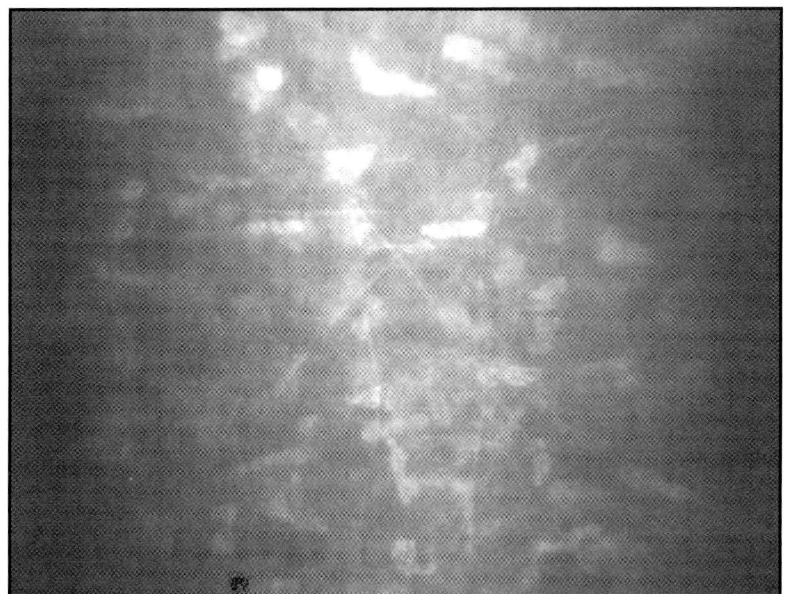

FIGURE 6-8: Confocal image of keratoconus. Small, spindle-like striae are seen here.

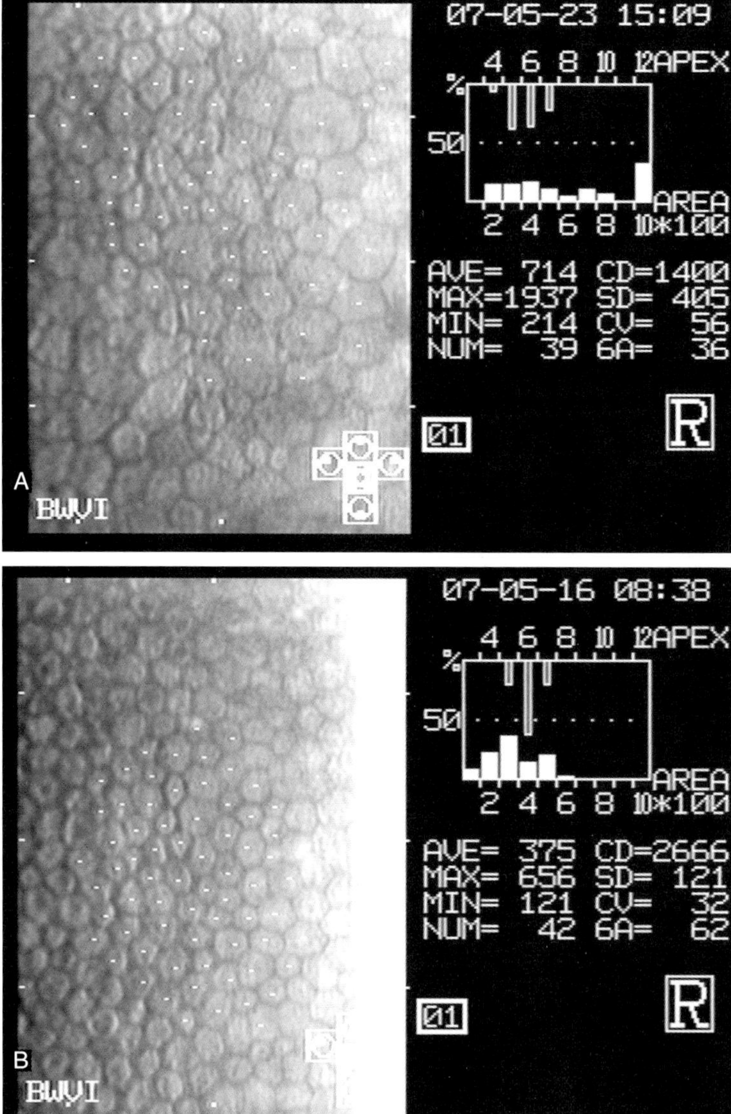

FIGURE 6-9: Specular microscopy photographs. Keratoconus endothelial patterns (A) show larger and irregular sized cells compared to a normal cornea (B). Coefficient of variation (CV) in keratoconic cornea (A) of 56 is significantly higher than 32 in the normal cornea (B) (Courtesy: Brian S Boxer Wachler, MD).

and then objectively measure or grade them. This may help us not only understand the disease better, but also it may provide a way to determine if certain combinations of these signs show an improved sensitivity and specificity to keratoconus.

Specular Microscopy Maps

As seen with confocal microscopy, specular microscopy of keratoconus shows signs of altered endothelium cell morphology **(Figure 6-9)**. There is a significant increase in polymegathism compared to normal controls and a significant decrease in hexagonality in the keratoconic cornea.[17] Higher pleomorphism (variation in endothelial cell shape such as percentage of hexagonal cells or coefficient of variation of endothelial cell shape) is seen in keratoconus. Pleomorphism is represented as coefficient of variation (CV) values **(Figure 6-9)**. One study noted that unaffected fellow eyes also had significant pleomorphic changes, suggesting latent forms of keratoconus (i.e. forme fruste keratoconus).

Conclusion

Clinicians have many available methods to screen for and diagnose keratoconus, many of which show exceptionally good results for sensitivity. However, high sensitivity alone is not sufficient. If the method is sensitive to peripheral cones, but consistently misses central keratoconus, this is problematic. If the method fails to grade severity of keratoconus correctly, this is not ideal. A screening method can have high sensitivity, but if it has low specificity, the clinician still has the burden of ruling out confounding conditions. Hopefully in the future, keratoconus screening will show continued improvements in current technology and better extraction of existing signs.

References

1. Belin MW, Litoff D, Strods SJ, Winn SS, Smith RS. The PAR technology corneal topography system. Refractive & Corneal Surgery 1992:8:88-96.
2. Sonmez B, Doan MP, Hamilton DR. Identification of scanning slit-beam topographic parameters important in distinguishing normal from keratoconic corneal morphologic features. American Journal of Ophthalmology 2007;143:401-8.
3. Quisling S, Sjoberg S, Zimmerman B, Goins K, Sutphin J. Comparison of Pentacam and Orbscan IIz on posterior curvature topography measurements in keratoconus eyes. Ophthalmology 2006;113:1629-32.
4. Thibos LN. Principles of Hartmann-Shack aberrometry. Journal of Refractive Surgery 2000;16(5):S563-5
5. Shah S, Naroo S, Hosking S, Gherghel D, Mantry S, Bannerjee S, Pedwell K, Bains HS. Nidek OPD-scan analysis of normal, keratoconic, and penetrating keratoplasty eyes. Journal of Refractive Surgery 2003;19(2 Suppl):S255-9.
6. Barbero S, Marcos S, Merayo-Lloves J, Moreno-Barriuso E. Validation of the estimation of corneal aberrations from videokeratography in keratoconus. Journal of Refractive Surgery 2002;18(3):263-70.
7. Schwiegerling J, Greivenkamp JE. Keratoconus detection based on videokeratoscopic height data. Optometry & Vision Science 1996;73(12):721-8.
8. Smolek M K. Tip and Tilt – lost prism components of Zernike analysis: clinical significance in refractive surgery planning. American Society of Cataract and Refractive Surgery (ASCRS) Annual Meeting. Washington, DC. April 18, 2005.
9. Smolek MK, Klyce SD. Zernike polynomial terms and corneal indexes as neural network inputs for videokeratography. Invest Ophthalmol Vis Sci Suppl 1997;38:S920.
10. Alio JL, Shabayek MH. Corneal higher order aberrations: a method to grade keratoconus. Journal of Refractive Surgery 2006;22(6):539-45.
11. Rabinowitz YS, Rasheed K, Yang H, Elashoff J. Accuracy of ultrasonic pachymetry and videokeratography in detecting keratoconus. Journal of Cataract & Refractive Surgery 1998;24(2):196-201.
12. Ambrosio R, Simonato Alonso R, Luz A, Guillermo Coca Velarde L. Corneal-thickness spatial profile and corneal-volume distribution: tomographic indicis to detect keratoconus. J Cataract Refract Surgery 2006;32:1851-9.
13. Luce DA. Determining in vivo biomechanical properties of the cornea with an ocular response analyzer. Journal of Cataract & Refractive Surgery 2005;31:156-62.
14. Ucakhan OO, Kanpolat A, Ylmaz N, Ozkan M. In vivo confocal microscopy findings in keratoconus. Eye & Contact Lens: Science & Clinical Practice. 2006;32:183-91.
15. Hollingsworth, Joanna G. Efron, Nathan. Tullo, Andrew B. In vivo corneal confocal microscopy in keratoconus. Ophthalmic & Physiological Optics 2005;25:254-60.
16. Erie JC, Patel SV, McLaren JW, Nau CB, Hodge DO, Bourne WM. Keratocyte density in keratoconus. A confocal microscopy study(a). Am J of Ophthalmology 2002;134:689-95.
17. Matsuda M, Suda T, Manabe R. Quantitative analysis of endothelial mosaic pattern changes in anterior keratoconus. American Journal of Ophthalmology 1984;98:43-9.

Section 3

Cornea Rehabilitation Treatments

Brian S Boxer Wachler, MD, ***Shawn Jalali,*** MD, ***Colin CK Chan,*** MD

7 C3-R® Corneal Collagen Crosslinking with Riboflavin

Introduction

Ever since keratoconus was first described by Burchard Mauchart in 1748, eye doctors had no means to stop the progression of this potentially devastating disease. When patients would ask, "Is there anything that can stop this from getting worse?" Often the answer was, "We do not even know what causes keratoconus, let alone understand how to stop it from progressing." Fortunately, we now have answers to both questions. Chapter 2 discussed the cause of keratoconus and this chapter will discuss C3-R®, the remarkable procedure that can stop keratoconus from progressing "dead in its tracks" as well as augment Intacs in improving corneal shape and visual quality.

Some eye doctors believe that wearing rigid gas permeable (RGP) contact lenses could stop keratoconus from progressing, however, this has never been proven. Logically, it does not seem possible that contact lenses could accomplish this. Keratoconus is a hernia (bulge) of the cornea much like an inguinal hernia that occurs in the groin. The keratoconus hernia results from weakened collagen tissue which bulges out in response to back pressure (intraocular pressure) inside the eye. Contact lenses float and are balanced on top of the cornea just like a surfer balances on top of a wave. Stating that contact lenses can stop the cornea from bulging is much like saying the surfboard can push back the wave. Another analogy is if someone's head (skull) was expanding, than wearing a hat will not prevent further head expansion. It is true that RGP contact lenses can cause temporary flattening of the outer corneal layer (epithelium), but this area has no structural contribution to corneal strength. Unfortunately, RGP lenses do not flatten the deeper corneal stromal layers which are the critical areas to address if there is to be structural enhancement of the cornea. C3-R® is the first and only proven method that has prevented further loss of vision and halted corneal steepening in patients with known keratoconus deterioration. Just as intraocular lenses and phacoemulsification revolutionized cataract surgery, we expect that the ophthalmic historians will likely consider C3-R® and Intacs® to have had an analogous impact on keratoconus treatment. There are many who already consider C3-R® and Intacs® to have fulfilled this analogy.

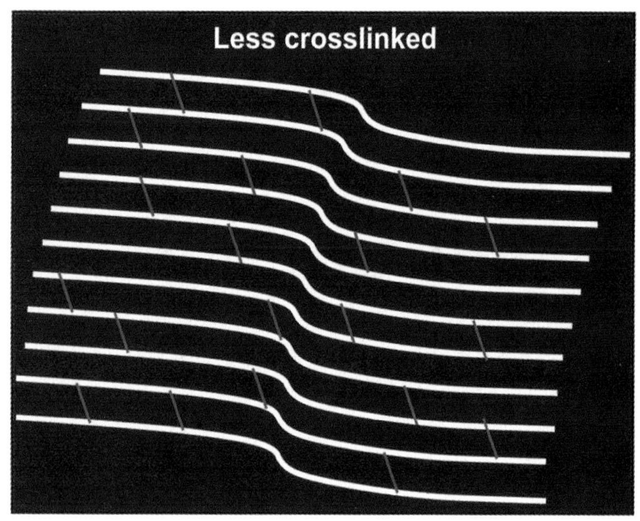

FIGURE 7-1: Diagram of reduced crosslinking in corneal stroma.

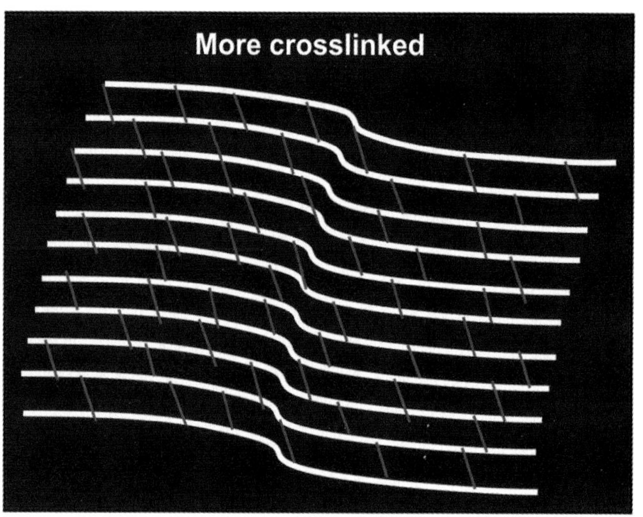

FIGURE 7-2: Diagram of enhanced crosslinking in corneal stroma.

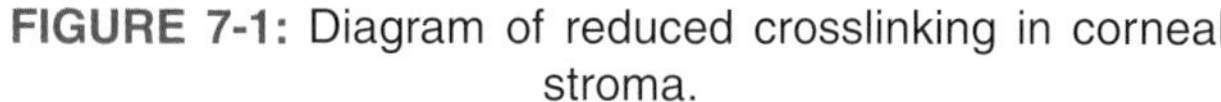

Basic Science Behind C3-R®

The biomechanical strength of the cornea in keratoconus is considerably reduced compared to a normal cornea with studies showing a 50% decrease in the stress necessary for a defined strain.[1,2] Progression of keratoconus typically slows with age possibly due to a reduction in free radicals generated in the cornea and/or increased tissue crosslinking that naturally occurs with age. Keratoconus is more common in younger patients because of high metabolic activity (and hence more free radical byproducts of metabolism) and low amount of natural crosslinking. It is interesting to note that patients with diabetes typically do not experience keratoconus presumably due to glucose-related glycation that results in accelerated crosslinking in the cornea and other tissues throughout the body.

The means of achieving corneal crosslinking from the C3-R® procedure is via a specialized riboflavin solution that is absorbed into the cornea which is simultaneously exposed to a controlled amount of ultraviolet A (UVA) light that directly leads to thicker collagen fibers and more crosslinking between collagen fibers **(Figures 7-1 and 7-2)**.

Once the collagen has absorbed the riboflavin solution, UVA light is required to activate riboflavin's strengthening effect on the collagen fibers **(Figure 7-3)**. This structurally reinforces the cornea much like enhancing weakened steel beams in a building that is tilting. The enhanced collagen integrity also makes the treated area of the cornea resistant to inflammatory and melting processes.

Laboratory Studies

In recent years, several studies have been published on the effect of UVA/riboflavin treatments on porcine, rabbit and human corneas. C3-R® increases the crosslinking between collagen fibers and leads to biomechanical strengthening of the cornea. There is an increase in collagen fiber diameter in rabbit corneas of 12.2% in the anterior stroma and 4.6% in the posterior stroma compared to control eyes after crosslinking.[3] Some scientists argue that the increase in collagen diameter may lead to loss of corneal transparency. This complication has not been reported in any clinical or laboratory studies. This theoretically should not occur since the critical threshold for corneal opacification is 150 nm and an increase of 12.2% would increase collagen diameter only to 25 nm to 28 nm,[4-6] which is far below the threshold for opacification.

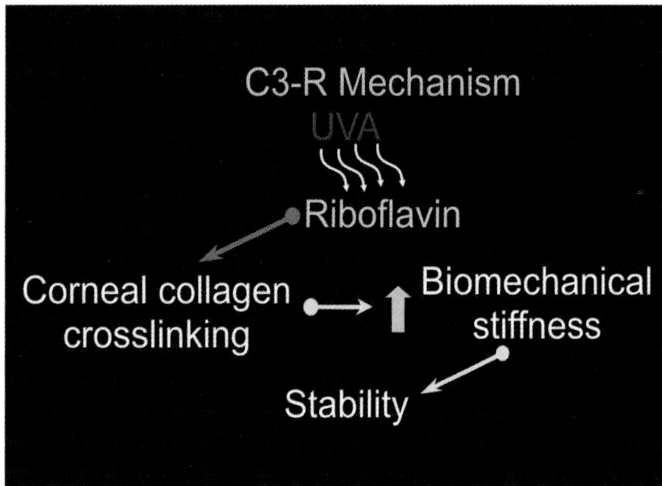

FIGURE 7-3: The mechanism of C3-R®.

Strong evidence of increased corneal biomechanical strength after C3-R® has been demonstrated by stress-strain measurements, thermal studies, and enzyme digestion studies. In porcine corneas, an increase of up to 71.9% in stress-strain measurements was reported across the entire cornea. This indicated an increase in biomechanical rigidity of 1.8 times. The change in donated human corneas was even more dramatic with a 328.9% increase in stress-strain values or an increase in rigidity of 4.5 times. The pre-treatment stress-strain values were not statistically different between porcine and human corneas which indicated a greater effect of treatment in human corneas.[7] Clinical biomechanical analyzers that measure hystersis may provide further insight.[8] Tests on the anterior 200 microns of the stroma compared to the posterior stroma post-crosslinking showed that in human corneas the stress-strain measurements post-treatment increased significantly more in the anterior stroma than the posterior stroma, though both increased significantly.[9]

Many studies show that the increase in rigidity appears to be mainly localized to the anterior stroma. In human corneas the anterior stroma is estimated to be 25% stiffer than the posterior stroma unlike porcine corneas where no such difference exists.[8,10] The difference may be due to the presence of Bowman's layer or more narrowly interwoven lamellae in the anterior one third of the stroma compared to the posterior stroma.[10,11]

Clinical Studies

Wollensak et al published the seminal study that showed that corneal crosslinking (exposure to UVA light at 3.0 mW/cm^2 and riboflavin 0.1% for 30 minutes) was able to stop progressive keratoconus in all 23 eyes of 22 eyes.[11] The patients ranged in age from 13 to 58 with the average age 34.7 ± 11.9 years. A reduction in steep keratometry values of 2.01 diopters was also seen in 70% of eyes with a refractive correction of 1.14 diopters. Over an average follow-up time of 23 months, no scarring in cornea, no lens opacities (i.e. no cataracts), and no endothelial cell loss were seen. There were no side effects from the minimal GVA eithar. Intraocular pressure did not change postoperatively.

The 5-year follow-up results to the 3-year study have been published in Wollensak's review of crosslinking.[12] Of their 150 eyes treated so far, 60 have 5-year follow-up and no progression of keratoconus has been seen in any of these patients. In 31 eyes (52%), a reduction in keratometry of 2.87 diopters was seen with best-spectacle corrected visual acuity (BSCVA) improving by 1.4 lines in these eyes. Other clinical studies in the United States, Italy, Brazil, and England have been smaller with shorter follow-up, but are consistent with the

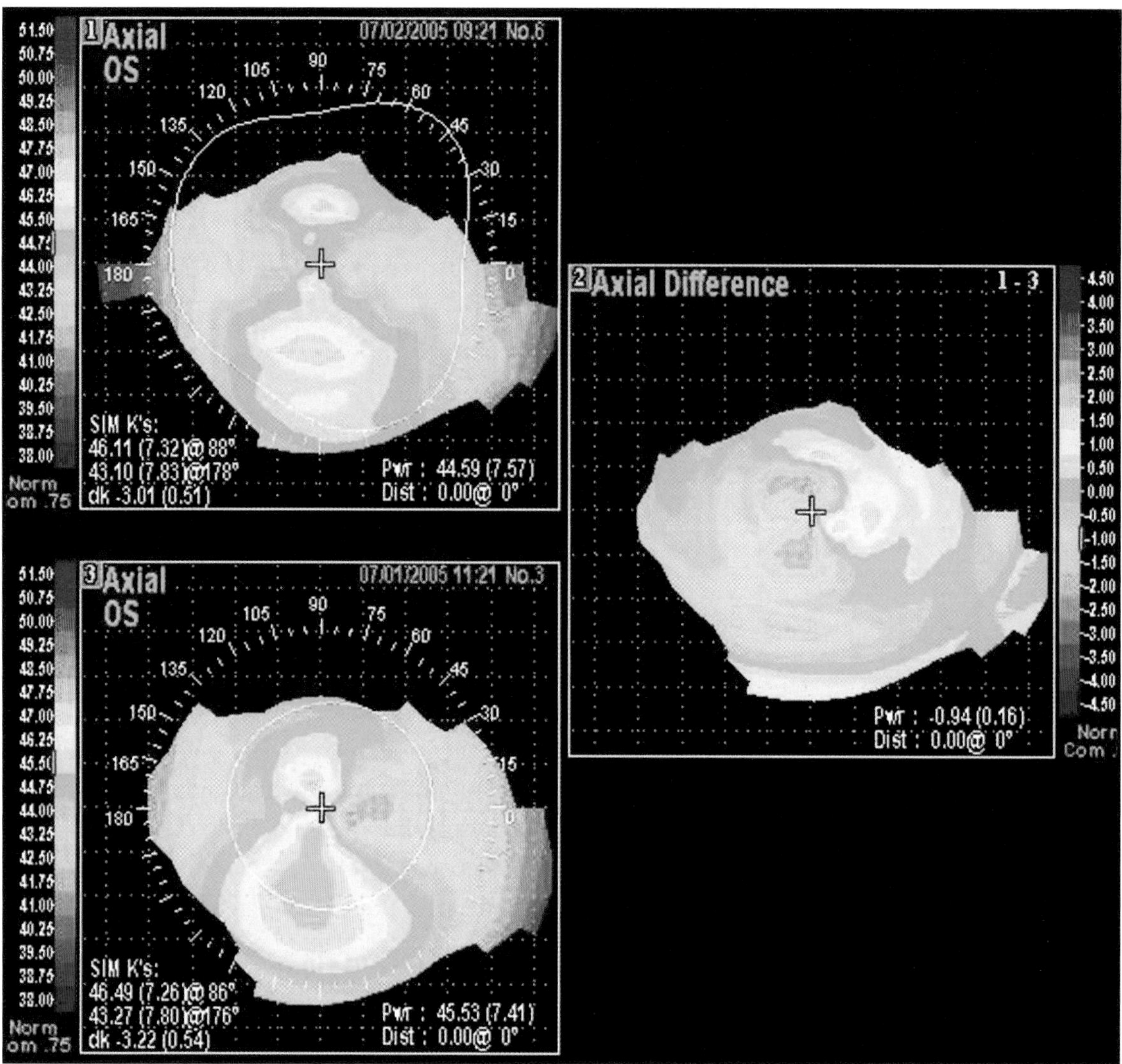

FIGURE 7-4: Corneal topography before and after C3-R®. Pre-C3-R® (lower left) and post-C3-R® (upper left) appear similar. Difference map (right) reveals preferential flattening (blue) over cone.

above cited studies in terms of efficacy and high safety profile. There have not been any side effects to the eye from the very small amount of UVA used for C3-R®.

In 2003, we performed our first C3-R® procedure which marked the first such procedure performed in North America. We observed that the corneal topography changes post-treatment indicated preferential flattening over the cone. Targeted flattening consistently occurs over the steepest part of the cone with less flattening on less steep areas **(Figure 7-4)**. Corneal coupling occurs in many patients after C3-R®, which is similar to, but less consistent than single segment Intacs® placement. With C3-R®, if the cone is located inferiorly, than flattening can occur inferiorly and superior steepening may occur as well **(Figure 7-5)**. This coupling effect (flattening below and steepening above) results in better corneal symmetry and BSCVA afterwards. There have been individual case reports of dramatic improvement in BSCVA without impressive changes in topography. These observations may be explained by the optical regularization of the cornea resulting from crosslinking.

It is worth noting that 99% of primary keratoconus and keratoectasia (LASIK-induced ectasia) patients treated to date have been stabilized after a one-time C3-R® procedure. There have been some patients with

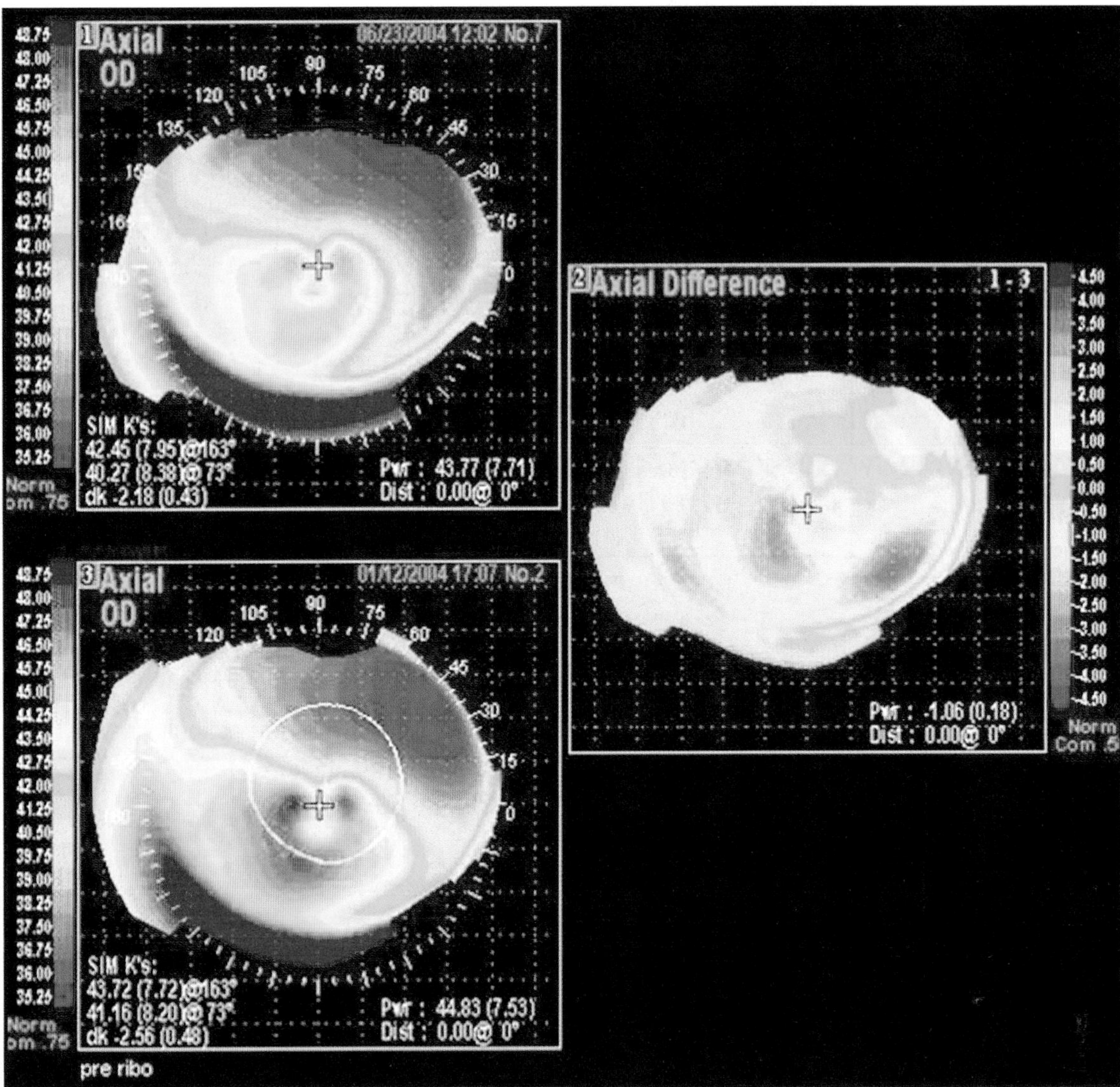

FIGURE 7-5: Corneal topography before and after C3-R®. Pre-C3-R® (lower left) and post-C3-R® (upper left) appear similar. The results are similar to case in Figure 7-4. Note in difference map the superior steepening (yellow) that occurred in upper flat area of cornea which signifies corneal coupling (flattening the steep area and steeping the flat area). This effect in the past was thought to only occur with single segment Intacs®.

very aggressive forms of ectasia that required a second C3-R® treatment to achieve stabilization. It almost seems too good to be true, but the results from multiple ophthalmologists around the world are remarkably consistent.

Our 10-step C3-R® Protocol

Treatments may be performed unilaterally or bilaterally at the same time if C3-R® is indicated for both eyes. If one eye is to be treated, the fellow eye is taped closed and covered. We performed the procedure per our protocol described below, which keeps the epithelium intact ("epi-on" technique). Dr Boxer Wachler is credited with inventing epi-on C3-R®. Although somewhat labor-intensive to perform (application of riboflavin solution every 3 minutes for a total of 30 minutes), this is the necessary means to achieve the desired effect for patients.

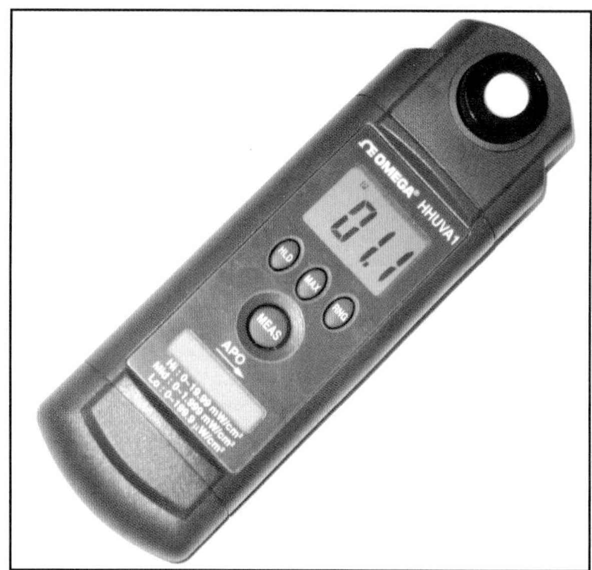

FIGURE 7-6: UVA meter.

1. The UVA device is periodically calibrated with a UVA meter to ensure that the irradiation is 3.0 mW/cm^2 ± 0.3 **(Figure 7-6)**.
2. Topical anesthesia is administered. Tetracaine 0.5% works well as it loosens the epithelial cell tight junctions to facilitate penetration of riboflavin into the stroma with intact epithelium.
3. Two surgical spear-type sponges are made "soppy wet": one sponge with 0.1% riboflavin solution and the sponge with tetracaine.
   Tetracaine is applied to the eye which is then closed for 5 minutes to allow preliminary superficial riboflavin absorption ("pre-soaking"). Note: when a procedure is not being performed, the bottle of riboflavin solution is stored in a refrigerator as it is prudent to avoid unnecessary external light exposure.
4. A speculum is inserted to expose the eye and the patient is instructed to look at the center of the lights.
5. The UVA light is positioned on the cornea at the proper distance from the eyes. The working distance varies according to the device used. The irradiation is performed for 30 minutes.
6. The "soppy wet" sponge soaked with riboflavin is wiped on the cornea every three minutes. The "soppy wet" sponge soaked with tetracaine is applied every 10 minutes for patient comfort.
7. After 30 minutes, the device is turned off and the speculum is removed.
8. Artificial tears are applied and the patient asked to keep eyes closed for 5 minutes to allow lubrication of the corneal surface.
9. The patient is advised to spend to rest of the day keeping his or her eyes closed.
10. Patients are given valium (or other benzodiazepine) to promote sleeping when arrival at home or the hotel room for out of town patients. A dilute bottle of anesthetic drops can be given to the patient that can be used every 20 minutes as needed. Often these drops are not used by patients because recovery is typically comfortable. This bottle should be discarded after two days because there are no significant amounts of preservatives.

Patients can expect some mild foreign body sensation for the remainder of the day. Pain does not occur with the epithelium-on technique, which is our technique (see below for more details on this technique compared to epithelium-off). On the next day examination after C3-R® with epithelium-on, slit lamp biomicroscopy of the cornea appears completely normal or rarely may reveal a few areas of scattered punctate epitheliopathy. Mild foreign body sensation or grittiness may be present on the first day that will resolve in a day or two.

Patients may be examined again at 3 months and again at 1 year. On occasion, patients may be examined at a more frequent basis.

If C3-R® is being performed with epithelial removal, initially a 7 mm corneal abrasion is created first after topical anesthetic is given. The procedure is then performed as described above. At the end of the procedure, a bandage contact lens is placed for 3 to 7 days while the epithelium heals. Analgesic medication is necessary as patients often experience pain during these days of epithelial healing.

Possible C3-R® Side Effects

It has been determined that the amount of UVA exposure is minimal and not clinically significant. The reason that the safety level of the procedure is so high because there is not a significant amount of UV penetration to structures posterior to 50% corneal depth. Thus structures such as the corneal endothelium, crystalline lens, and retina do not experience any clinically significant amount of UV exposure. To put the UV amount in perspective, the level of UV exposure from C3-R® is less than spending one hour at the beach.

- C3-R® with "epi-on" (epithelium not removed) has not had any complications reported
  - Rare mild foreign body sensation from transient corneal epitheliopathy is the only side effect ever reported
  - No infection
  - No cataracts or crystalline lens opacities
  - No endothelial cell loss
  - No retinal pathology
  - No corneal haze.
- C3-R® with "epi-off" (7 mm central area of epithelial removal) can have adverse experiences
  - Pain related to corneal abrasion
  - Haze in areas of epithelial removal
  - Delayed epithelial healing
  - No infection
  - No cataracts or crystalline lens opacities
  - No endothelial loss
  - No retinal pathology.

Epi-on vs Epi-off

C3-R® with epi-on has considerable benefits in terms of no postoperative pain and full patient recovery on the following day. If patients were wearing contact lenses up to the procedure day, they can resume all forms of contact lens wear the day after epi-on C3-R®. With epi-off C3-R®, patient needs to wait until they are comfortable enough to resume wearing of prior contact lenses.

Some doctors assert that not removing the epithelium leads to inadequate penetration of riboflavin and therefore increased UV penetration and possible cell damage or no effect on corneal stabilization. In our studies, we found similar results as Wollensak in terms of safety and efficacy for corneal stability. Robert Pinelli, MD from Italy reported his 6 month results and found equivalent results of epi-on C3-R® in terms of changes in keratometry and vision compared to epi-off C3-R®.[13] Endothelial cell count did not change significantly. We have taken serial slit lamp photographs of the riboflavin prior to and during the procedure. We observed that prior to starting the procedure, fluoroscein diffusely covered the epithelium at the slit lamp microscope using cobalt blue filter. After 6 minutes into the procedure, subepithelial fluoroscein (riboflavin) was seen **(Figure 7-7)**. At 15 minutes, greater depth of fluoroscein penetration was observed **(Figure 7-8)**. At the conclusion

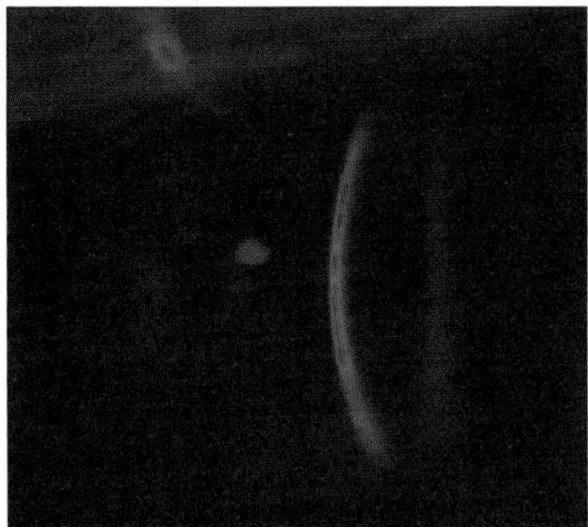

FIGURE 7-7: Six minutes of C3-R®. Riboflavin solution shows fluorescence of anterior stroma which demonstrates absorption with intact epithelium at slit lamp microscope.

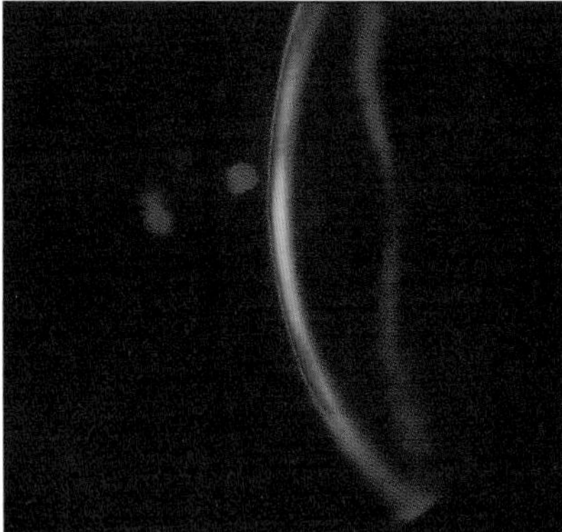

FIGURE 7-8: Fifteen minutes of C3-R®. Deeper fluorescence confirms further riboflavin penetration into corneal stroma at slit lamp microscope.

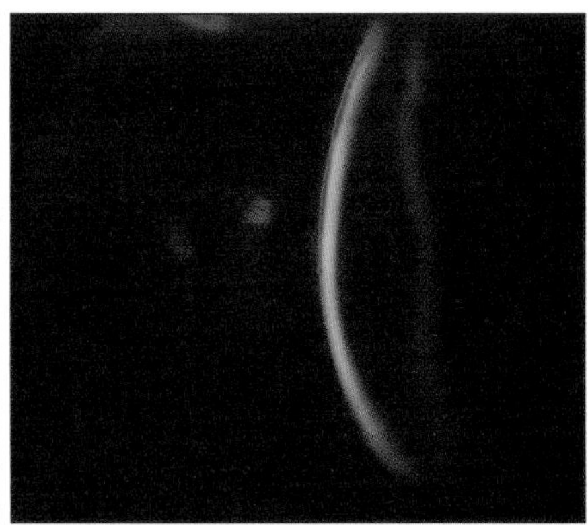

FIGURE 7-9: Thirty minutes at completion of C3-R®. Near complete stromal penetration is evident at slit lamp microscope.

of 30 minutes, fluoroscein was diffusely observed at 50% corneal depth **(Figure 7-9)**. These results demonstrate that riboflavin is sufficiently absorbed with intact epithelium which is consistent with the same clinical outcomes achieved with epithelial removal.[14]

Roberto Pinelli, MD conducted another study comparing outcomes of epi-on C3-R® vs epi-off C3-R® (Pinelli R. Corneal collagen crosslinking with riboflavin: C3-R opens new frontiers for keratoconus and ectasia. Eyeworld 2007; May). He found identical results between the two groups for improvements in BSCVA, uncorrected visual acuity (UCVA), corneal topographic flattening, and higher order aberrations. Endothelial cell counts were unchanged in both groups. Therefore, safety and effectiveness was the same between the groups. Patient satisfaction was dramatically higher with epi-on C3-R®. This study confirms our initial study and current practice of epi-on C3-R®. It seems that nothing is gained with epi-off C3-R® except causing discomfort to patients.

Age Limit for C3-R®

Keratoconus onset typically occurs in the teenage years and early 20s. Some concerns have been raised regarding what should be the youngest age limit for treatment. Crosslinking a young cornea is not expected to have any adverse side effects; older patients or diabetic patients with significant crosslinking in the corneal stroma do not have any adverse effects.

Perhaps the most practical concern is whether the C3-R® works and lasts in young patients with aggressively progressive keratoconus. The youngest patient treated in the published literature is 13 years old in the original study by Wollensak et al. [11] The follow-up of this patient was 47 months with no changes in endothelial cell count, lens and corneal transparency. Our youngest treated patient is also 13 years old. He had aggressively progressing keratoconus and following the treatment, complete stabilization was achieved. As corneal and refractive specialists, we have seen thousands of patients with varying degrees of keratoconus, including severe end-stage disease that require corneal transplant. A young patient with progressive keratoconus can in a short period of time dramatically progress **(Figures 7-10 and 7-11)** and result in lost the ability to function in glasses or soft contact lenses due to visual distortions and required RGP contact lenses that were not comfortable. With further progression, this patient may require a cornea transplant to help improve vision function and after healed will still require corrective lenses.

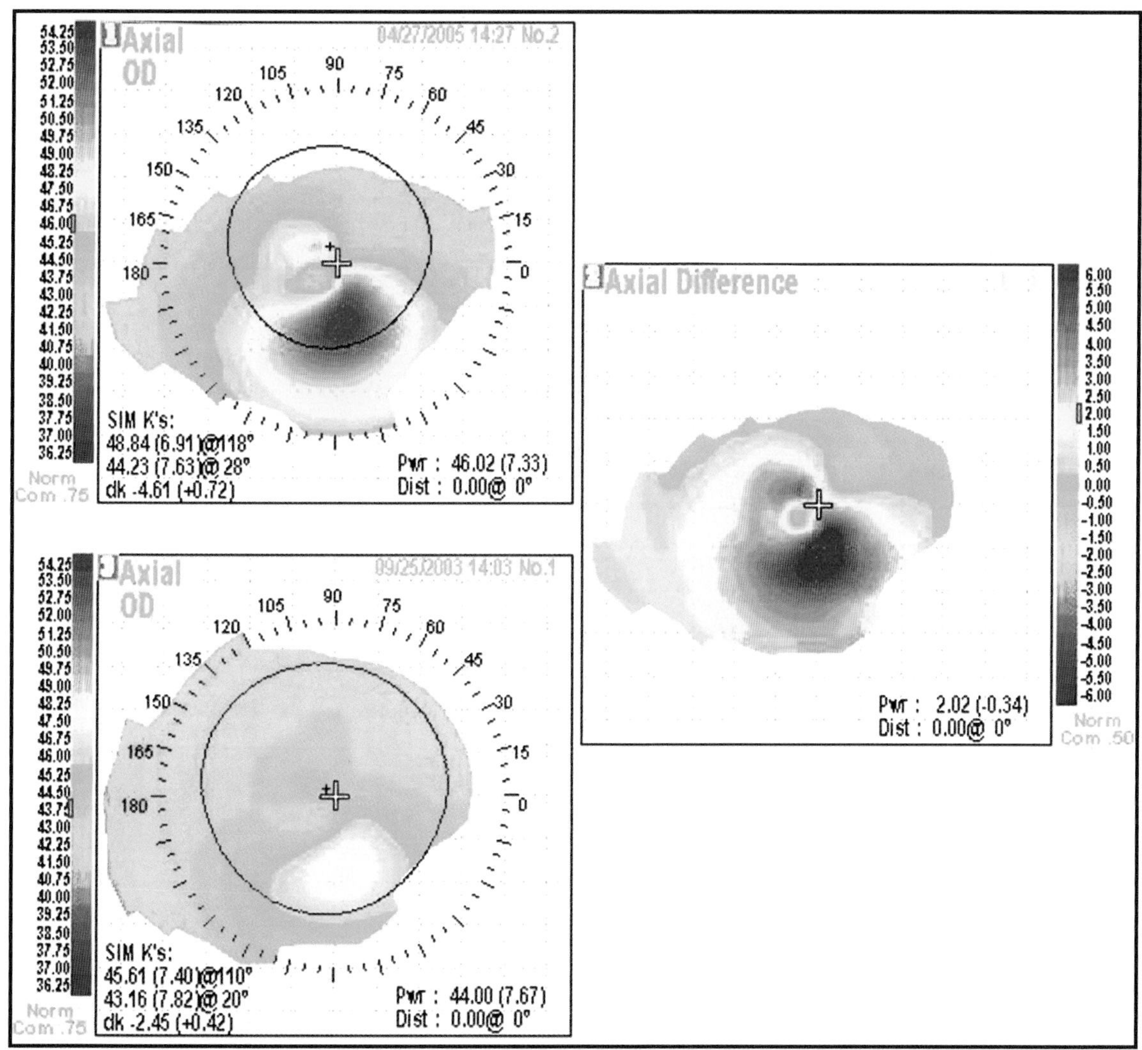

FIGURE 7-10: Rapid natural progression in right eye during 1.5 years. Right eye topography at initial diagnosis of keratoconus (lower left) and 1.5 years later (top left). Manifest refraction astigmatism increased from 0.75 D to 4.25 D during this time.

Given this very real scenario just described, imagine if young children or young adults with newly diagnosed keratoconus could have the disease halted? It would save them from all the visual complications of the disease that were waiting to happen in the near future. That means preventing loss of quality of vision, preempting all the doctor visits, saving the costs of those visits and contact lenses, eliminating lost income due vision difficulties, and preventing the impairment of quality of life and depression that can accompany such vision difficulties. Therefore, it seems reasonable that younger patients with newly diagnosed keratoconus are ideally suited for C3-R®. The power and impact of C3-R® cannot be overemphasized.

Combining C3-R® with Intacs®

Intacs® enable targeted flattening of the cornea. However, they do not treat the underlying structural problem, which is weakened collagen. Therefore, we surmised that it might make intuitive sense to combine C3-R® with Intacs® in patients with keratoconus for maximal effect. Our recently published study showed an additional reason for combining the two therapies.[15]

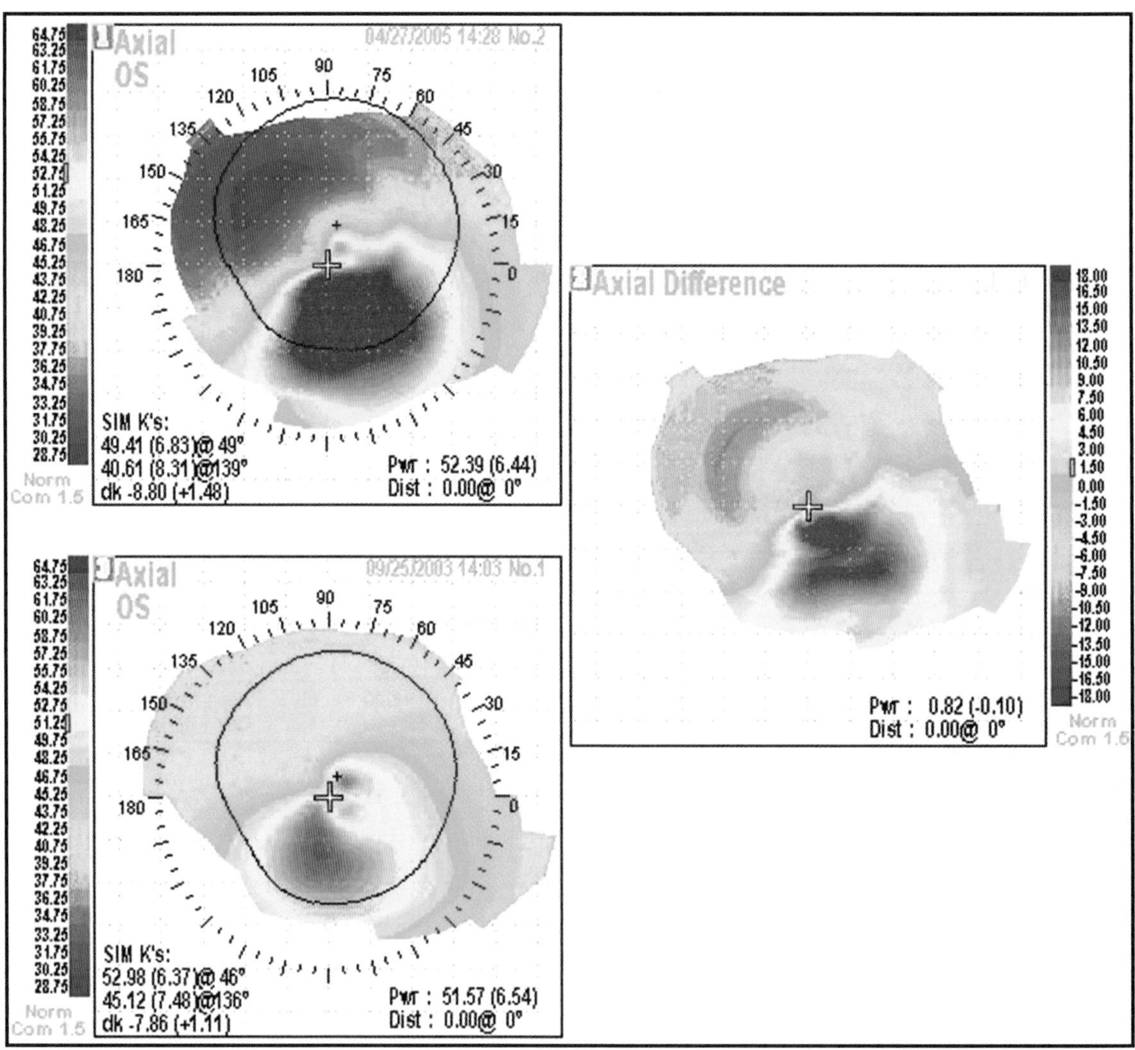

FIGURE 7-11: Rapid natural keratoconus progression in left eye of patient in Figure 7-10. Rapid natural progression in right eye during 1.5 years. Right eye topography at initial diagnosis of keratoonus (lower left) and 1.5 years later (top left). Note increase in red (steep) area in lower cornea which corresponds to manifest refraction astigmatism change from 2.25 D to 8.75 D during this time.

We conducted a retrospective nonrandomized, matched comparative study of 25 eyes with keratoconus. 12 eyes of 9 patients who had inferior segment Intacs® placement without C3-R® (Intacs Only group) and 13 eyes of 12 patients who had inferior segment Intacs® placement combined with C3-R® (Intacs with C3-R group). All patients had inferior segment Intac placed with the entry in the steep axis of manifest refraction. C3-R® was performed immediately after the Intacs® were inserted on same day. Outcome measures were vision, refraction, topographic keratometry values, and the L-U (lower-upper) index, which is a topography irregularity measure of the degree of keratoconus (see Chapter 5 for details on L-U index). Preoperative data were compared to the last postoperative visit, which on average was 3 months.

There was a statistically greater reduction in cylinder (astigmatism) and K values in the Intacs with C3-R group compared to the Intacs-only group **(Table 7-1)**. In particular, there was a greater than two-fold reduction in steep and average keratometric values in the Intacs with C3-R group **(Figure 7-12)**. Most importantly, we found the corneal irregularity (as measured by L-U index) had twice as much improvement in the Intacs® with C3-R group compared to the Intacs-only group **(Table 7-1)**.

Table 7-1: Preoperative and postoperative results comparing Intacs® with C3-R® and Intacs® alone groups

	Mean Change ± SD		
Value	Intacs with C3-R	Intacs only	P value
UCVA (logMAR)	0.76 ± 0.80 (6.5 lines)	0.93 ± 0.89 (9.5 lines)	0.65
BCVA (logMAR)	0.11 ± 0.12 (1 line)	0.13 ± 0.20 (1 line)	0.73
Sphere	0.12 ± 1.72	0.25 ± 2.12	0.66
Cylinder	2.73 ± 1.87	1.48 ± 1.17	0.04*
K steep (D)	1.94 ± 1.32	0.89 ± 2.07	0.03*
K flat (D)	1.05 ± 1.31	0.64 ± 2.40	0.16
K average (D)	1.34 ± 1.27	0.21 ± 2.70	0.04*
MRx L–U (D)	11.23 ± 24.40	6.87 ± 14.90	0.04*

BCVA = best correct visual acuity, C3-R = corneal collagen crosslinking with riboflavin; I-S = inferior-superior; L–U = lower-upper; MRx = manifest refraction; UCVA = uncorrected visual acuity; * Statistically significant

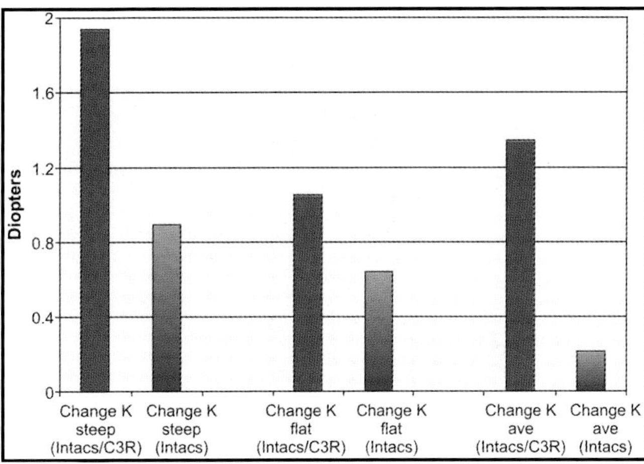

FIGURE 7-12: Greater keratometry flattening occurred with Intacs/C3-R compared to Intacs along.

There are several possible reasons for the increased effect seen with the addition of crosslinking. First it may be a simple additive effect as both procedures independently cause corneal flattening. Second, the channel created for Intacs® insertion may result in localized pooling and concentration of the riboflavin around the Intacs® segment. This may produce an area of locally increased riboflavin concentration and hence may increase collagen crosslinking at that site. Third, corneal collagen change after crosslinking increased overall biomechanical rigidity by 4.5 times, and the placement of an Intacs® segment may modify the pattern and distribution of collagen changes for an enhanced effect. Fourth, new collagen formation was observed in rabbit corneas around Intacs® segments.[16] These new fibers may become thicker over time as C3-R® leads to collagen fiber thickening that may contribute to greater contracture and "pulling back" of the cone. Further research may elucidate the mechanism.

Case Report

A 25-year-old male with a history of worsening vision in both eyes due to keratoconus. He elected to undergo Intacs in both eyes, but deferred C3-R®. The patient was explained that Intacs can help reverse keratoconus, but they cannot make the collagen stronger and therefore would not be able to halt the progression. Initially after Intacs only, he had excellent results with UCVA of 20/25 in the right eye and BSCVA of 20/20 with MRx of –0.25 sphere. In the left eye with more advanced keratoconus, BSCVA was 20/25 with MRx of +1.00 – 6.00 × 135. One year later, the patient returned with complaints of decreased vision in both eyes. In the right eye, UCVA dropped to 20/50 and BSCVA worsened to 20/30 with MRx of -0.25 – 2.50 × 27 and in the left eye BSCVA decreased to 20/40 with -0.75 – 5.75 × 158. Topography in the left eye showed progression of keratoconus **(Figure 7-13)**. The patient was motivated to do C3-R®, which was performed in both eyes. One year after bilateral C3-R®, the refractions were stable. In the right eye, UCVA improved to 20/25 and MRx was -0.25 – 1.00 × 030 producing 20/20 and MRx was -0.75 –4.75 × 145 yielding 20/25, reflecting an improvement in BSCVA and astigmatism. Topography in the left eye showed stability **(Figure 7-14)**.

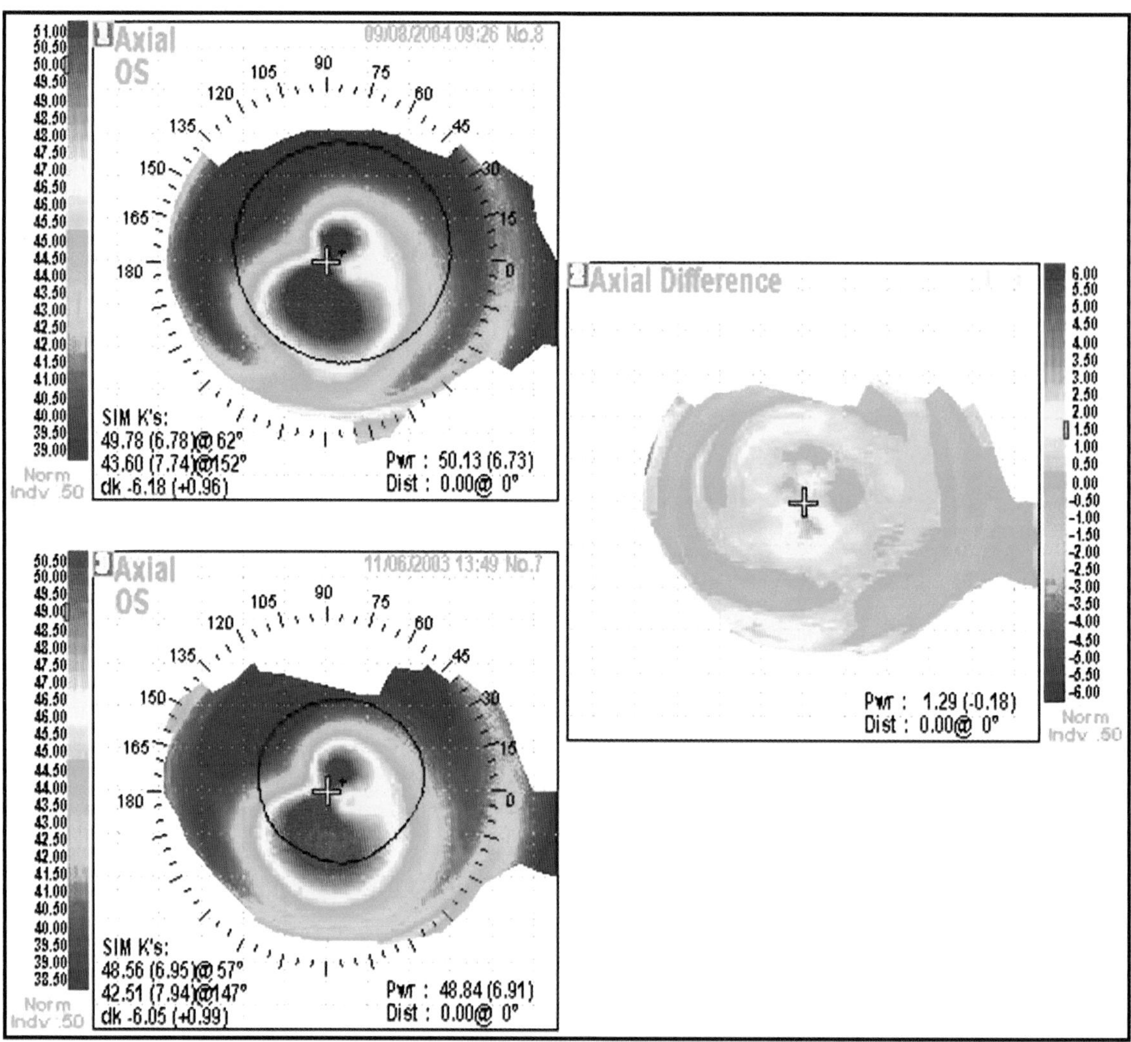

FIGURE 7-13: Progression of keratoconus. The difference map (right) shows continued steepening after Intacs only.

Keratoectasia

Keratoectasia (post-LASIK ectasia) is one of the most feared complications of modern refractive surgery. There are similarities between keratoconus and keratocectasia, but there are biomechanical differences. The flap after LASIK has been shown not to contribute to the biomechanical strength of the cornea. [17,18] It was shown that in porcine eyes that had a flap created, the majority of crosslinking occurred in the anterior stroma or first 200 µm.[19] Given this, the depth of the initial flap and depth of ablation will affect the effectiveness of crosslinking. For example if the LASIK flap was 250 µm in thickness and crosslinking only occurred in the flap, this may result in less of an increase in rigidity and therefore reduce the chance of stopping progression. A thicker than expected flap is one of the postulated causes in cases of ectasia where topography was normal preoperative and an adequate calculated residual stromal bed was thought to have been left.

We have used C3-R® to treat patients with keratoectasia. Three patients required a repeat C3-R® procedure 3 months postoperatively. Two of these patients had very thick flaps and were stabilized with the second C3-R® treatment. The third patient had undiagnosed keatoconus prior to LASIK and subsequently developed severe keratoectasia. Although this patient was stabilized with a second C3-R®, the patient went on to have

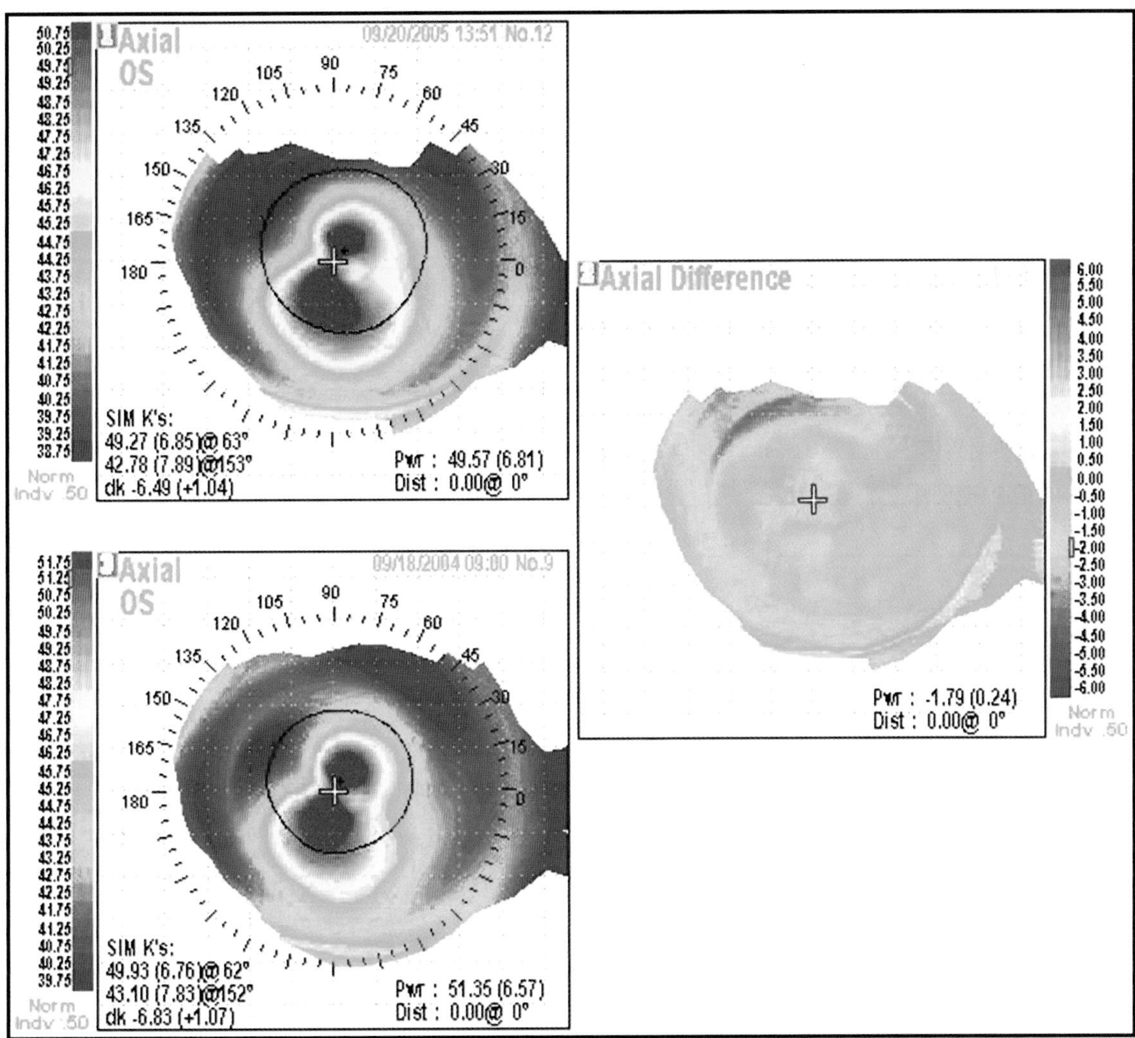

FIGURE 7-14: Stability of keratoconus after C3-R®. One year after, stability was achieved along with mild flattening evident on difference map (right).

a corneal transplant due to contact lens intolerance that was never achieved from C3-R®. Therefore, it seems that almost all keratoectasia patients can be stabilized with a single C3-R® treatment, while a select few may require a second treatment. Corneal transplantation seems preventable in almost all of these patients.

C3-R® Pretreatment in Eyes with Keratoconus or Keratoectasia with Planned Future Surface Ablation (PRK)

While surface laser vision correction (PRK) results in less biomechanical corneal stress than LASIK, keratoconus is still regarded as relative contraindication. "Relative contraindication" means that it is not routinely performed, but may be in certain circumstances. Keratoconus patients who do not undergo Intacs®, do not desire contact lenses, are considering a corneal transplant, and/or desire improved uncorrected visual acuity may be candidates for this PRK. It is prudent to pretreat such patients with C3-R® 1-2 months before PRK to add additional corneal strength. This improves the biomechanical strength of the cornea and reduces risk of triggering progressive ectasia from PRK. To illustrate this process, we describe a case that we treated (see Chapter 15 for more details).

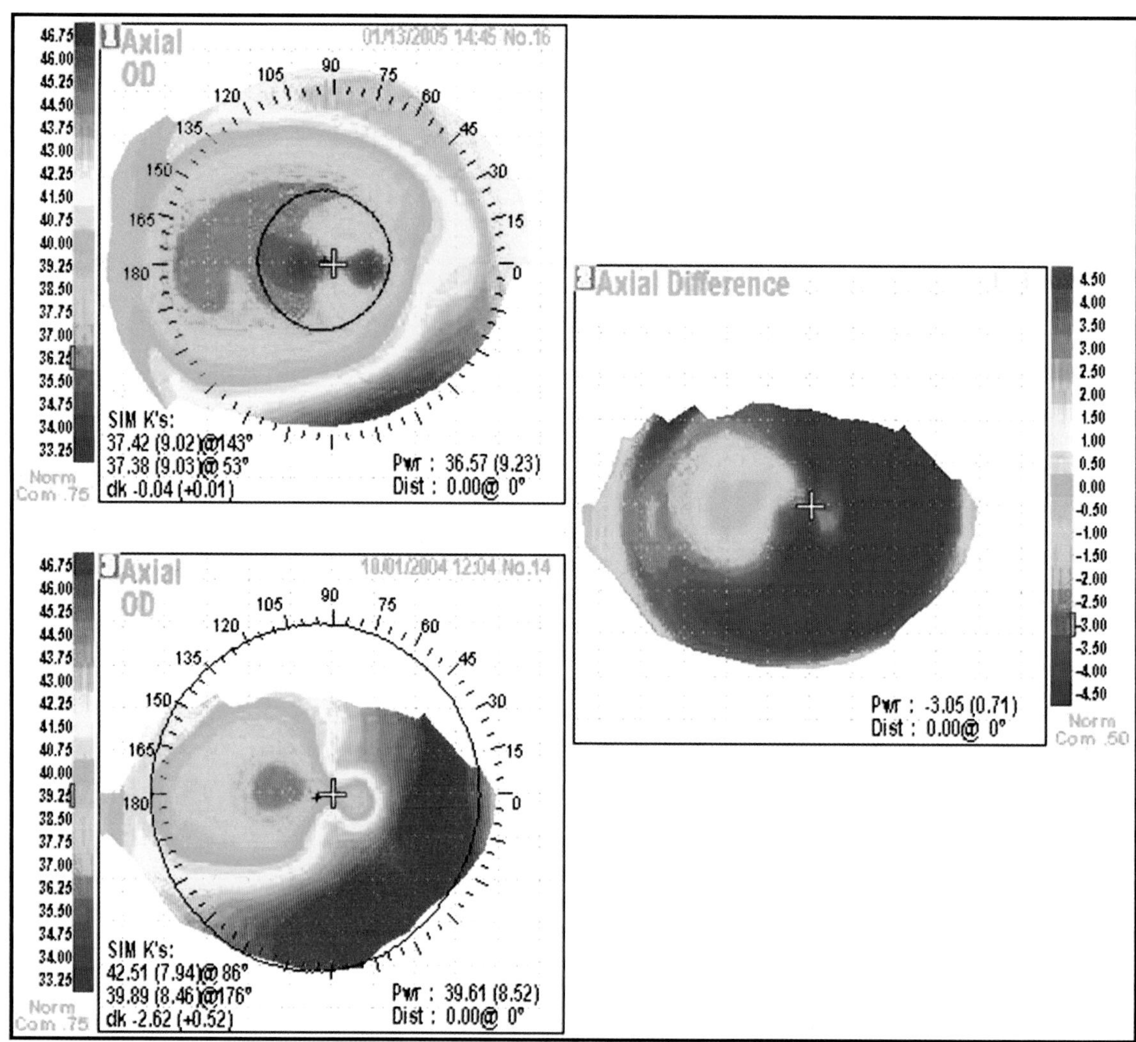

FIGURE 7-15: Wavefront-guided PRK for keratoectasia after C3-R®. Pre-PRK (bottom left) and post-PRK (top left) show flattening of nasal cornea which is reflected in difference map (right).

Case Report

A 43-year-old lady underwent LASIK in both eyes in 1999. The microkeratome used at the time was not calibrated and inadvertently made excessively thick flaps as the keratectomy approached Descemet's layer in each eye. Keratoectasia resulted in both eyes; the left eye required a corneal transplant. The right eye had less ectasia and we were able to stabilize the progression with a single C3-R® treatment. Manifest refraction stabilized at –1.25 –3.50 × 005 yielding blurry, distorted 20/30. The patient desired improved UCVA. Fortunately the corneas were thick as the source of ectasia was deep keratectomy. Wavefront-guided PRK with mitomycin C (0.02% applied for 2 minutes after laser ablation then copiously rinsed) was performed with CustomCornea on the Alcon LADARVision 4000 system. At 3 months postoperatively, the manifest refraction was +1.25 –1.25 × 159 which yielded 20/20 which was good visual quality **(Figure 7-15)**.

Table 7-2: Results of C3-R® in RK eyes with progressive hyperopia

	Preoperative	*Postoperative*	*Change*
UCVA	0.47 ± 0.11	0.49 ± 0.18	−0.03 ± 0.19
BCVA	0.01 ± 0.02	0.13 ± 0.18	−0.02 ± 0.70
Sphere	2.04 ± 1.78	2.04 ± 2.18	0.00 ± 0.67
Cylinder	−1.88 ± 1.55	−1.83 ± 1.71	0.04 ± 0.53
Spherical equivalent	1.10 ± 1.73	1.13 ± 1.94	0.02 ± 0.70
K steep	41.03 ± 4.39	41.20 ± 4.03	0.18 ± 0.97
K flat	39.00 ± 4.40	38.78 ± 4.11	−0.25 ± 1.27
K average	40.01 ± 4.27	39.98 ± 3.87	−0.03 ± 1.09
Endothelial cell count	2447 ± 210	2711 ± 206	−264 ± 358

C3-R® for Progressive Hyperopia (Farsightedness) after Radial Keratotomy (RK)

At the 2006 American Academy of Ophthalmology Annual Meeting, we presented a small, consecutive series of 6 eyes who had undergone C3-R® for the treatment of progressive hyperopia from radial keratotomy (RK). RK was the predecessor procedure to LASIK and PRK that was used to treat myopia. RK involved creation of multiple radial, spoke-like incisions in the cornea to cause flattening. Some eyes experienced continued, uncontrolled flattening that in turn led to increasing hyperopia. In our study, all eyes had undergone previous laser ablation (3 eyes had LASIK, 3 eyes had PRK) to treat the hyperopia after RK. Even though the hyperopia was initially treated, it recurred since the corneas were not stable. The RK incisions are the source of progressive corneal flattening. Our hypothesis to use C3-R® was that crosslinking would result in tightening within the RK incisions and lead to a more stable cornea and stop the progressive flattening and hyperopia. The results were that all eyes were treated with crosslinking and experienced improved stability **(Table 7-2)**. At 7 months following C3-R®, there was a trend in manifest refraction and keratometry values towards no change but with individual variation (Boxer Wachler BS, Chan CC. C3-R for Stabilization of Progressive Hyperopia after Radial Keratotomy and Laser Ablation. American Academy of Ophthalmology meeting 2006).

Corneal Melts

Successful use of crosslinking for corneal melts has been reported in the literature.[20, 21] Four patients with corneal melts were treated with crosslinking, but with a lower surface irradiation than standard treatments (2.5 mW/cm^2). This lower amount was presumably to compensate for a thinner cornea. In three of four patients the melting was arrested. The proposed mechanism is that crosslinking increases the cornea's resistance to digestive enzymes such as collagenases which are part of the inflammatory melting process. In another study, corneal melts from rheumatoid arthritis were controlled with C3-R®.[20, 21]

Infectious Corneal Ulcers

Jes Mortensen, MD of Sweden has treated 4 recalcitrant cases of infectious corneal ulcers with C3-R® (personal communication). One case was presumed to be *Acanthamoeba* in origin, the other two cases were confirmed to be due to *Pseudomonas*. The fourth case was due to *Propionibacterium* acnes. In all cases, despite standard intensive anti-infective topical drop therapy, the ulcers did not improve. After a single C3-R® treatment, the infections began to slowly resolve ending with complete resolution and epithelial healing.

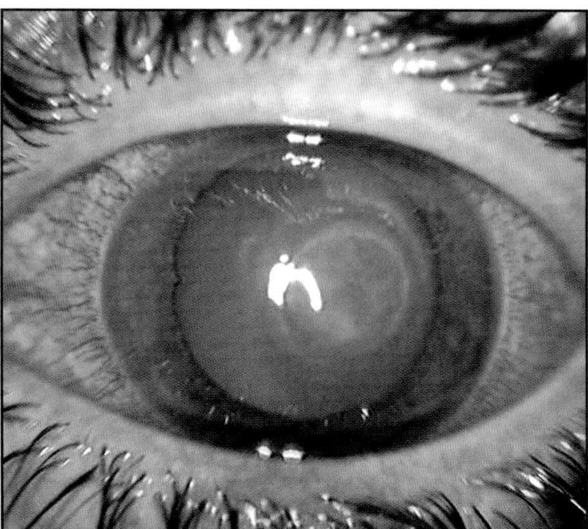

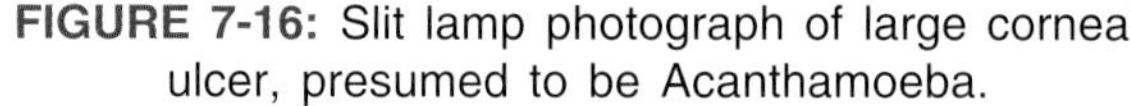

FIGURE 7-16: Slit lamp photograph of large corneal ulcer, presumed to be Acanthamoeba.

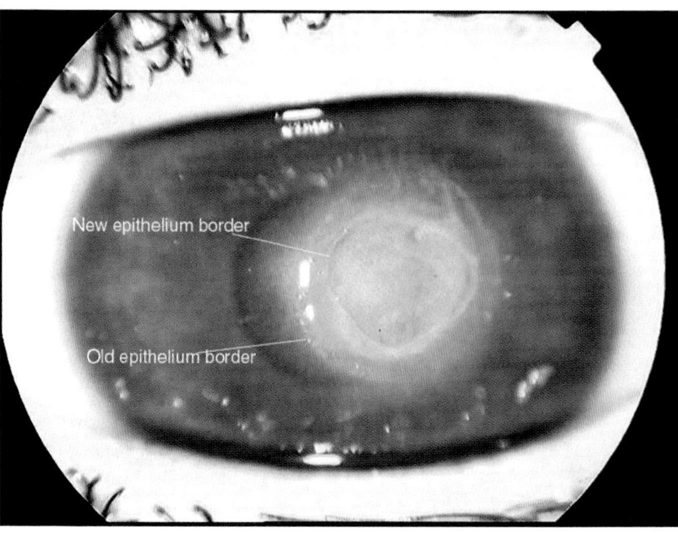

FIGURE 7-17: Slit lamp photograph of corneal ulcer two weeks after C3-R. Note dramatic epithelium healing.

Case Report

Dr Mortensen's first case is described. A 25-year-old woman wearing "day/night" contact lenses developed a large corneal ulcer which was culture negative for *Acanthamoeba* and herpes simplex. The ulcer was presumed to be from *Acanthamoeba* from clinical assessment, but bacterial or fungal etiologies could not be ruled out. She was treated with levofloxacin, polyhexametylbiguanide, brolene, chloramfenicol, ketoconazol. After 1 month of intensive therapy with, there was no improvement in the ulcer **(Figure 7-16)** and stromal tissue loss approached 50% corneal thickness. The patient had extreme eye pain which was not improved with analgesic medication and she required medication for sleep. C3-R® was performed. Within 1 day, the patient's pain was much less which allowed her to sleep without medicaition for the first time since the infection occurred. Slit lamp examination was noteworthy for less corneal edema and the epithelium began to close. Two weeks later the cornea continued to heal and the epithelium was closing with peripheral stromal clearing of the infiltrate **(Figure 7-17)**. After another two weeks, only a smaller epithelial defect remained and the stromal infiltrate was resolved **(Figure 7-18)**.

This case demonstrates the ability of C3-R® to sterilize even the most resistant corneal infections. However, questions remain: was it the ultraviolet light, riboflavin, or combination? Can C3-R® be effective for other types of infectious corneal ulcers including viruses such as herpes? Further research will be needed to address these important questions.

Conclusion

C3-R® may represent one of the most important advances in ophthalmology in the last decade. The laboratory and clinical studies indicate a safe, effective, and elegant treatment for a disease which commonly causes significant morbidity and reduction of vision throughout the world. Combining C3-R® with Intacs® provides synergistic results. In the future, we expect C3-R® to have an even greater impact at saving newly diagnosed patients from future years of vision loss and the problems that accompany such losses. By locking in mild keratoconus, such patients would ideally continue to be correctable with glasses and soft contact lenses for the rest of their lives.

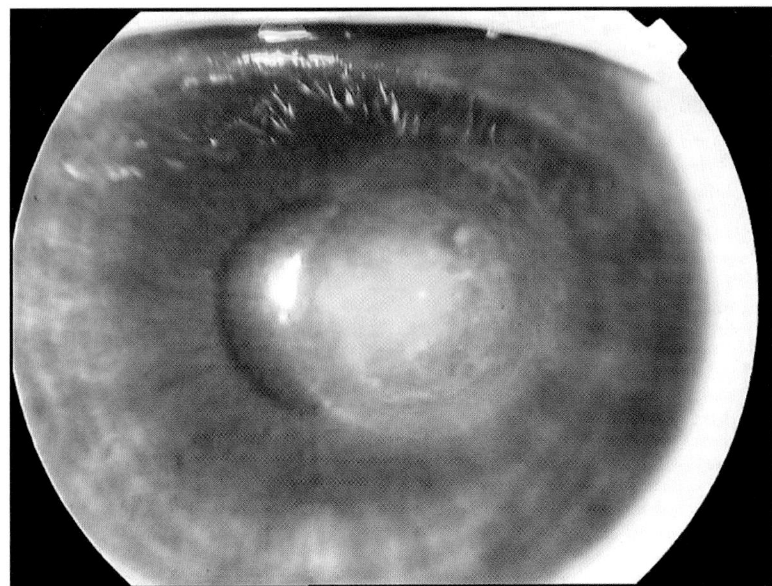

FIGURE 7-18: Slit lamp photograph of corneal ulcer one month after C3-R. A pinpoint epithelial defect remains and the ulcer is resolved.

References

1. Andreassen TT, Simonsen AH, Oxlund H. Biomechanical properties of keratoconus and normal corneas. Exp Eye Res 1980;31:435-41.
2. Nash IS, Greene PR, Foster CS. Comparison of mechanical properties of keratoconus and normal corneas. Exp Eye Res 1982;35:413-24.
3. Cho KS, Lee EH, Choi JS, Joo CK. Reactive oxygen species-induced apoptosis and necrosis in bovine corneal endothelial cells. Invest Ophthalmol Vis Sci 1999;40:911-9.
4. Wollensak G, Wilsch M, Spoerl E, Seiler T. Collagen fiber diameter in the rabbit cornea after collagen crosslinking by riboflavin/UVA. Cornea. 2004;23:503-7.
5. Daxer A, Fratzl P. Collagen fibril orientation in the human corneal stroma and its implication in keratoconus.Invest Ophthalmol Vis Sci 1997;38:121-9.
6. Komai Y, Ushiki T. The three-dimensional organization of collagen fibrils in the human cornea and sclera. Invest Ophthalmol Vis Sci 1991;32:2244-58.
7. Kohlhaas M, Spoerl E, Schilde T, Unger G, Wittig C, Pillunat LE. Biomechanical evidence of the distribution of cross-links in corneas treated with riboflavin and ultraviolet A light. J Cataract Refract Surg 2006;32:279-83.
8. Luce DA. Determining in vivo biomechanical properties of the cornea with an ocular response analyzer. J Cataract Refract Surg 2005;31:156-62.
9. Lee D, Wilson G. Non-uniform swelling properties of the corneal stroma. Curr Eye Res 1981;1:457-61.
10. Kim WJ, Helena MC, Mohan RR, Wilson SE. Changes in corneal morphology associated with chronic epithelial injury. Invest Ophthalmol Vis Sci 1999;40:35-42.
11. Wollensak G, Spoerl E, Seiler T. Riboflavin/ultraviolet-A-induced collagen crosslinking for the treatment of keratoconus. Am J Ophthalmol 2003;135:620-7.
12. Wollensak G. Crosslinking treatment of progressive keratoconus: new hope. Curr Opin Ophthalmol 2006;17:356-60 (Review).
13. Pinelli R. The Italian Refractive Surgery Society (SICR) results using C3R. 2nd International Congress on Crosslinking, Zurich 2006.
14. Sharma M, Boxer Wachler BS. Corneal collagen crosslinking with riboflavin for corneal stabilization. American Academy of Ophthalmology Annual Meeting October, 2005.
15. Chan CC, Sharma M, Boxer Wachler BS. Effect of inferior-segment Intacs with and without C3-R on keratoconus. J Cataract Refract Surg 2007; 33:75-80.
16. Twa MD, Ruckhofer J, Kash RL, Costello M, Schanzlin DJ. Histologic evaluation of corneal stroma in rabbits after intrastromal corneal ring implantation. Cornea 2003;22:146-52.
17. Stonecipher K, Ignacio TS, Stonecipher M. Advances in refractive surgery: microkeratome and femtosecond laser flap creation in relation to safety, efficacy, predictability, and biomechanical stability. Curr Opin Ophthalmol 2006;17:368-72 (Review).

18. Schmack I, Dawson DG, McCarey BE, Waring GO 3rd, Grossniklaus HE, Edelhauser HF. Cohesive tensile strength of human LASIK wounds with histologic, ultrastructural, and clinical correlations. J Refract Surg 2005;21:433-45.
19. Kohlhaas M, Spoerl E, Schilde T, Unger G, Wittig C, Pillunat LE. Biomechanical evidence of the distribution of cross-links in corneas treated with riboflavin and ultraviolet A light. J Cataract Refract Surg 2006;32:279-83.
20. Spoerl E, Wollensack G, Seiler T. Increased resistance of crosslinked cornea against enzymatic digestion. Curr Eye Res 2004;29: 35-40.
21. Schnitzler E, Spoerl E, Seiler T. Irradiation of cornea with ultraviolet light and riboflavin administration as a new treatment for erosive corneal processes, preliminary results in four patients. Klin Monatsbl Augenheilkd 2000; 217:190-3.

Brian S Boxer Wachler, *MD*, ***Shawn Jalali,*** *MD*

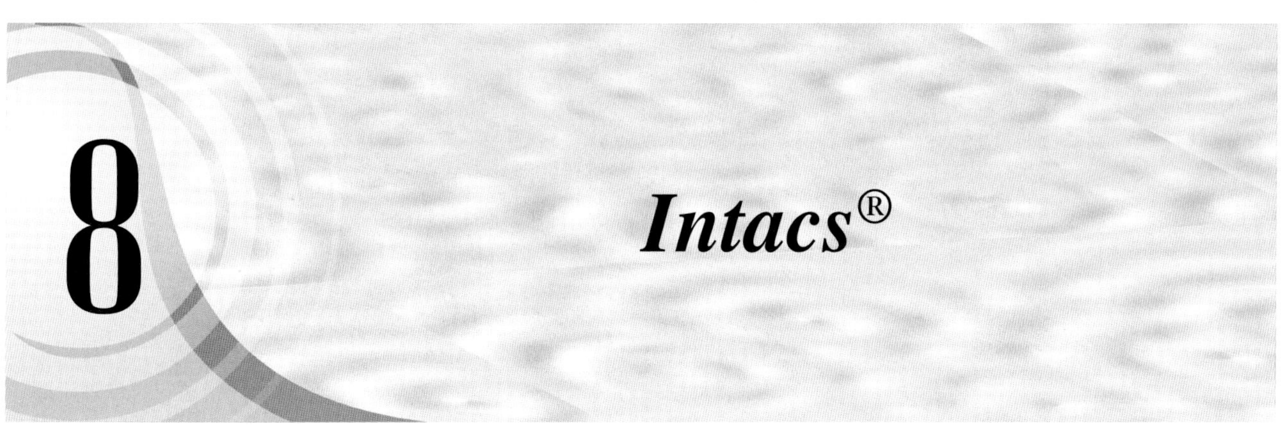

8 Intacs®

Introduction

Intacs® (Addition Technology Inc, Des Plaines, IL, USA) are one type of intrastromal corneal ring segment available to patients with keratoconus and keratoectasia. The idea of using an alloplastic material to correct refractive errors was first suggested by Barraquer in 1949. Since then many intracorneal implants made of various materials have been used for correction of aphakia, myopia or presbyopia. Intacs® are tiny ring segments made of biocompatible polymethylmethacrylate (PMMA). Each Intacs® segment has an arc length of 150 degrees and has a hexagonal cross-section with an outer diameter of 8.1 mm and an inner diameter of 6.8 mm. Each segment has a small hole at each end to assist with surgical insertion or removal of the segment **(Figure 8-1)**.

Intacs® are implanted in the peripheral cornea at approximately 2/3 depth below the surface **(Figure 8-2)** and cause localized flattening adjacent to the inner border of the segment by shortening of the arc length of the anterior corneal curvature. The degree of flattening is directly related to the thickness of the product.

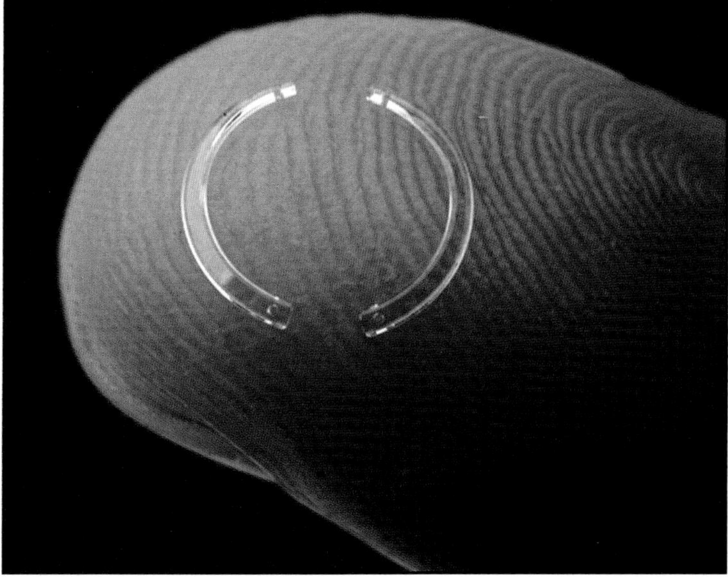

FIGURE 8-1: Two Intacs® segments are shown on the finger tip.

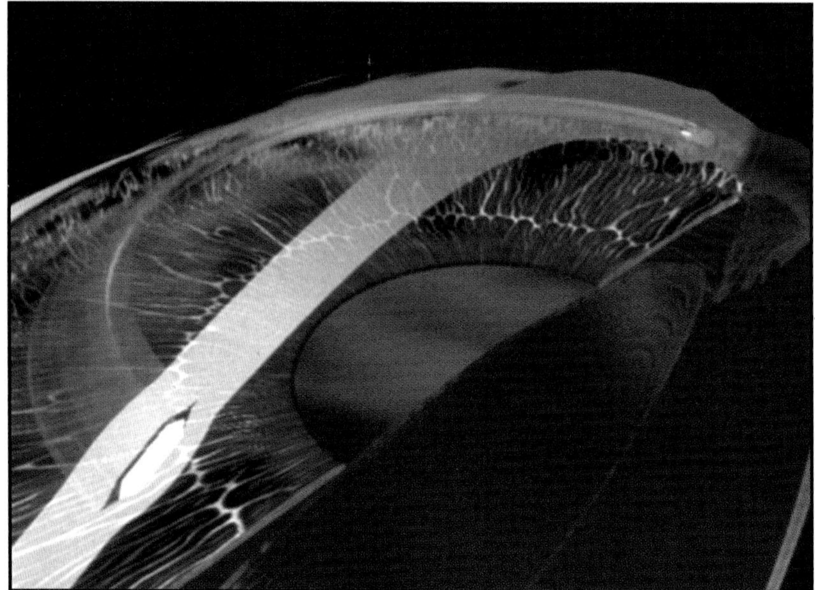

FIGURE 8-2: Diagram of Intacs® placed in mid-stromal depth between corneal lamellar layers.

Originally, Intacs® were developed for flattening the cornea to treat low myopia (–1 to –3 D) and were shown to be safe and effective. They are maintenance-free and can be removed or exchanged if needed.

Intacs® are available in the United States in five different thicknesses, 0.25, 0.275, 0.30, 0.325 and 0.35 mm. In Europe and some other countries outside the United States, Intacs® are also available in thicknesses of 0.40 and 0.45 mm. Because of limited range of correction and possibility for induced astigmatism, Intacs® have declined in popularity for the initially intended correction of myopia, but their specific design makes them an integral and common surgical treatment of keratoconus and keratoectasia.

The goal of Intacs® is to improve vision by reducing the irregular corneal shape caused by the cone. Depending on the level of keratoconus prior to Intacs® placement, patients can expect improvement ranging from (i) enhanced uncorrected vision without any lenses, (ii) better vision in contacts and glasses, (iii) moving out of one type of contact lens into another (e.g., being able to switch from rigid gas permeable (RGP) lenses to soft contact lenses), or (iv) improved fitting and vision with current RGP or SynergEyes® lenses being worn. Chapters 14 to 17 discuss contact lens fitting after Intacs® in detail.

Procedure Technique

An experienced surgeon can perform the Intacs® procedure in less than 10 minutes which is typically painless. While the patient is sitting upright, topical anesthetic (Propracaine Hydrochloride 0.5%) is given and a sterile marking pen is used to make 3 and 9 o'clock reference marks at the limbus. The patient is placed under the microscope in the supine position and the eye is given additional topical anesthesia. The periorbita is prepped and draped in the usual sterile fashion with povidone iodine followed by a drop of Naphazolin hydrochloride 0.025% to constrict conjunctival blood vessels to reduce post-suction subconjunctival hemorrhage. A lid speculum is used to expose the eye. The patient fixates on the operating microscope light.

The center of the pupil is marked with an inked Sinskey hook. With an astigmatism axis marker (we use the Menedez axis marker), the I & P (incision and placement) marker is aligned in the proper axis for the entry incision, and then used to mark the cornea. Ultrasonic pachymetry measures the cornea thickness over the incision mark. The diamond knife is set at 70% of this pachymetry and used to make a 1.0 mm radial

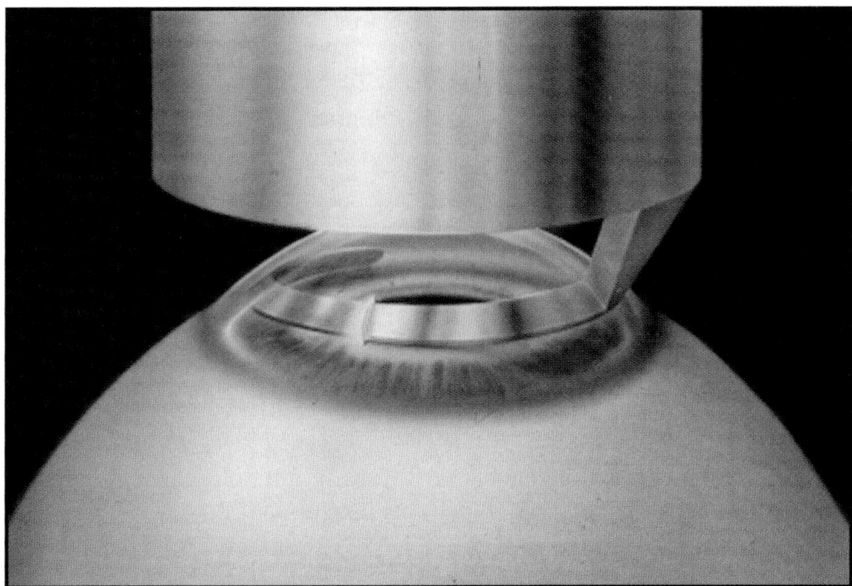

FIGURE 8-3: The manual channel separator initiates channel creation.

entry at the marked site. Using the spreader instrument, the pocket(s) are created which initiates channel separation. Glides may be subsequently used to confirm proximal channel, but with experience, glides are not necessary for this step. The vacuum centering guide (VCG) and I & P marker are used for centration and suction is initiated to hold the eye stable. The glide is placed in the incision and the channel separator is rotated under the glide and rotated a 1-2 clock hours into the channel and the glide is removed. The separator is rotated to simply separate the channel **(Figure 8-3)**, then removed. If a second channel is planned, the above steps are repeated while the VCG is still on the eye. Suction is released and the VCG is removed and Intacs® are inserted into the channel(s) **(Figure 8-4)**. We do not place a suture. If a suture (10-0 nylon) is placed in the incision, it may be removed any time after 1 week. Failure to remove the suture can lead to suture loosening and subsequent corneal thinning and chronic foreign body sensation until the suture is removed.

Postoperatively, we use a 4th generation fluoroquinolone, such as Vigamox (Moxifloxacin) four times a day for a week, prednisolone acetate four times a day for one week, and non-steroidal anti-inflammatory drug (NSAID) such as nevanac (Nepafenac) twice a day for two weeks. Artificial tears are used four times a day for the first month and continued if needed afterwards.

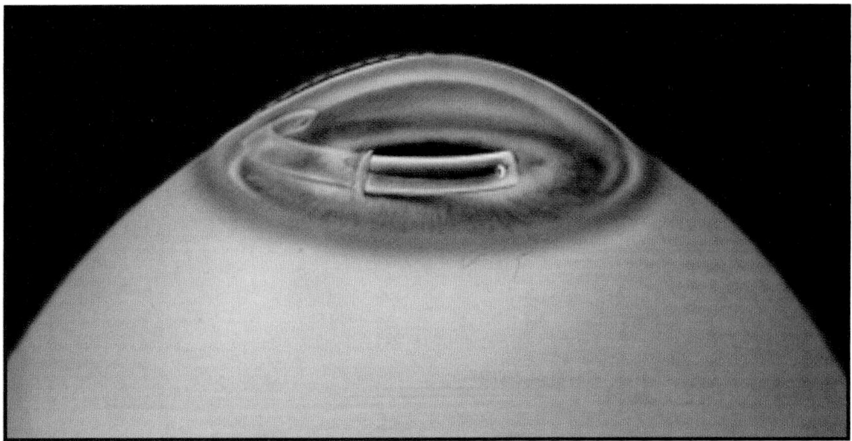

FIGURE 8-4: Segment insertion into channel.

Femtosecond Laser to Create Channels

For beginner surgeons, the femtosecond laser can simplify the process of creating channels for Intacs®. It is recommended to create inner (6.8 mm) and outer (7.8 mm) channel parameters similar to mechanical instruments to create a 0.9 mm channel. The laser can also be programmed for 1.0 mm entry and energy set at 1.5 millijoules. If the channels are made narrower than 0.9 mm, there is increased risk of segment migration and extrusion of the segments out of the channel due to excessive pressure from a channel that is too narrow. In this case, the segment can be squeezed out of the channel by the high tension of the narrow channel much like toothpaste is squeezed out of the tube under pressure from fingers. Care must be taken with the femtosecond laser as there is a higher risk of decentered Intacs® due to compression of the cornea by the applanation plate which distorts the pupil center.[1] Marking the pupillary center before the applanation plate is applied might prevent such decentrations.

As the femtosecond laser penetrates (effectively cuts) across multiple corneal lamellae, it is unknown if this will compromise corneal strength in the future. With mechanical channel creation, the potential space between lamellae is separated, not cut, and respects the natural lamellar plane. There is no penetration of the lamellae and corneal strength is not compromised.

Intacs® Selection

Internationally, Joseph Colin, MD initially described Intacs® for keratoconus[2,3] and Brian S Boxer Wachler, MD was the first to report the use of Intacs® for keratoconus in the United States.[4] The first technique used two asymmetrical segments—a thicker Intacs® segment below the cone and a thinner Intacs® segment above the cone **(Figure 8-5)**.

Colin described making the entry incision at 180 degrees and Boxer Wachler described the technique of placing the incision on the steep, plus cylinder axis of manifest refraction.

Later Boxer Wachler discovered that using only a single segment yielded a unique result: flattening of the cone adjacent to the segment and steepening of the cornea 180 degrees away in the area that was relatively too flat **(Figure 8-6)**. In a follow-up study, it was found that for peripheral cones, which are the vast majority

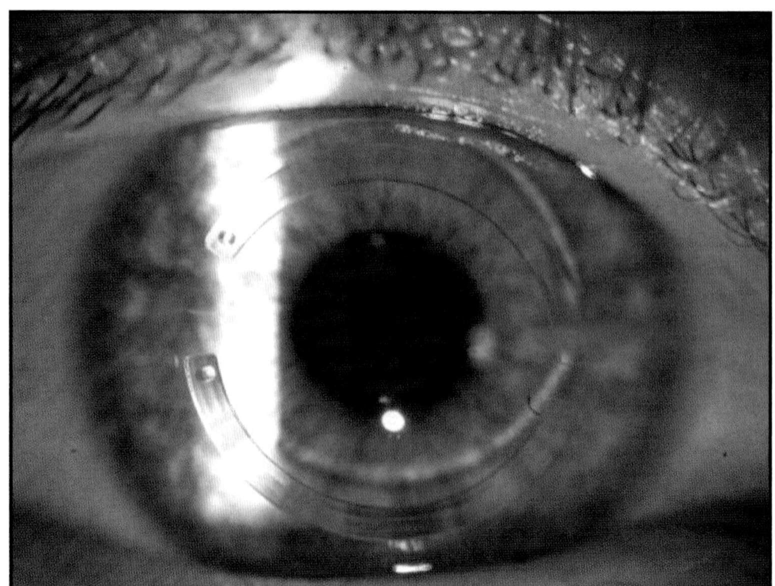

FIGURE 8-5: Two Intacs® segments in the cornea that were placed through a horizontal entry.

of patterns of keratoconus and keratoectasia, single segments had superior results compared to double segment implantations.[5] Use of two segments cause global flattening which includes unnecessarily flattening the already flat upper part of the cornea **(Figure 8-7)**.

Given the pathological shape of the cornea **(Figure 8-8)**, it is ideal to steepen the upper cornea (that is too flat) and flatten the lower cone (that is too steep). Placement of a single segment gives this ideal result **(Figure 8-6)**. A single segment effect is just like sitting in a bean bag chair which causes flattening under the person sitting, while the top of the bean bag pops up.

Contraindications

Uncontrolled Autoimmune, Collagen Vascular or Immunodeficiency Diseases

It is possible in context of these uncontrolled conditions that there could be corneal wound healing problems. There is a low likelihood of increased risk in patients if these conditions are under control. Uncontrolled immunodeficiency diseases may have increased risk of infection.

Pregnant or Nursing Patients

Due to potential unstable refractions that can occur often in pregnancy and during nursing, it is recommended to wait until after pregnancy or breastfeeding before proceeding with Intacs®.

Considerations

Central/Paracentral Corneal Scarring or Hydrops

Scarring in the central cornea is a sign of a more advanced degree of keratoconus and typically the size of the scar correlates with the amount of reduced BSCVA (best spectacle corrected visual acuity with manifest refraction). Intacs® have been shown to be effective in patients with corneal scarring, but appropriate preoperative expectations are important. In patients with large (> 4 mm), dense scars that completely obstruct the pupillary area, Intacs® are unlikely to be effective. Reticular scarring **(Figure 8-9)** does not preclude Intacs®. Hydrops (breaks in Descemet's layer with stromal edema) needs to be resolved before considering Intacs® as the corneal shape will change once the edema is resolved and degree of corneal scarring emerges.

Pachymetry at Incision Site <400 Microns

If Intacs® are inserted when the incision site pachymetry is less than 400 microns, the cornea may not be strong enough to keep the Intacs® in place and there may be anterior corneal thinning of stroma on top of the segment.

Progressive Disease

Keratoconus and keratoectasia result from compromised collagen strength. Intacs® mechanically change the shape of the cornea and do not make the collagen stronger. C3-R® is the only means to strengthen the cornea. If the condition is progressive, Intacs® will improve the corneal shape, but the condition will continue to progress unless the collagen is reinforced with C3-R®.

Pupil Diameter >7.0 mm in Dim Light

Such patients can be at higher risk of glare and halos from light rays passing through the Intacs® entering the eye through the larger sized pupil. Even in patients implanted with large pupils who were preoperatively

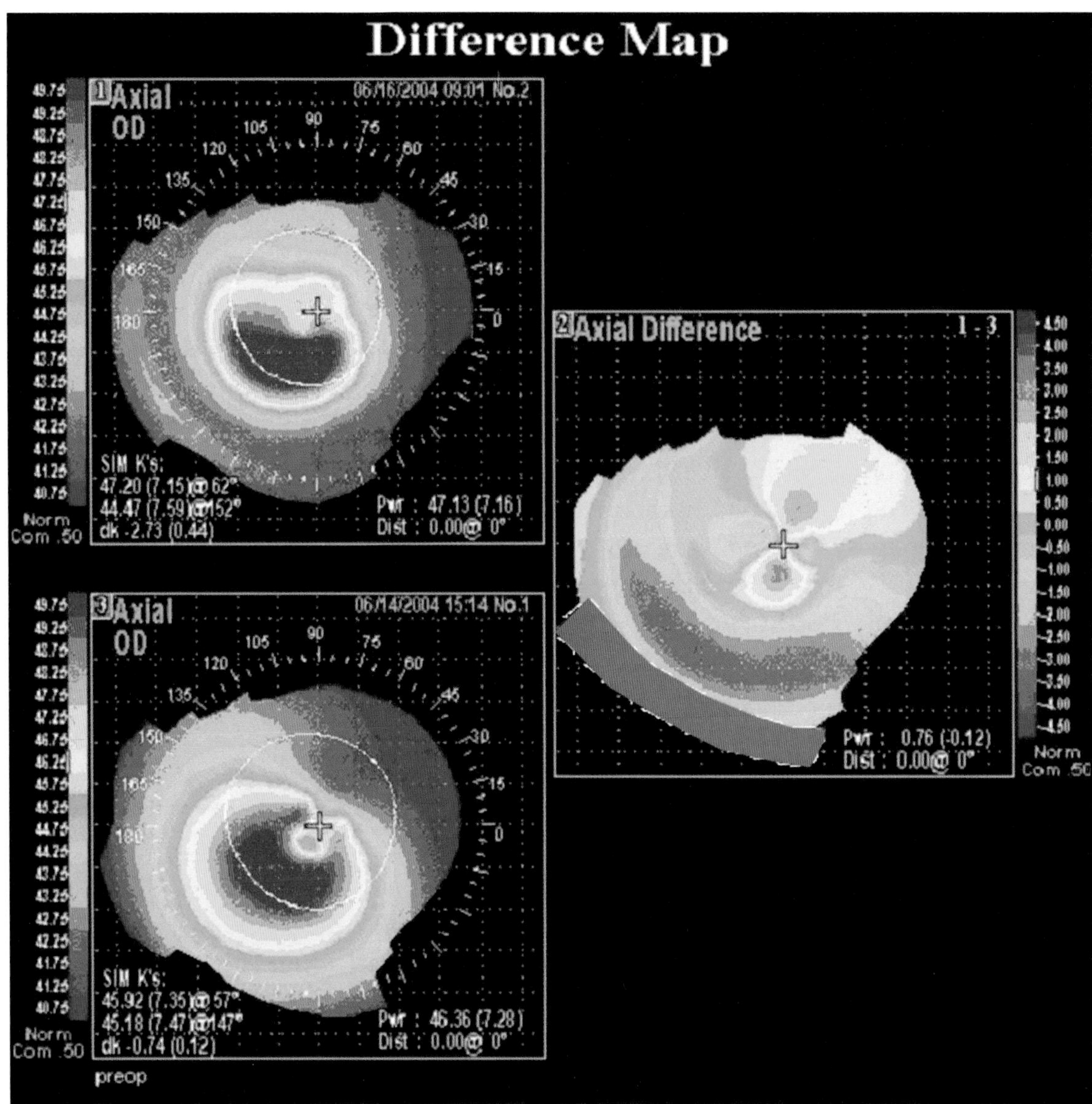

FIGURE 8-6: Topographical changes associated a single segment inferiorly placed below. Preoperative map (lower left) and postoperative map (upper left) show effect. Note the inferior flattening and superior steepening, evident on difference map (right).

counseled of increased glare or halos at night, it is very rare for them to request Intacs® removal because the vision improvements from Intacs® outweigh the mild halos or glare. If patients are symptomatic, use of Alphagan P 0.15% eye drops (brimonidine tartrate) to constrict the pupil at night time is an option. Intacs® removal (explant) is always a definitive solution option.

History of Ophthalmic Herpes or Herpes Zoster

If the patient has a history of herpes in the eye, any corneal surgery can trigger a recurrence. It is prudent to consider pretreating patients 2 weeks before surgery with oral acyclovir 400 mg BID and to continue for 1 month postoperatively to reduce the risk of recurrence.

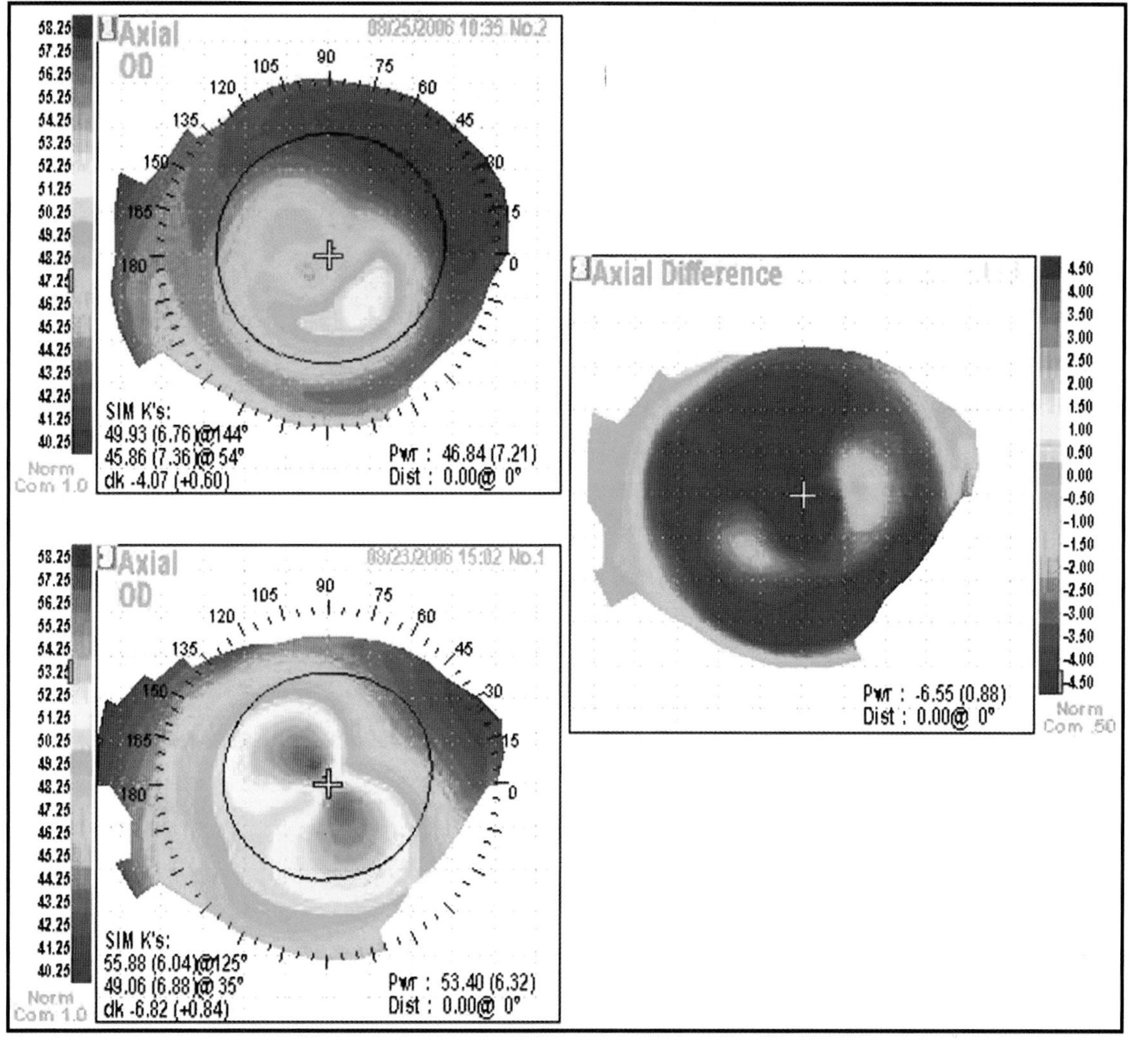

FIGURE 8-7: Topographical changes associated with double segment Intacs®. Preoperative map (lower left) and postoperative map (upper left) show global flattening effect, which is also shown on difference map (right).

Potential Side Effects

Intacs® is a very safe procedure and has stood the test of time.

The following side effects are rare, but have been reported after Intacs®:

Infectious Keratitis

Symptomatic patients present with pain and light sensitivity. Examination reveals diffuse conjunctival injection and slit lamp examination shows a dense, light blocking infiltrate in the channel with scattered polymorphonuclear cells (PMNs) in the stroma **(Figure 8-10)**.

The borders of the infiltrate are "fuzzy" and not distinct (which is in contrast to sterile keratitis from epithelium in incision which has well-demarcated borders). There is no epithelial defect. There may be associated iritis. Cases typically respond to empiric fourth generation fluroquinolone, fortified cefazolin or fortified vancomycin antibiotic treatment over 2 to 3 weeks. If a patient is not responding to empiric therapy, than Intacs® explant and culturing of segment is advised. Once infection is healed, a new Intacs® segment can be reimplanted.

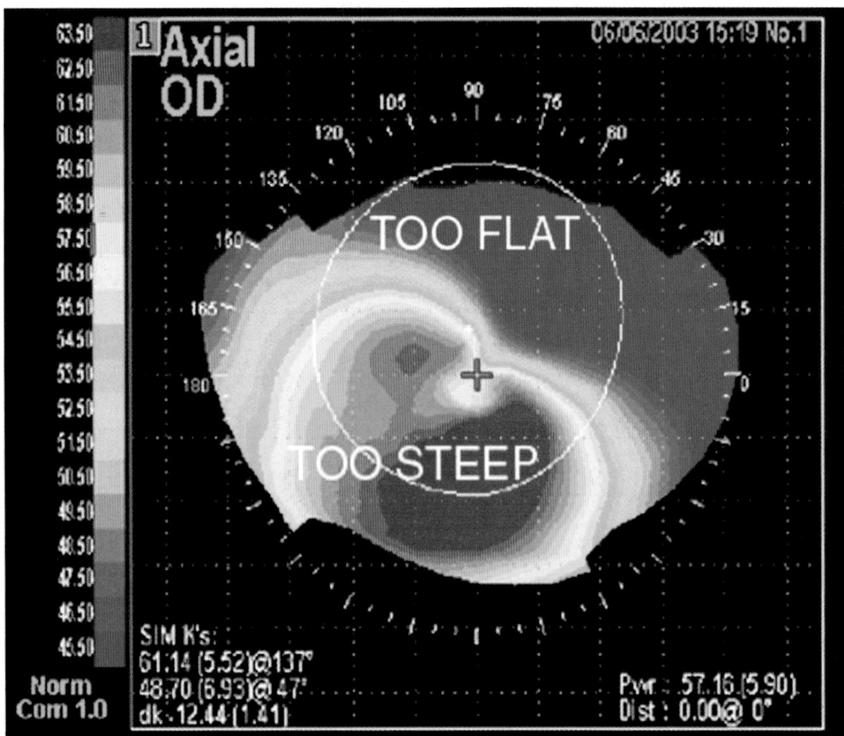

FIGURE 8-8: Typical keratoconus topography. The cornea is too steep inferiorly and too flat superiorly.

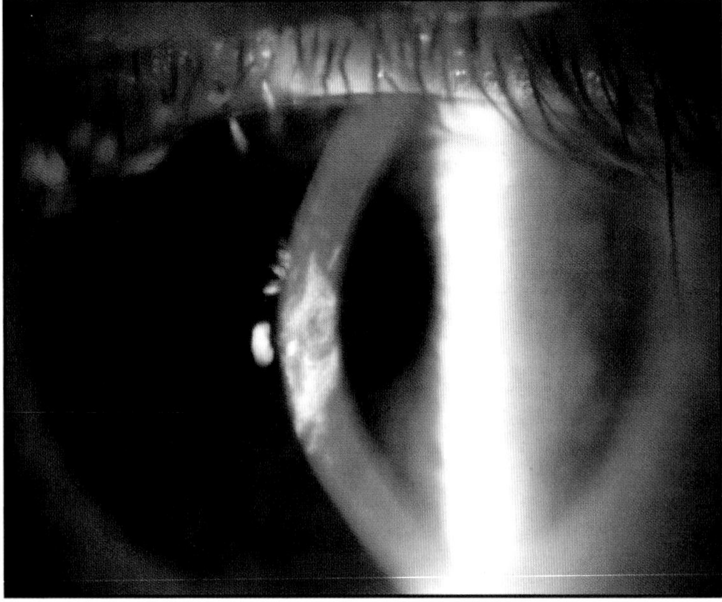

FIGURE 8-9: Subepithelial scarring at the cone apex.

Sterile Keratitis

Sterile keratitis may present with a delayed onset at 1 to 2 weeks after surgery. Sterile keratitis can result from epithelium within the channel that incites a self-limited sterile, non-infectious, inflammatory reaction. Sometimes this can be confused with infectious keratitis, but patients with sterile keratitis usually are not in frank pain, but usually note photophobia and mild irritation. Examination can be similar to infectious keratitis, but in

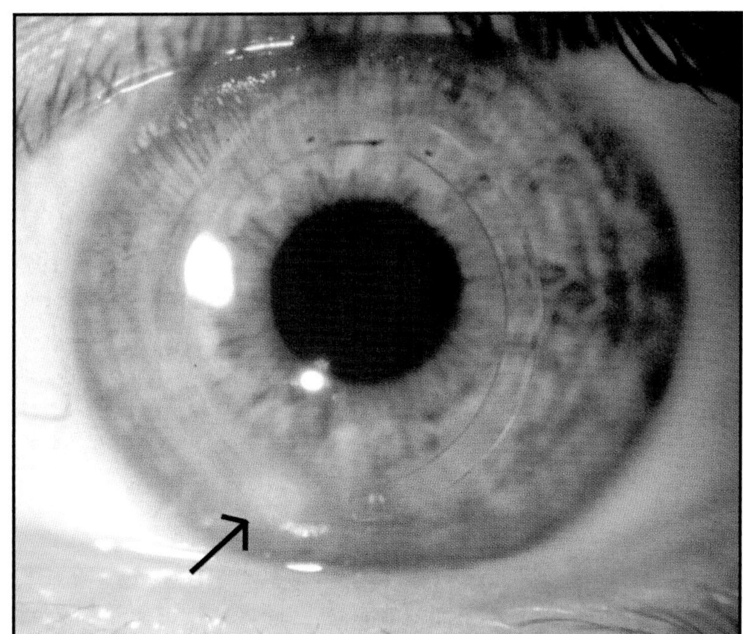

FIGURE 8-10: Stromal infection (arrow) at inferior end of temporal Intacs® segment.

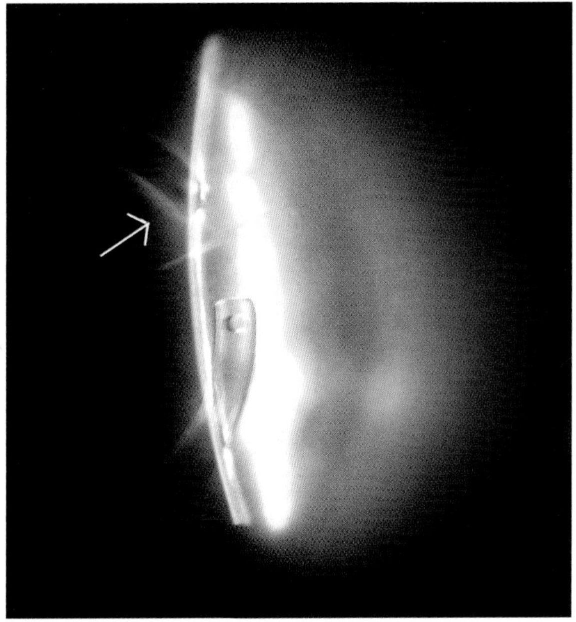

FIGURE 8-11: Epithelial ingrowth in the channel. Note the epithelium is wrapped around the tip of the upper segment (arrow).

sterile keratitis the epithelium can be seen in the channel to wrap around tip of segment **(Figure 8-11)** with surrounding PMNs in the stroma. Patients typically respond to a 2-week taper of a topical NSAID such as Nevanac qid for 1 week and bid for another week. This side effect can be prevented by making the incision relatively short (1.0 mm) to reduce the risk of epithelium migrating into the channel. If there is difficulty with using a short incision, a longer incision can be used, but we recommend placing a temporary 10-0 nylon suture to keep the wound apposed for these longer incisions.

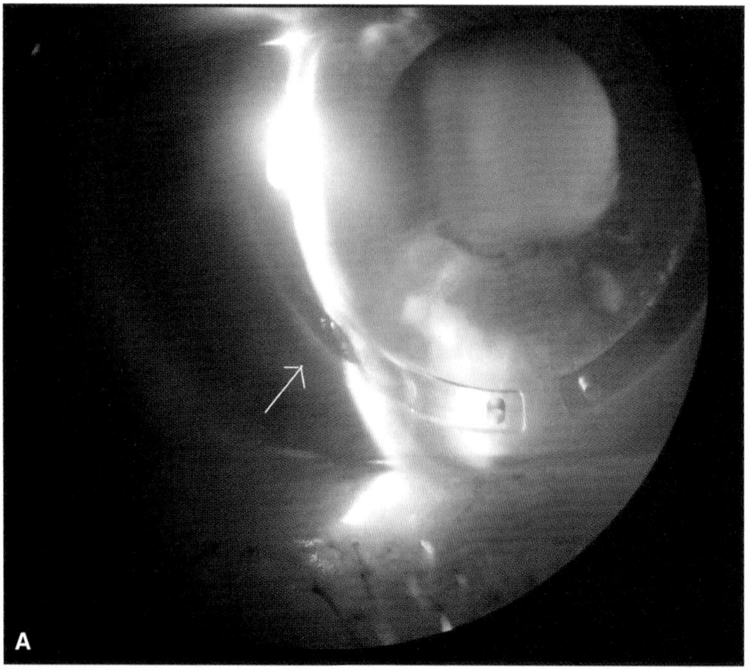

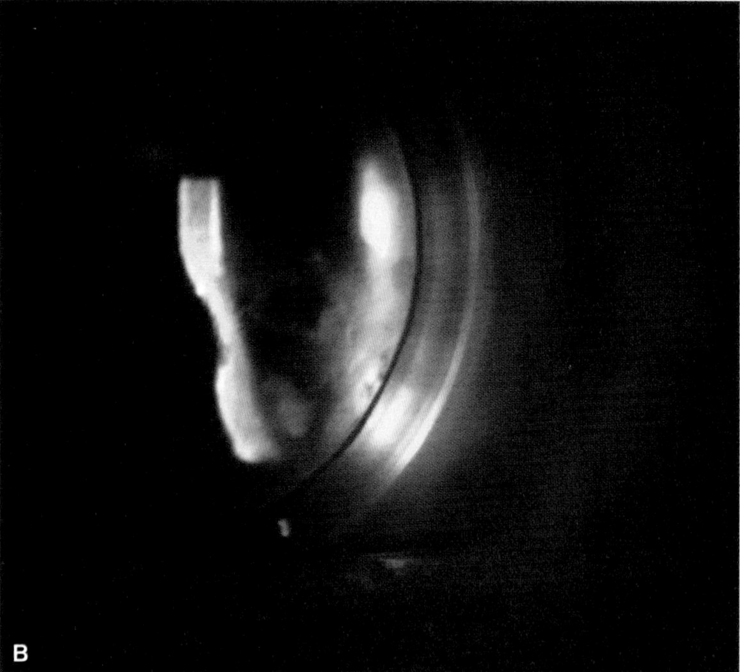

FIGURE 8-12: Corneal melting due to patient NSAID abuse. Note exposure of mid-section of Intacs® segment (arrow) (A). In the same patient there is 50% tissue loss at the center of the cornea. This condition necessitated explant of both Intacs®. The patient healed well with aggressive lubrication after the NSAID was discontinued.

It is important to note that prolonged use of a topical NSAID can lead to epithelial breakdown and stromal melting **(Figure 8-12)**. It is important to emphasize to patients who are being treated for sterile keratitis that patient abuse of NSAID drops can be associated with significant side effects. If NSAIDs are being prescribed for a period longer than 2 weeks, patients should be followed closely in case NSAID toxicity occurs.

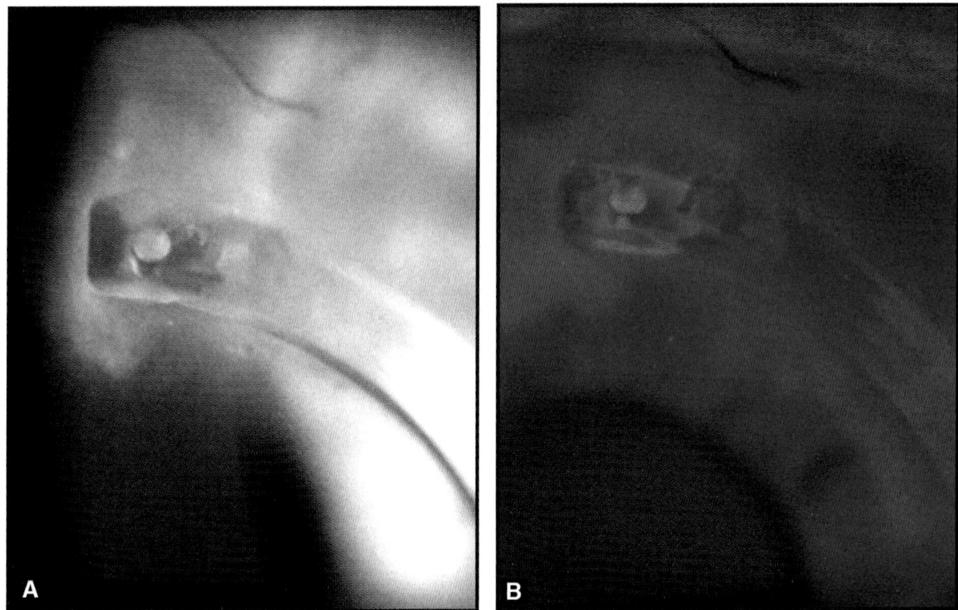

FIGURE 8-13: Corneal thinning due to shallow segment placement. Stromal breakdown is not always obvious (A), but fluoroscein makes the diagnosis easy (B).

Shallow Intacs® Placement and Corneal Thinning

Unintended superficial channel creation with the channel separator instrument is usually the cause of shallow channels. However, if the channel was initially dissected at the proper depth, it is still possible to create a shallow channel. After VCG and suction are turned on, the glide may not have been placed at the base of the incision, but inadvertently inserted at a shallow depth between stromal fibers. The separator is then used to create an unintended shallow channel. Most times shallow Intacs® placement will not cause a problem. Sometimes it will lead to corneal thinning perhaps years after surgery, which can lead to exposure and possible extrusion of the segment. Patients will complain of chronic foreign body sensation, and fluoroscein staining will be helpful to reveal this condition **(Figure 8-13)**. If there is a concern about channel depth, the surgeon can simply remove the segment, make a deeper channel, and reinsert segment.

Perforation into Anterior Chamber

Perforation of Descemet's layer can occur if the incision is made too deep or if the separator is rotated too quickly that causes the tip to dive deeper than the intended lamellar plane. In this situation, the segment should be removed and incision then sutured. After 1 month, Intacs® surgery with the incision at relatively shallower depth can be performed.

Intacs® Migration and Extrusion

Has the Intacs® migrated and is the tip under the incision **(Figure 8-14)**? If so, this can lead to non-inflammatory corneal melting and thinning at the incision site. If the end of the Intacs® is exposed due to stromal thinning, the segment can be removed under topical anesthesia at the slit lamp using the Intacs® forceps. Depending on the cause of extrusion, it may not be advisable to replace the segment.

If the segment is completely absent from the channel due to complete extrusion, Intacs® can be replaced using the technique for initial implantation described above as long as there is no thinning of the cornea in

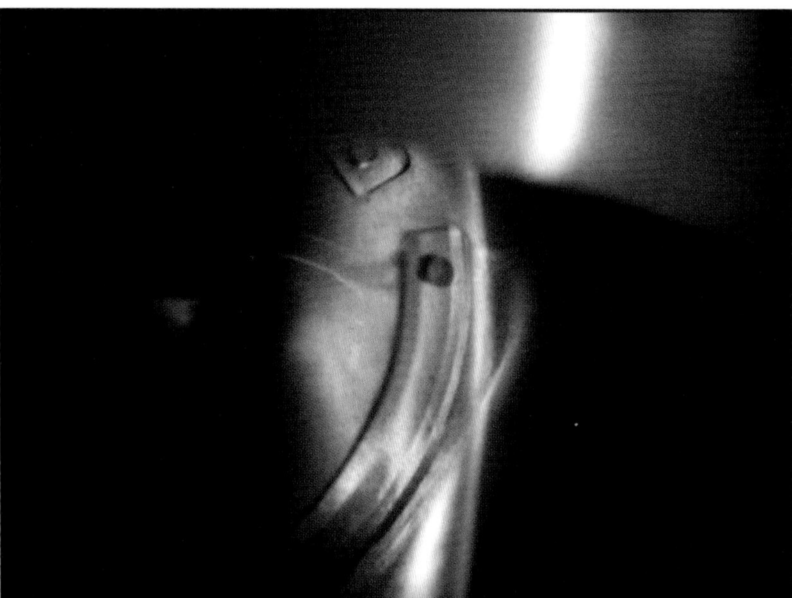

FIGURE 8-14: Migration of the Intacs® segment with the tip externalized outside the incision.

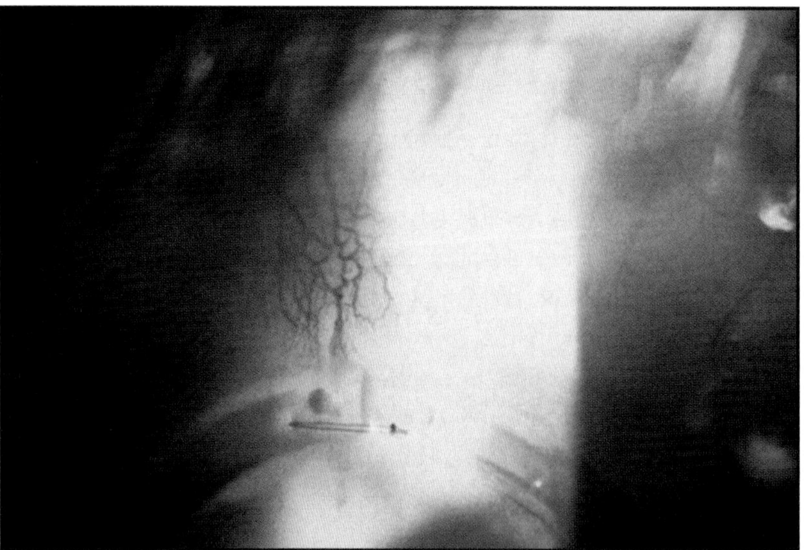

FIGURE 8-15: Corneal neovascularization at the incision site. This can result from a long-standing cornea suture that should have been removed earlier.

the channel area. It is prudent though to consider the cause of the extrusion: too tight channel or too shallow channel? Plan appropriately to avoid the factor that led to extrusion. This is also the reason that patients are advised not to touch their eyes for the first several months after Intacs® insertion to avoid patient-induced Intacs® migration. After several months, the Intacs® are very stable.

Neovascularization at the Incision Site and into the Channel

Superficial or deep neovascularization may occur if a suture was placed and not removed **(Figure 8-15)**. Sometimes neovascularization results from an incision too close to the limbus. A segment that has migrated under the incision can cause deep stromal neovascularization and diffuse lipid deposits in the stroma **(Figure 8-16)**. If the suture is present, it should be promptly removed. A short course of topical steroids can be used

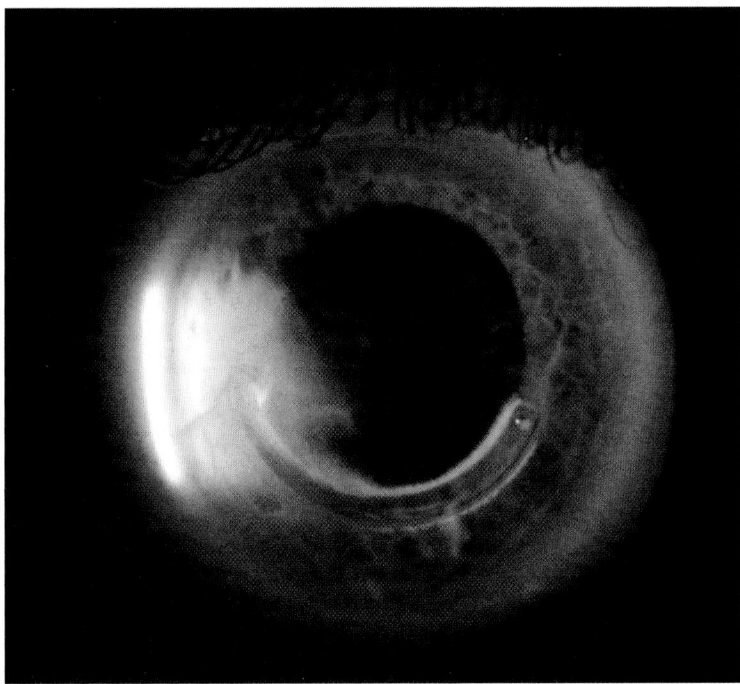

FIGURE 8-16: Deep stromal neovascularisations and lipid deposits in the stroma as a result of Intacs® migration under the incision. This condition can only occur after several months of the segment resting under the incision; it does not occur immediately.

to help partially regress the blood vessels. The patient should be followed periodically (every 1-2 months). If the neovascularization is progressing, Intacs® removal may be considered.

Photophobia

Photophobia is typically a delayed-onset symptoms occurring 1 to 2 weeks after implantation. There is usually sterile inflammation within the channel (see Sterile Keratitis section above for cause and management details).

Glare and Halos

In patients with pupils diameters >7 mm, glare and halos can occur, which tend to be mild. These symptoms can also occur if the Intacs® are decentered relative the pupil. Often these symptoms are not problematic. If so, patients can respond well to Alphagan P 0.15% to be used at night time. For recalcitrant cases, the Intacs® can be removed to resolve symptoms.

It is important to understand the source of the glare and halos. Such symptoms are common in keratoconic patients due to the abnormally shaped cornea. Glare and halos specific to Intacs® are usually crescent-shaped in the same meridian as the Intacs® themselves and are described more often as a shimmering halos around light sources.

Improper Intacs® Planning

Placing wrong sized segments in the improper areas of the cornea can induce loss of BSCVA in some patients. From earlier studies on double segment Intacs®, placing a thicker segment below the cone and a thinner segment above the cone can lead to improvement even in peripheral cones (which do not require an upper segment at all as described below).

Some surgeons place a thinner segment below the cone and a thicker segment above the cone which gives excessive and unnecessary flattening to the already flat corneal area. This can result in untended exacerbation of adverse visual symptoms and loss of BSCVA.[6] Fortunately, this can be remedied as the upper segment can be explanted and the lower segment can be exchanged for a thicker segment (see section below on Explant and Exchange). If the initial axis was incorrect, a new entry axis and channel can be created for a new Intacs® insertion as long as the old incision will not be on top on the Intacs® segment. If the segment is located under the incision, it can lead to corneal thinning (see above Intacs® Migration and Extrusion section). For this reason, we do not recommend placing Intacs® in corneas with a history of radial keratotomy.

Dry Eyes

Dry eyes are rare after Intacs®.[7] If this condition occurs postoperatively, artificial tears four times a day for the first month is routinely recommended. Oral flaxseed oil capsules (1000 mg/capsule), three capsules a day can help relieve dry eyes. The best quality flaxseed oil capsules are organic and cold-pressed. Punctal plugs and Restasis (cyclosporin) eyedrops can also be effective.

Incidental Findings

1. *Channel deposits*—After a few months, fine white deposits may appear within the channels after Intacs® placement **(Figure 8-17)**. The incidence and density of the deposits increase with the duration of implantation, then are stable. Deposits usually do not have any negative effect on vision.
2. *Channel haze*—Sometimes a light haze may be seen in the channel outside of the Intacs® **(Figure 8-18)**. There are no adverse sequelae from this.
3. *Subepithelial incision haze*—There may be a strong healing response at the incision site as evidenced by haze under the epithelium at the incision site **(Figure 8-19)**.
4. *Epithelial plug in incision*—There are no adverse effects to this condition **(Figure 8-20)**. If epithelium migrates along channel and surrounds tip of segment, sterile inflammation may occur that can be treated with topical NSAIDs.
5. *Segment tips touching*—If the segments ends touch (180 degrees from incision site), there are no adverse effects from this **(Figure 8-21)**.

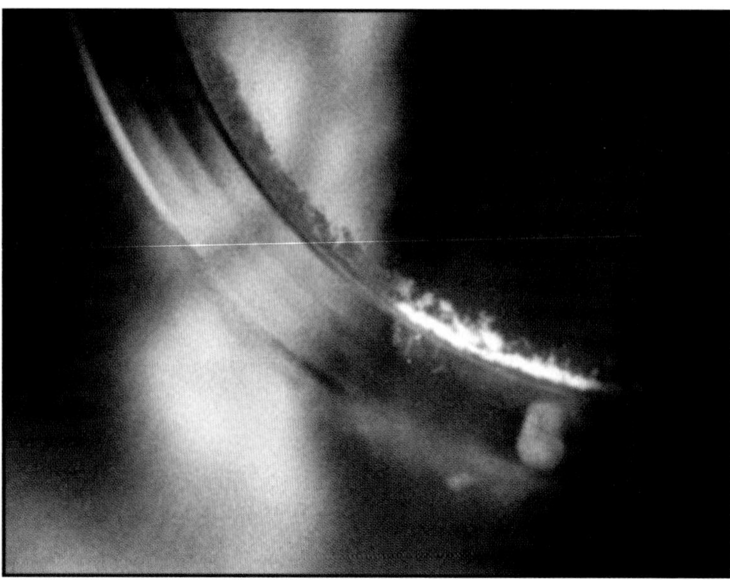

FIGURE 8-17: Lamellar channel deposits.

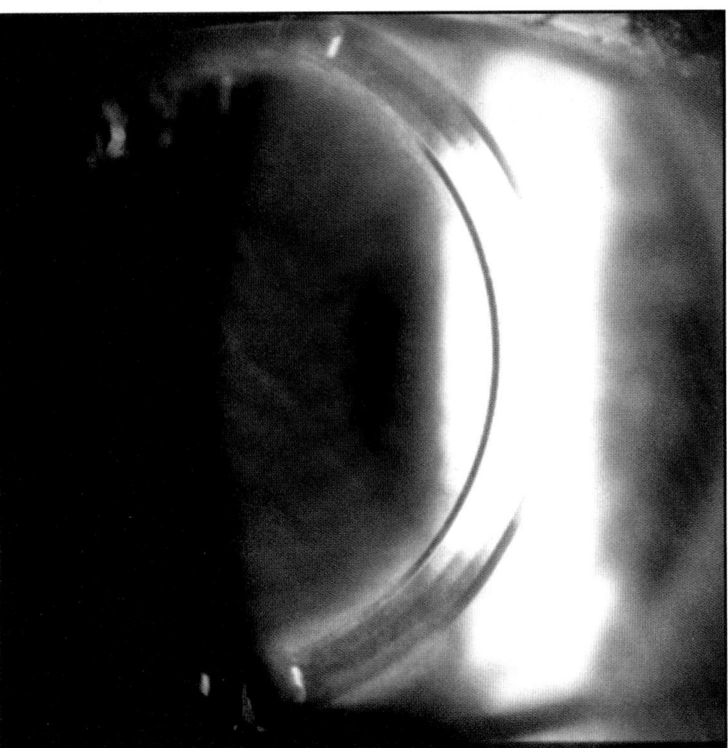

FIGURE 8-18: Mild channel haze.

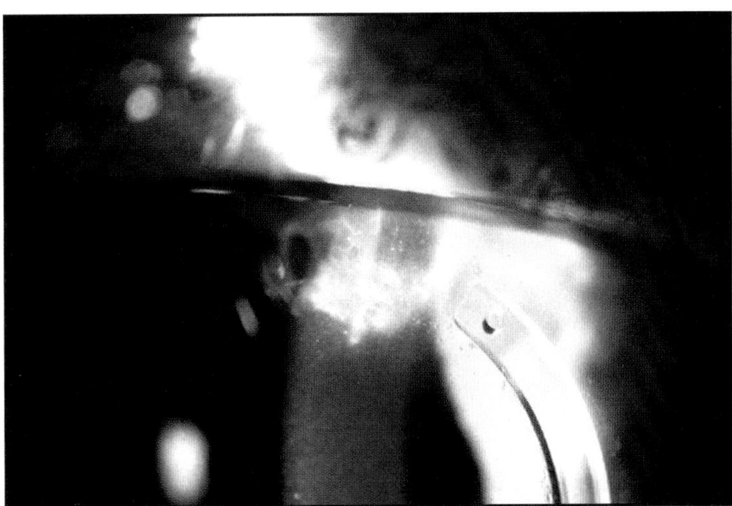

FIGURE 8-19: Subepithelial haze under the epithelium at the entry site as result of a strong healing response.

Case Report

A 13-year-old boy presented with his parents with a history of progressive vision loss due to keratoconus in both eyes. He was a gifted hockey player and his performance was beginning to suffer from his vision loss. UCVA was 20/40 in each eye and MRx in the right eye was plano – 4.25 × 040 giving 20/20– and in the left eye was plano –2.25 × 104 producing 20/20–. As he was a minor, he and his parent consented to Intacs® and C3-R®. In both eyes, a single segment Intacs® was first inserted in the lower cornea to surround the cone which was followed by C3-R® on the same day. The patient experienced improved UCVA of 20/25 in each eye. One year later, stability of the disease was shown (**Figures 8-22 and 8-23**). He also regained his confidence as a hockey player and continues to excel in the sport.

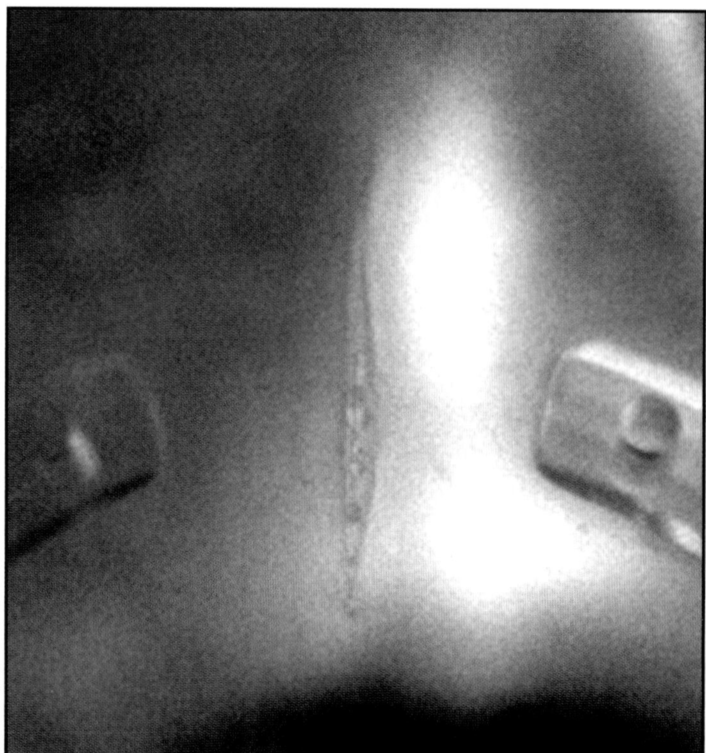

FIGURE 8-20: Clear epithelial plug in the incision site. This is best visualized by retroillumination.

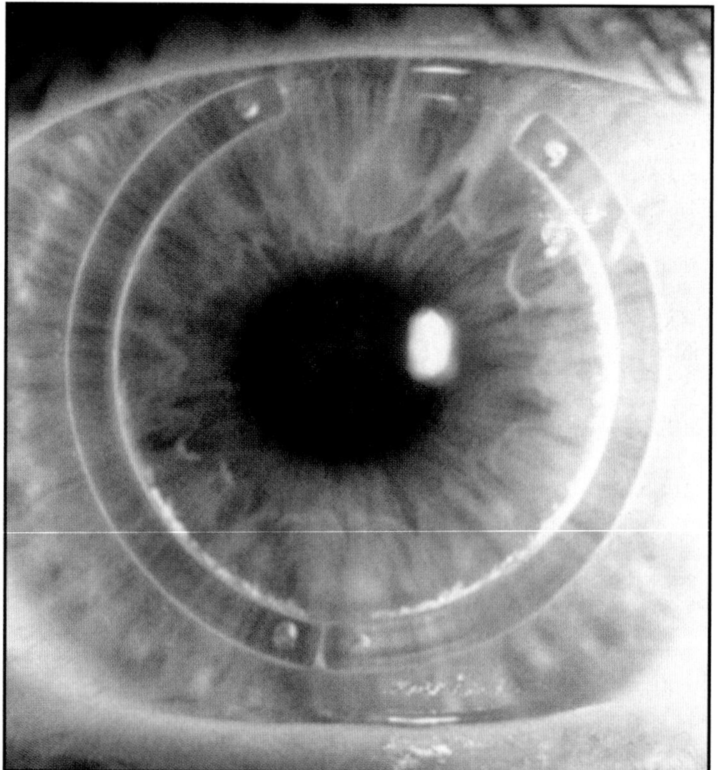

FIGURE 8-21: Touching segment ends. This slit lamp picture shows that the inferior ends of the Intacs® segments are touching 180 degrees from the incision site. There are no side effects from this.

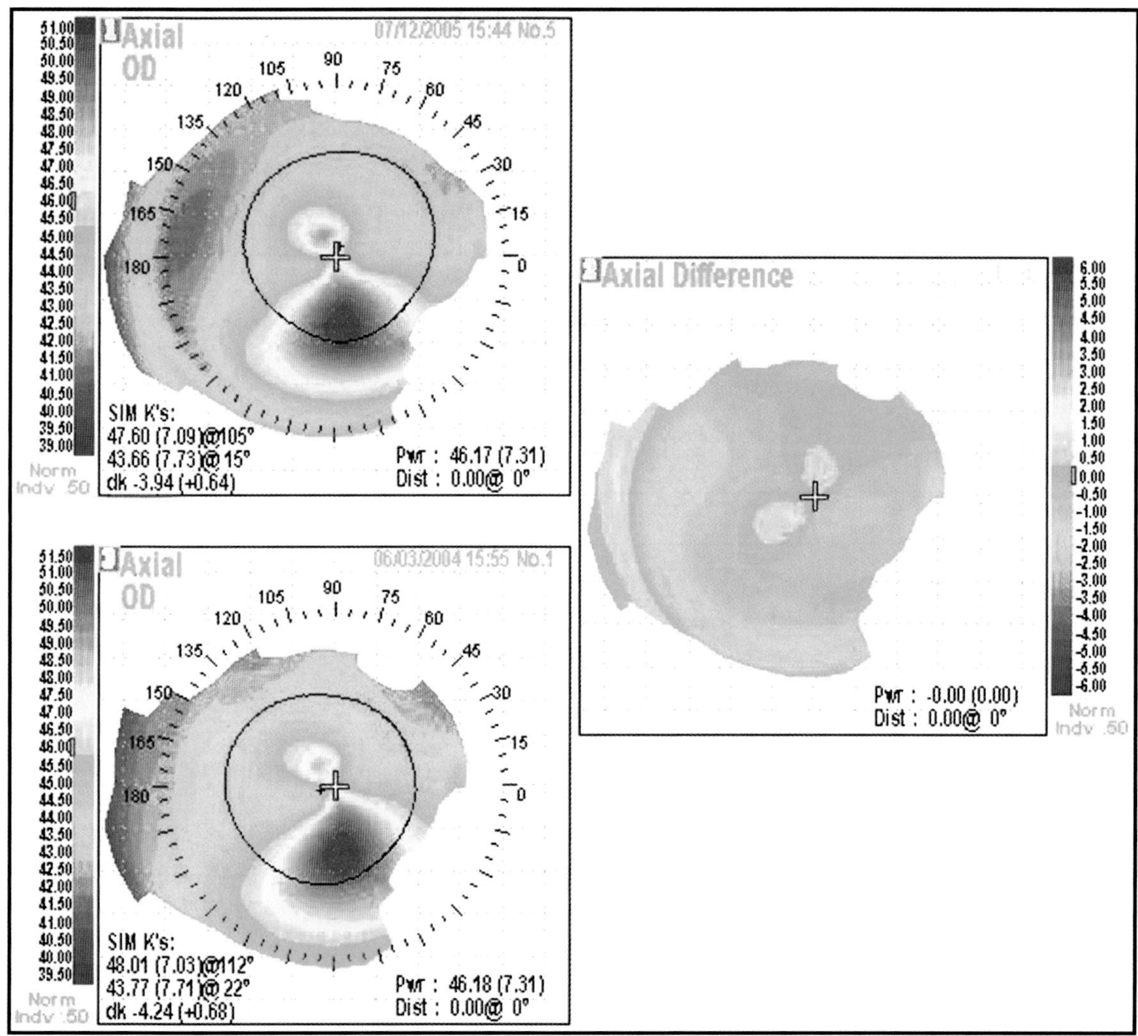

FIGURE 8-22: Effect of Intacs® and C3-R® on right eye. Preoperative topography (lower left) compared to postoperative topography (upper left) shows no change after one year. Difference map (right) indicates inferior flattening from a lower Intacs® segment and no progression of keratoconus.

Single vs Double Segments Intacs®

After we first reported the comparative results of single vs double segments, there has been an increasing trend for surgeons to use a single segment Intac below the cone. In our study comparing single segment to double segments[5], we reported more improvement in UCVA in the single-segment group (9 lines) than the double-segment group (2.5 lines), more improvement in BSCVA in the single-segment group (2.5 lines) than the double-segment group (<1 line), more improvement in steep K values in single-segment group (2.76 diopters +/– 2.68) than the double-segment group (0.93 diopters +/– 2.01), and more than twice as much improvement in I-S index in the single-segment group (9.51+/– 7.49) than the double-segment group (4.22 +/– 4.82) **(Table 8-1)**.

We achieved greater cylinder decrease as measured with Holladay vector analysis in the single- segment group (5.69 diopters +/– 3.10) than the double-segment group (1.58 diopters +/– 3.09) and concluded that single segment Intacs® for peripheral keratoconus achieved significantly better results double segment Intacs®. **Figure 8-6** shows the preferential effect of flattening the lower, steep area and steepening the upper, flat area compared to **Figure 8-7** that shows global flattening including the already flat upper cornea.

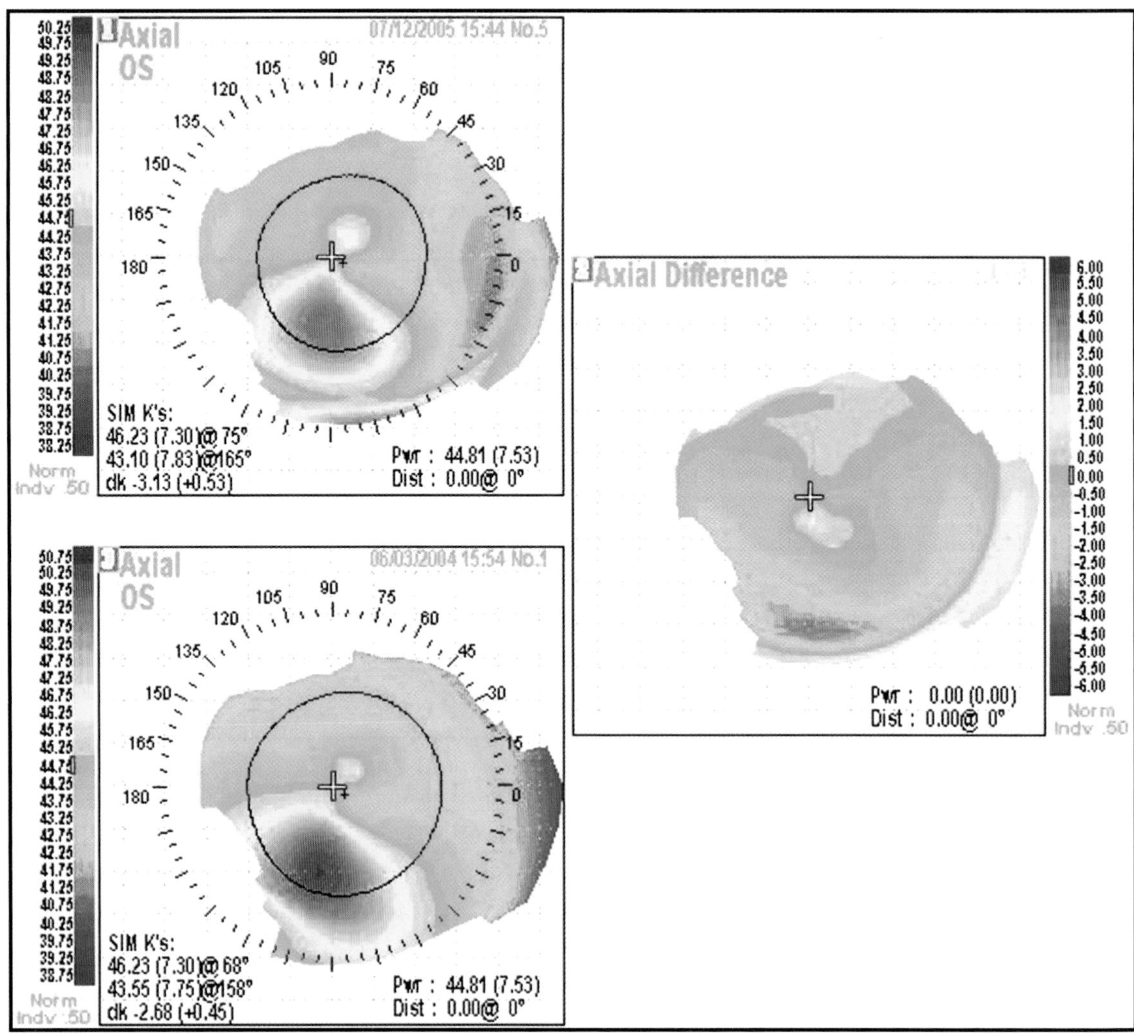

FIGURE 8-23: Effect of Intacs® and C3-R® on left eye. The fellow eye of patient in Figure 8-22 shows similar effect of the combined treatment: improvement in lower cone and stability after one year.

TABLE 8-1: Comparison of I-S values in single-segment and double-segment groups

	K values (D)		
Variable	*Single-segment group*	*Double-segment group*	*P value**
Preoperative I-S value	20.49 ± 14.33	27.78 ± 13.07	0.16
Postoperative I-S	10.98 ± 10.24	23.56 ± 11.04	< 0.01
Change I-S	9.51 ± 7.49	4.22 ± 4.82	0.01

*Change in single-segment vs double-segment group

Intacs® Explant

In patients with previous double segment Intacs® implantation for peripheral keratoconus, it is possible to still achieve the same result as for single segment placement. In these cases, the upper segment can be explanted to relieve the unnecessary flattening in the upper cornea. This will lead to steepening in the upper cornea coupled with flattening in the lower cornea. In effect, this selective explant can achieve the same result as if a single segment was originally placed. There may be an increase in myopia due less flattening in the upper

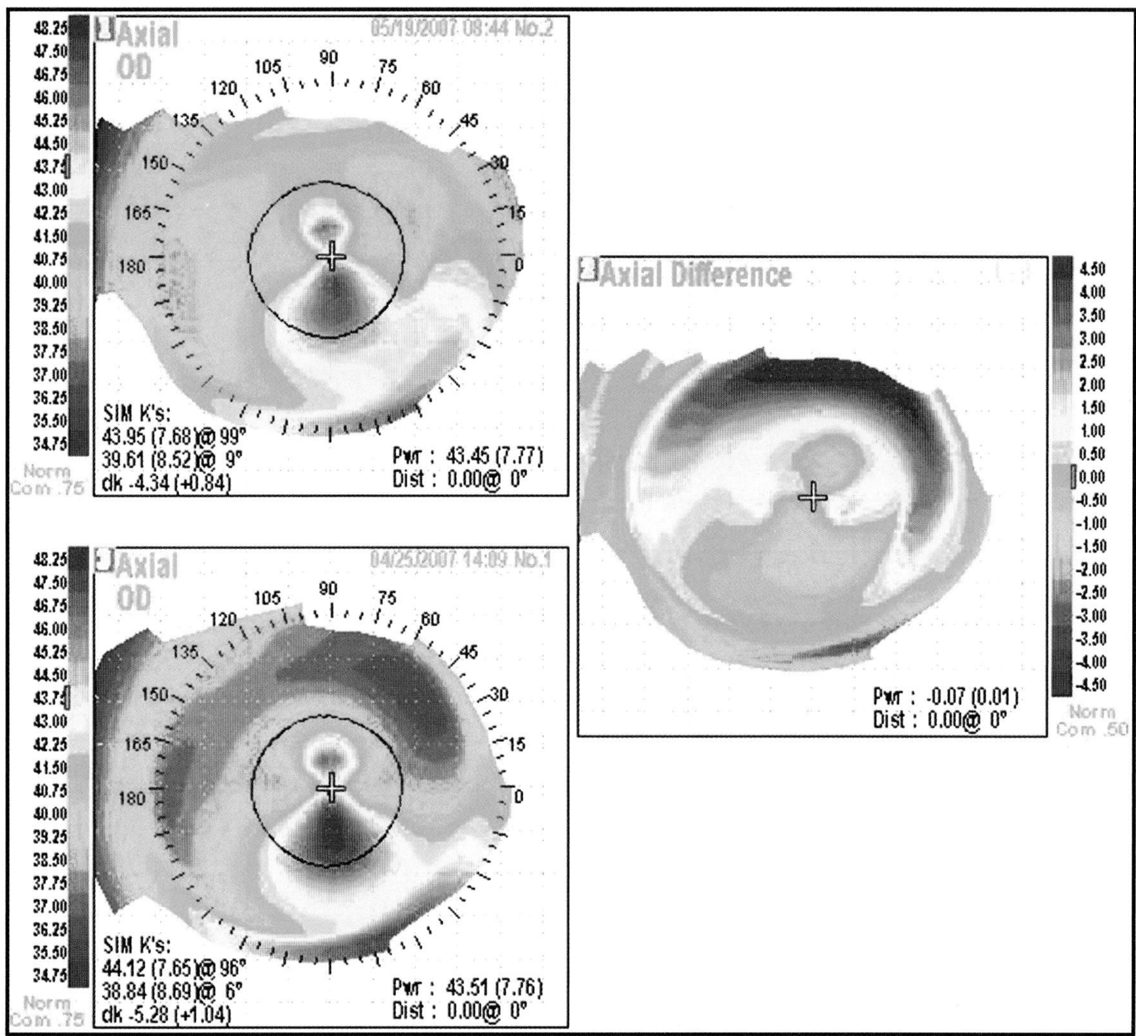

FIGURE 8-24: Topography analysis after superior segment explant of another patient. The same effects are seen in Figure 8-22 example with the exception of significant central flattening as well.

cornea which may reduce UCVA in the process of improving BSCVA. On occasion, the upper segment explant can also lead to central flattening in addition to superior steepening **(Figure 8-24)**.

Case Report

A 52-year-old male patient with keratoconus was treated with double segment Intacs® several years ago. The upper Intacs® segment was removed to improve quality of vision by removing unneeded flattening in upper cornea **(Figure 8-25)**. Pre-explant UCVA was 20/40 and MRx was +0.50 –3.0 × 176 yielding 20/40. After the explant, UCVA was 20/80 due to increased myopia from superior steepening. The benefit was in quality of vision as BSCVA improved to 20/30 with MRx of –0.50 –3.0 × 10.

Surgical Technique

After the eye is anesthetized, prepped, and draped in the sterile fashion, a wire lid speculum is applied for exposure. A Sinskey hook is used to bluntly open the prior incision, extending the opening down to the base of the incision. The hook is then used to separate the closed channel between the incision site and distal tip of segment. The hook is then used to separate the stroma that encompasses the tip of the segment. Use an

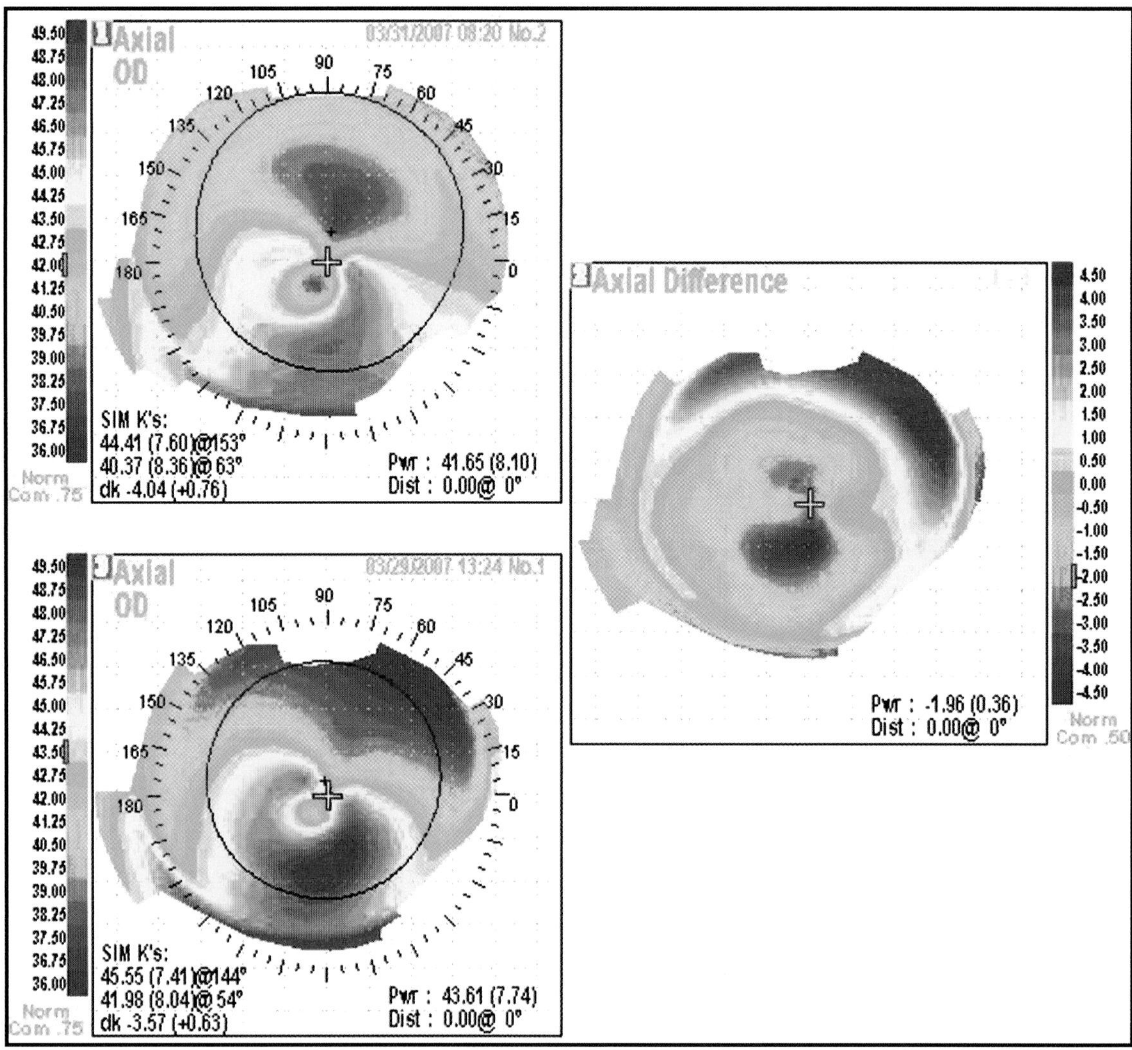

FIGURE 8-25: Topography analysis after superior segment explant. Preoperative topography (lower left) compared to postoperative topography (upper left) shows steepening in upper cornea. Difference map clearly shows this change along with flattening in the lower cornea.

anterior approach when placing the hook in the segment hole prior to pulling out the segment. Avoid placing the hook in the hole from the posterior side of the segment as this makes it harder to initiate the segment from being dislodged from the tunnel. Using counter traction from a forceps grasping the sclera with the other hand, the Intacs® segment is carefully pulled from the channel **(Figure 8-26)**. Expect some resistance from the tissue, but the segment can be removed in all cases. Once the segment tip is externalized, the hook can then anteriorly be placed in the hole to further extract the segment. A forceps can also be used to remove the segment from the channel. The channel will immediately collapse. No sutures are required. Antibiotic, steroid, and NSAID drops are used for 1 week.

Alternative Technique

1. If the previous Intacs® implantation was performed more than 1 year prior to day of explant, it may not be possible to bluntly enter the channel with Sinskey hook through the initial incision due to incision fibrosis. It is recommended to make a new incision directly at the site of the prior incision; diamond blade should be set at same depth as prior incision. If prior incision depth is not known, pachymetry can be measured

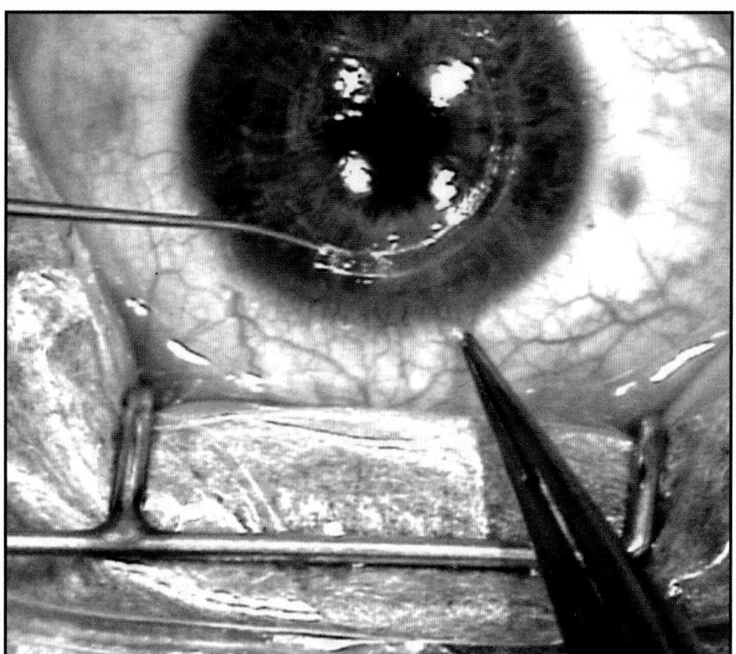

FIGURE 8-26: Segment explant. Once the Sinkey hook is used to separate the stroma from the tip of the segment, the segment is partially removed before using a forceps to completely remove segment.

over incision site and diamond knife is set at 70% of the cornea thickness. After the incision is made, the procedure is performed according to protocol detailed above.

2. If the Intacs® will not be replaced (i.e., explant only), then the diamond knife can be extended to 400 microns and used to incise the cornea directly over the distal tip of the segment. The diamond will contact the Intac segment and the diamond can be used to incise the cornea over the width of the segment. A Sinskey hook can then be placed under the posterior tip of the segment and also placed in the hole followed by removal. This technique is not recommended for exchanges, since the incision will be over the tip of the new segment placed.

Intacs® Exchange

There are conditions where a patient with Intacs® placed in past may require exchange of segments. One condition is if a different nomogram was used that advises placing a thicker upper segment and thinner lower segment for a peripheral cone. In such a case, it would be desirable to explant both segments and implant a thicker segment below. The surgical technique for explant described above can be applied to exchange the Intacs®. Once the segment is removed, the desired size segment can be immediately reinserted into the channel. Sutures are optional.

Conclusion

After initial reports, many studies have subsequently been conducted to evaluate Intacs® for keratoconus.[8-19] Intacs® provide a unique ability to modify the shape of the keratoconus. This in turn can lead to improvement in vision and reduction of astigmatism and myopia. The goal of Intacs® is to improve patients' ability to function in corrective lenses such as soft lenses, hybrid lenses, RGP lenses, or glasses. The goal of each patient depends on the degree of keratoconus being treated. Patients should be given realistic expectations from Intacs® procedures. Some patients with very mild keratotoconus can expect to improve their UCVA without the use of corrective lenses.

References

1. Ertan A, Kamburoglu G. Analysis of centration of Intacs® segments inserted with a femtosecond laser. J Cataract Refract Surg 2007; 33:484-7.
2. Colin J, Cocherner B, Savary G, Malet F. Correcting keratoconus with intracorneal rings. J Cataract Refract Surg 2000; 26(8):1117-22.
3. Colin J, Cochener B, Savary G, Malet F, Colmes-Higging D. Intacs® inserts for treating keratoconus: one-year results. Ophthalmology; 2001; 108 (8):1409-14
4. Boxer Wachler BS, Christie JC, Chou B, Chandra N, Korn T. Intacs® for the treatment of keratoconus. Ophthalmology 2003;110:1031-40.
5. Sharma M, Boxer Wachler BS. Comparison of single segment and double segment Intacs® for keratoconus and post-LASIK ectasia. Am J Ophthalmol 2006;141:891-95.
6. Chan CCK, Boxer Wachler BS. Reduced best corrected visual acuity from surgical technique of inserting a thicker Intac above and thinner Intac below the cone. J Refract Surg 2007; 23:93-5.
7. Kessler D, El-Shiaty AF, Wachler BS. Evaluation of tear following Intacs® for myopia. J Refract Surg 2002;18:127-9.
8. Hustler A, Manna A, Morris S, Obi A, Horgan S. Intacs for the correction of keratoconus. J Cataract Refract Surg 2007;33(8):1354.
9. Rodríguez LA, Guillén PB, Benavides MA, Garcia L, Porras D, Daqui-Garay RM. Penetrating keratoplasty versus intrastromal corneal ring segments to correct bilateral corneal ectasia: preliminary study. J Cataract Refract Surg 2007;33(3):488-96.
10. Kymionis GD, Siganos CS, Tsiklis NS, Anastasakis A, Yoo SH, Pallikaris AI, Astyrakakis N, Pallikaris IG. Long-term follow-up of Intacs in keratoconus. Am J Ophthalmol 2007;143(2):236-44. Epub 2006 Nov 30.
11. Samimi S, Leger F, Touboul D, Colin J. Histopathological findings after intracorneal ring segment implantation in keratoconic human corneas. J Cataract Refract Surg 2007 Feb;33(2):247-53.
12. Colin J, Malet FJ. Intacs for the correction of keratoconus: two-year follow-up. J Cataract Refract Surg 2007;33(1):69-74.
13. Pokroy R, Levinger S. Intacs adjustment surgery for keratoconus. J Cataract Refract Surg 2006;32(6):986-92.
14. Alió JL, Shabayek MH, Belda JI, Correas P, Feijoo ED. Analysis of results related to good and bad outcomes of Intacs implantation for keratoconus correction. J Cataract Refract Surg 2006;32(5):756-61.
15. Kanellopoulos AJ, Pe LH, Perry HD, Donnenfeld ED. Modified intracorneal ring segment implantations (INTACS) for the management of moderate to advanced keratoconus: efficacy and complications. Cornea 2006;25(1):29-33.
16. Tan BU, Purcell TL, Torres LF, Schanzlin DJ. New surgical approaches to the management of keratoconus and post-LASIK ectasia. Trans Am Ophthalmol Soc 2006;104:212-20.
17. Hellstedt T, Mäkelä J, Uusitalo R, Emre S, Uusitalo R. Treating keratoconus with intacs corneal ring segments. J Refract Surg 2005;21(3):236-46.
18. Alió JL, Artola A, Hassanein A, Haroun H, Galal A. One or 2 Intacs segments for the correction of keratoconus. J Cataract Refract Surg 2005;31(5):943-53.
19. Siganos CS, Kymionis GD, Kartakis N, Theodorakis MA, Astyrakakis N, Pallikaris IG. Management of keratoconus with Intacs. Am J Ophthalmol 2003;135(1):64-70.

Carlo F Lovisolo, MD, Paulo Ferrara, MD

9 Ferrara Rings

Introduction

The Ferrara rings™ (Ferrara Ophthalmics, Belo Horizonte, Brazil)[1-3] also manufactured and commercialized under the trade name of Keraring™ (Mediphakos, Belo Horizonte, Brazil) are computer-lathed PMMA CQ-acrylic arc segments **(Figure 9-1)**, designed for being implanted in the intermediate-to-deep corneal stroma. The most commonly used segment is the 5.0 mm optical zone with an internal and external diameter of 4.4 mm and 5.6 mm, respectively. The segment cross-section is triangular **(Figure 9-1C)**, with a constant 600 μm base for every thickness which varies from 100 to 350 μm. Wider optical zone segments (6.0 mm with 5.4 mm internal and 6.6 mm external diameter) and segment arcs (longer and shorter than the standard 160°, i.e. 210°, 140°, 120°, 90°, 60°) are available on special order. Two positioning holes are located at both ends to allow manipulation inside the tunnel.

The Ferrara rings obtained the CE mark in 2003 and since are commercially available in Europe. In the United States they are not commercially available since they are not approved by the Food and Drug Administration (FDA).

The goals of Ferrara rings are similar to Intacs as discussed in first section of Intacs description (Chapter 8).

Mechanism of Action

Like Intacs®, Ferrara rings are placed within the mid-peripheral corneal stroma. Their effect is consistent with the Barraquer and Blavatskaya theories[4] that indicate that such corneal inserts result in a centripetal flattening of both anterior and posterior surfaces by preserving their physiological asphericity **(Figures 9-2 and 9-3)**.

In ectatic corneal diseases such as keratoconus and keratoectasia, Ferrara rings have been shown to have the potential to result in a more physiological central corneal shape of the cone and to reduce the values of irregular astigmatism.[5-9] This can improve both uncorrected visual acuity (UCVA) and best spectacle-corrected visual acuity (BSCVA). Postoperatively, all the indices of topographic regularity improve with lower power variance and minimal change of asphericity.[3] Improved corneal optics are due to the remodeling of the epithelium that thickens in the flattened areas and thins on the top of the segments themselves **(Figure 9-4)**,[10] along

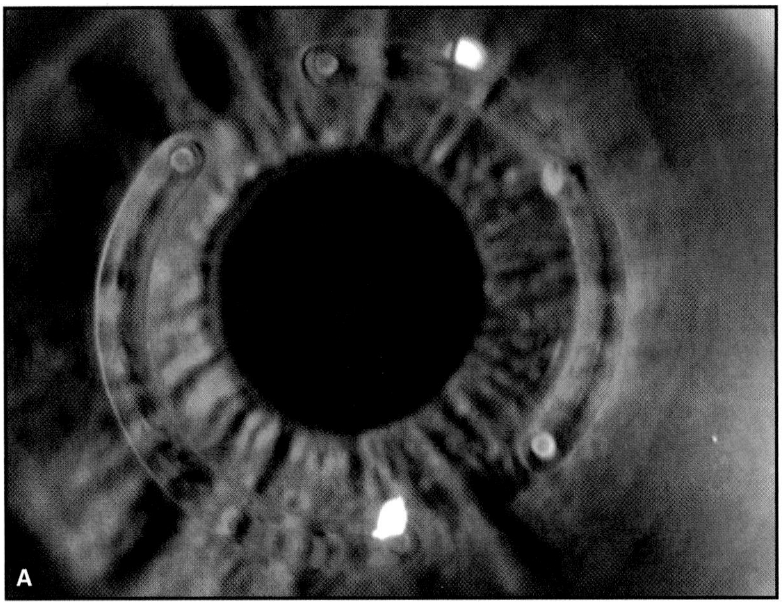

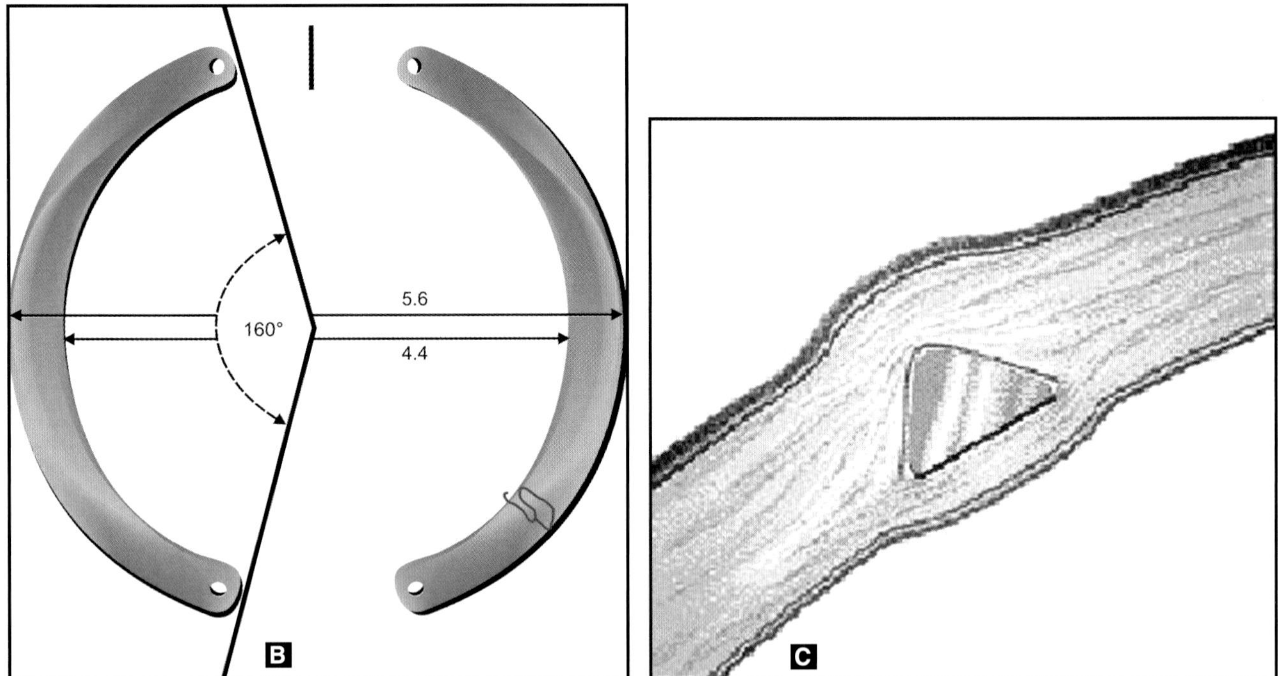

FIGURE 9-1: As compared to the Intacs, Ferrara ring segments (A) have 160° (instead of 150°) of arc, 5.0 mm (instead of 6.8 mm) optical zone (B) and a triangular (instead than hexagonal) shape (C).

with reduction of the anterior chamber depth.[3] Anecdotal evidence of other benefits have been reported such as influencing the natural history of keratoconus evolution, diminishing the opacity on the cone apex, improving the postoperative tolerance of contact lens, improving the overall aberrations generated by the new corneal surface and the reduction of symptoms like itching, photophobia and ocular discomfort.[3, 11] Further study is necessary to corroborate these reports.[12, 13]

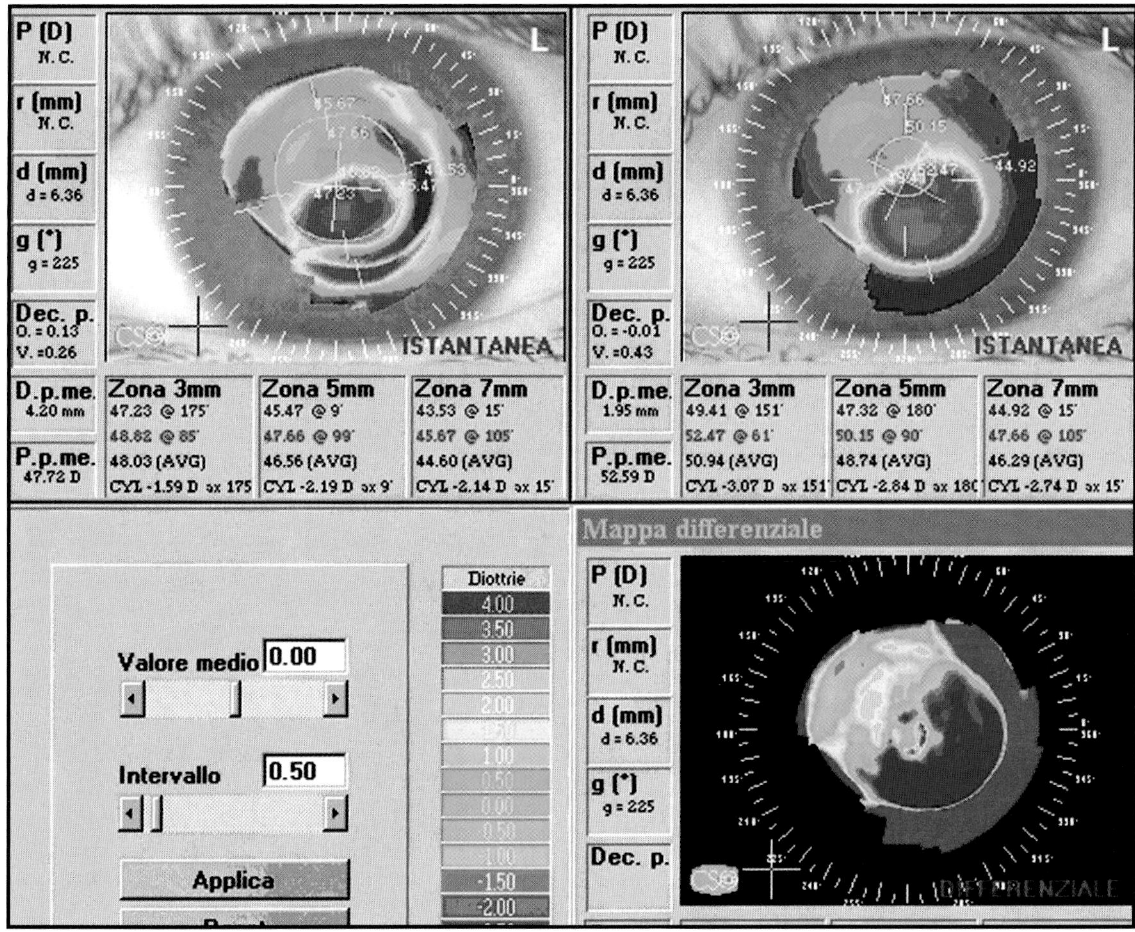

FIGURE 9-2: Tangential topography difference maps (bottom right) show the effect obtained on the anterior corneal surface after implantation of 1 inferior-temporal segment in a stage I (Apud Amsler). Note inferotemporal flattening and superonasal steepening.

Indications

The goal of surgery is mainly "orthopedic" in nature to improve the corneal shape; Ferrara rings are not intended to be performed for refractive purposes. The common indications are the unstable ectatic corneal disorders such as keratoconus;[3,5-7,12] pellucid marginal degeneration,[9,14] and keratectasia.[8] Patients who are best suited are those with contact lens intolerance and irregular astigmatism induced by traumatic scars, infections, complicated corneal surgeries (penetrating keratoplasty in particular)[3] which are not amenable to topography-guided or wavefront-guided excimer laser procedures. As compared to Intacs® and other intrastromal segments,[3,15] the smaller the optical zone allows a more direct and effective correction on keratoconic corneas.

Nomograms

Initially, surgeons implanted a pair of symmetrical segments in every case. The method of selecting the segment thickness was based on the degree spherical equivalent of the manifest refraction and on the cone evolution, by staging the ectasia with the Amsler-Ferrara classification[3,16] **(Table 9-1)**. The incision was always placed on the steep meridian to take advantage of the coupling effect achieved by the space-occupying devices.

When the benefits of single segment or asymmetrical implantations were shown,[17,18] alternative approaches were proposed for Ferrara rings that took into account purely refractive data **(Table 9-2)**.

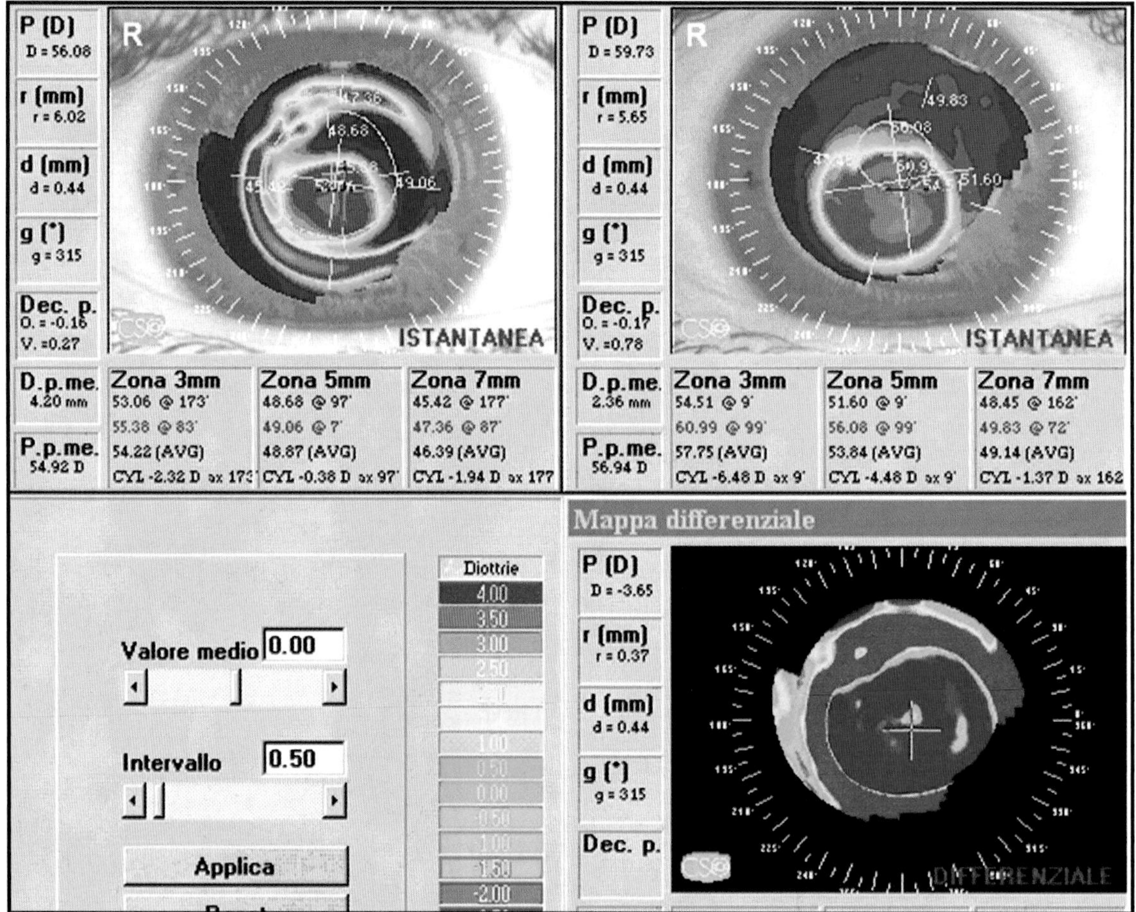

FIGURE 9-3: Tangential topography difference maps (bottom right) after two asymmetrical segments (infratemporal of 250 µm and the superonasal segment of 150 µm) in a stage II (Apud Amsler) keratoconus. Global flattening occurs between the segments, while the surface steepens on segments themselves.

Table 9-1: Paulo Ferrara original nomogram (1999) for double segment Ferrara ring implantation for keratoconus.

Segment thickness	*KC stage (Amsler-Ferrara)*	*Refraction (Sph.Eq.)*
150 µm	Fruste	–2.0 to –4.0
200 µm	I	–4.0 to –6.0
250 µm	II	–6.0 to –8.0
300 µm	III	–8.0 to –10.0
350 µm	IV	–10.0 to –12.0

With the current knowledge about placing segments on coma axis **(Figure 9-5)**, we developed a refined nomogram for segment thickness and number of segments to be used. This is based on the topographic astigmatism value from elevation maps and the pattern of keratoconus. For the symmetric bow-tie patterns, two equal-thickness segments are selected as per nomogram in **Table 9-3**. For the central cones, a single 210 μm is chosen based on **Table 9-4** nomogram.

For peripheral cones, the most common form type, asymmetrical segments are selected based on a topographic asymmetry index **(Figure 9-6)** that is used for nomograms in **Tables 9-5 and 9-6**. We use a pachymetry map to assure that the segment thickness used does not exceed 50% of the thickness of the cornea where the channel will be located.

Table 9-2: Albertazzi's nomogram (2004) for asymmetrical Ferrara Ring segment implantation for classic inferotemporal located keratoconus. Amount of myopia and astigmatism in diopters are on the X-axis and on the Y-axis, respectively. The entry incision is made in the steep meridian.

–6	— 250	150 250	150 250	200 300	200 300	250 350	250 350	250 350	300 350	350 350	350 350
–5	— 200	150 250	150 250	200 300	200 300	200 300	250 350	250 350	300 350	350 350	350 350
–4	— 150	150 250	150 250	200 300	200 300	200 300	250 350	250 350	300 350	350 350	350 350
–3	— 150	150 200	150 250	200 250	200 250	250 300	300 350	300 350	300 350	350 350	350 350
–2	— 150	150 150	150 200	200 200	200 250	250 250	250 300	300 300	300 350	350 350	350 350
–6	— —	— —	150 150	150 150	200 200	200 200	250 250	300 300	300 300	350 350	350 350
	0	**–2**	**–3**	**–4**	**–5**	**–6**	**–7**	**–8**	**–9**	**–10**	**–12**

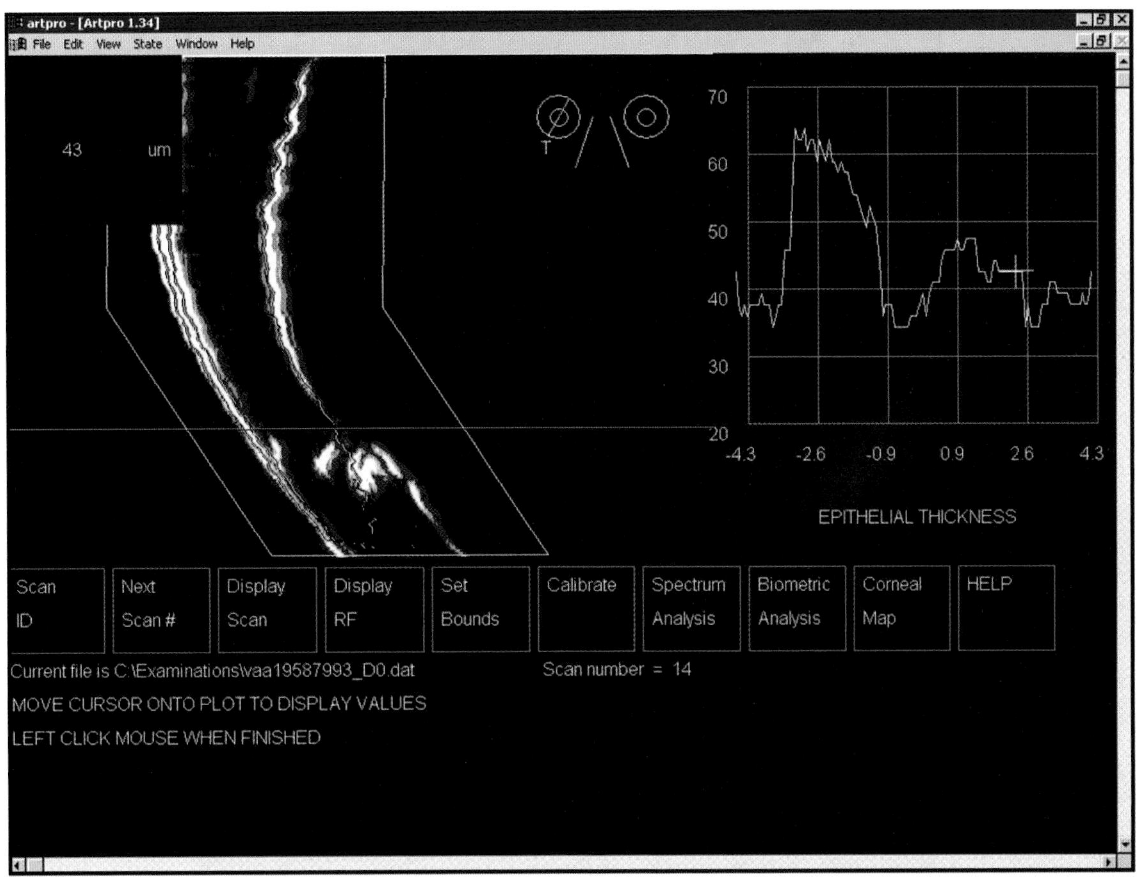

A

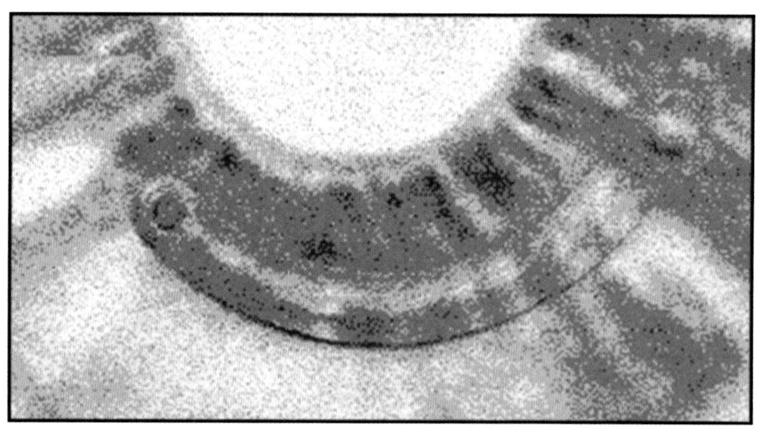

B

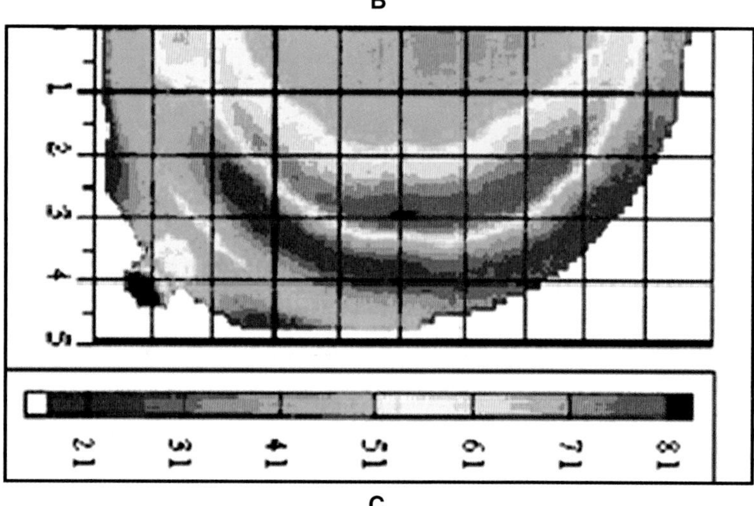

C

FIGURE 9-4: Very high frequency ultrasound with Artemis 2 (Ultralink) (A) of eye implanted with a single 5.0 mm, 250 μm Ferrara ring segment in the lower cornea (B). The epithelial thickness map of a keratoconic cornea after Ferrara ring (C) shows the compensating behavior of the epithelium. The thickest points of the epithelium are near the inner edge of the segment where the corneal surface shows the maximum flattening effect; the thinnest points of epithelium are above the segments and maximum steepening is observed directly on to of the implants.

Table 9-3: Segment thickness choice in symmetric bow-tie keratoconus

Topographic astigmatism (D)	*Segment thickness (μm)*
≤ 1.00	150 / 150
1.25 to 2.00	200 / 200
2.25 to 3.00	250 / 250
≥ 3.25	300 / 300

Table 9-4: Single 210°-segment thickness choice in central nipple and iatrogenic corneal ectasia

Topographic astigmatism (D)	*Segment thickness (μm)*
≤ 2.50	150
2.75 to 4.00	200
4.25 to 3.00	250
≥ 6.00	300

Table 9-5: Asymmetrical segment thickness choice in sag cones with 0/100% and 25/75% of asymmetry index (patterns in Figures 9-6A and B)

Topographic astigmatism (D)	*Segment thickness (μm)*
≤1.00	None / 150
1.25 to 2.00	None / 200
2.25 to 3.00	None / 250
3.25 to 4.00	None / 300
4.25 to 5.00	150 / 250
5.25 to 6.00	200 / 300

Table 9-6: Asymmetrical segment thickness choice in sag cones with 33/66% of asymmetry index (pattern in Figure 9-6C)

Topographic astigmatism (D)	*Segment thickness (μm)*
≤1.00	None / 150
1.25 to 2.00	150 / 200
2.25 to 3.00	200 / 250
3.25 to 4.00	250 / 300

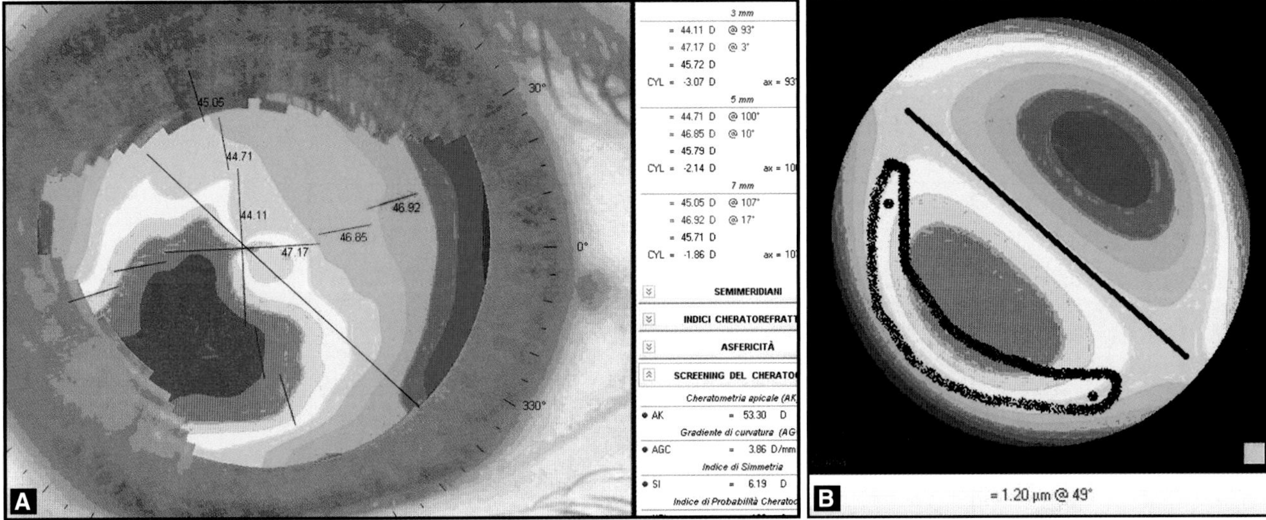

FIGURE 9-5: After the original observations of Luis Cadarso, the most effective optical correction occurs when the incision site is placed on the coma axis and it often does not correspond to the steep topographic axis. Corneal aberrometry-based software developed by Calossi A, Versaci F, Cadarso L and Lovisolo C is commercially available with the CSO corneal topographer. In this patient the topographic steep axis was 7° (A), while the coma axis was 49° (B). Implantation on the steep axis would have resulted in undercorrection and displacement of the coma axis. Corneal topography alone can be used to estimate the coma axis by drawing a line parallel to the cone (A).

Surgical Technique

While outside the procedure room, the patient's corneal limbus is marked with two dots at 3 and 9 o'clock positions with marker at the slit lamp, and then a topography and a corneal wavefront map are obtained.

Surgery is performed under topical anesthesia after miosis achieved with 2% pilocarpine. An eyelid speculum is used to expose the eye. The ocular surface is cleaned with with 2.5% povidone iodine eyedrops. The segments are centered on the visual axis by marking it with a Sinskey hook. This axis is easily identified by asking the patient to fixate on the corneal light reflex of the microscope light. The light reflex closely approximats the visual axis. The segments are not centered on the pupil.

Map	Ectasia Distribution	Description
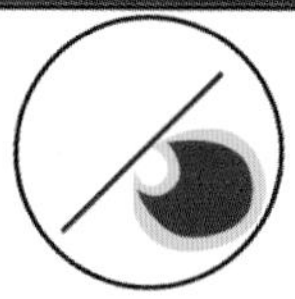	0% / 100%	A. All ectatic area located at one side of the cornea
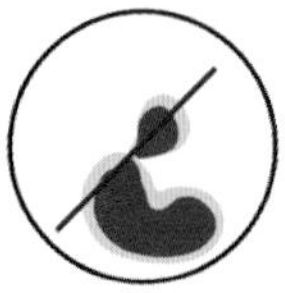	25% / 75%	B. 75% of the ectatic area located in one corneal side
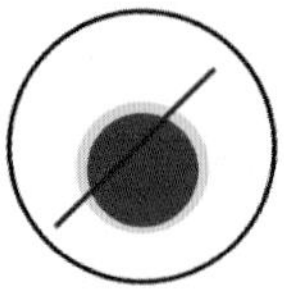	33% / 66%	C. 66% of the ectatic area located in one corneal side
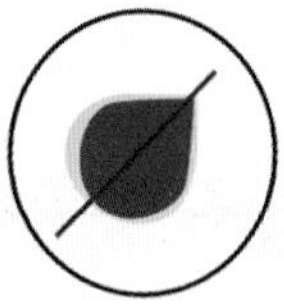	50% / 50%	D. Ectatic area symmetrically distributed

FIGURE 9-6: Evaluation of topographic distribution of corneal ectasia as per percentage of asymmetry. A and B correspond to nomograms in Table 9-5. Figure 9-6C corresponds to nomogram in Table 9-6.

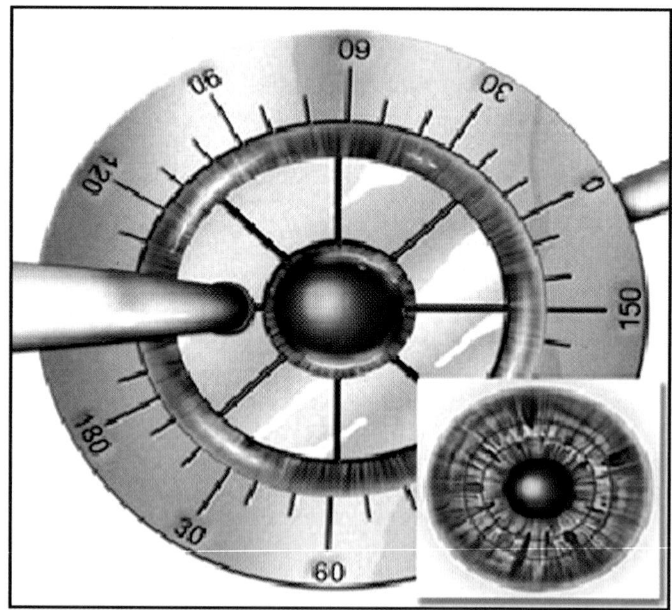

FIGURE 9-7: Marking the site of incision and the segment placement locations. The Mendez axis marker (right) is used to align the 0 and 180 degrees axes. The Ferrara ring marker (left) is oriented to the desired axis based on the axis marking on the Mendez marker. In this example, the desired axis is 150 degrees.

Using a Mendez marker to orient the 3 and 9 o'clock limbal marks, the gentian-violet marked, 5.0 mm optical zone and incision site marker is aligned to the desired axis based on the steepest topographic axis or the coma axis **(Figure 9-7)**.

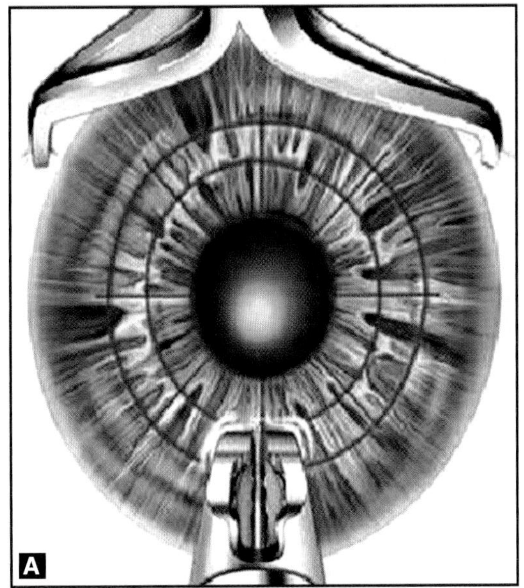

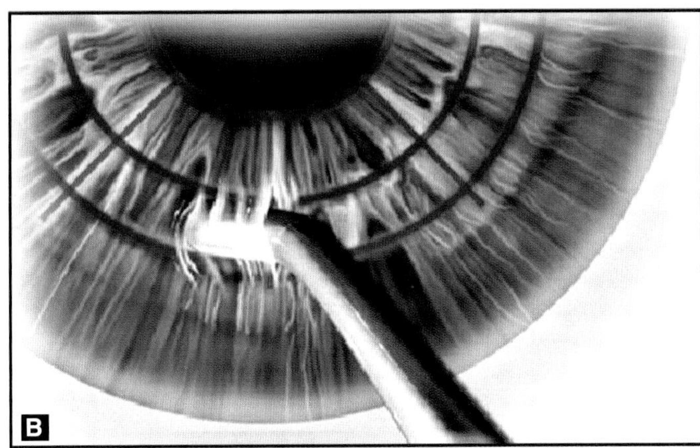

FIGURE 9-8: 1.0 mm incision is made with a diamond knife (A) and pocketing of the channel is created with the stromal spreader (B).

Ultrasonic pachymetry is measured over the incision site. The depth of a 1.0 mm, square diamond blade is set at 80% of the mean ultrasound pachymetry reading at the incision site. The blade is used to make the incision **(Figure 9-8A)**. The channel of incision is initiated using a Soarez stromal spreader **(Figure 9-8B)**, which creates a double pocket. **Figure 9-9** shows a how these steps are used to create the pockets of the channel.

Two (clockwise and counter clockwise) 270° semicircular dissecting spatulas **(Figure 9-10)** are consecutively inserted through the incision and gently pushed with some, quick, rotary "back and forth" tunneling movements. In the original free-hand technique, globe fixation is achieved by using Kremer forceps and asking the patient to keep fixing the light of the microscope. Adequate expertise and skill are required for maintaining appropriate depth, centration and symmetry during tunnel creation. Alternative options for channel creation are the use of the Lovisolo vacuum suction system (Janach) or the femtosecond laser. The clinical advantages of using

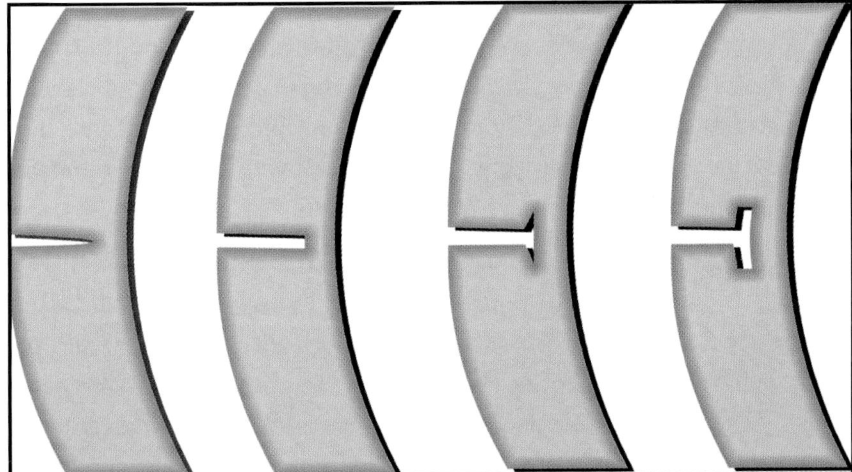

FIGURE 9-9: Evolution of stromal pockets of the channel. Initial incision after diamond blade (left) and final shape of the pockets after stromal spreader (right).

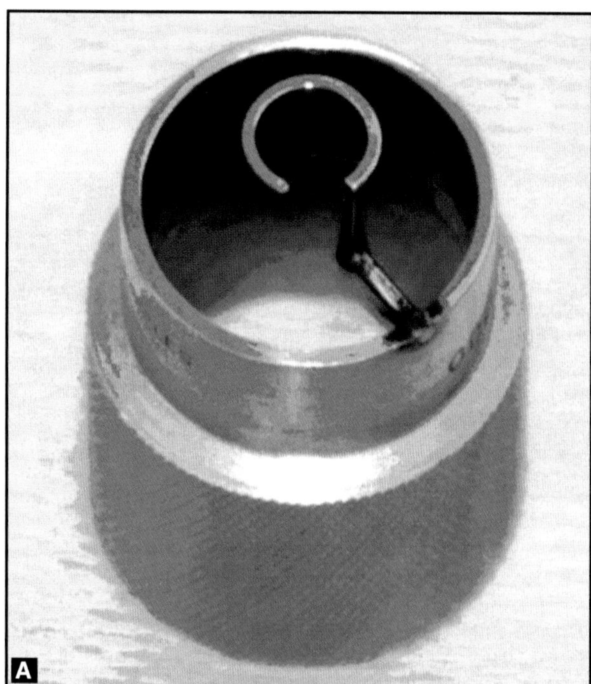

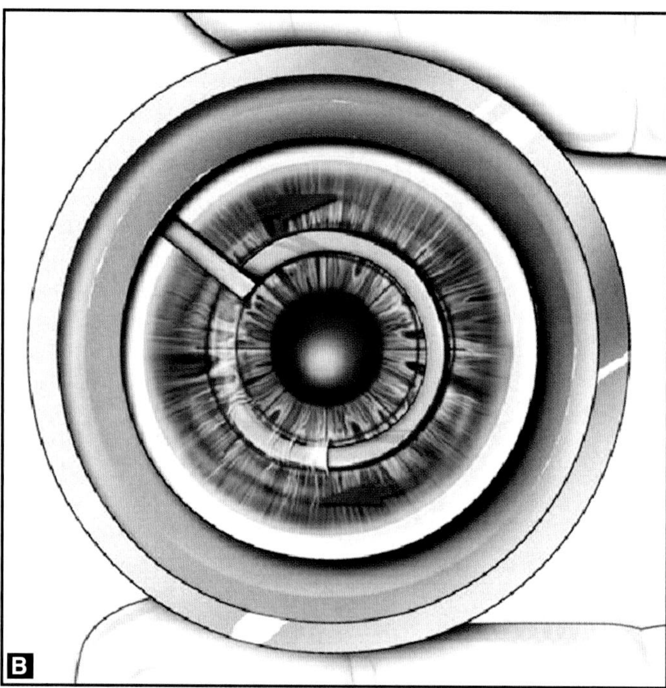

FIGURE 9-10: The channel dissecting spatula shown upside down (A). The spatula is shown after being placed in the channel pocket and partially rotated in clockwise fashion (B). Note a portion of the spatula has created part of the channel.

the vacuum system or the femtosecond laser for channel creation versus free-hand surgical technique included safety, consistency and flexibility and may be advisable for beginner surgeons.

Following channel creation, the channels are rinsed with 0.5% vancomycin. The segments are then inserted by using special instruments (Lovisolo Ferrara Ring Instrument Set, Janach, Como, Italy). Wound hydration and incision edge apposition is assessed. In most cases, the incision edges are apposed and a suture is not needed. The inked marks of the corneal marker that were initially placed are used to check rings are in proper position.

Results

We have placed Ferrara rings for keratoconus in more than 2200 eyes between 1996 and 2007. Interpreting the results is not always straightforward because of the wide range of keratoconus clinical characteristics.[19,20] Statistical analysis was performed on the most homogeneous group of 606 eyes with more advanced (stage IV with significant apex opacity). Central cones were excluded. The average and the minimum follow-up periods were 46 and 24 months, respectively.

Efficacy

The following percentages of BCVA equal or better than 20/50 were observed at two years postoperatively (cases are staged along with the Amsler-Ferrara classification[3,16]): phase I (mild keratoconus): 84%; phase II (moderate keratoconus): 77%; phase III (advanced keratoconus): 46%. These percentages support our belief that surgery should be applied at its early stage if possible **(Figure 9-11)**. In general, patients satisfaction was high. Psychologically, patients appreciate the chance to postpone corneal transplantation.

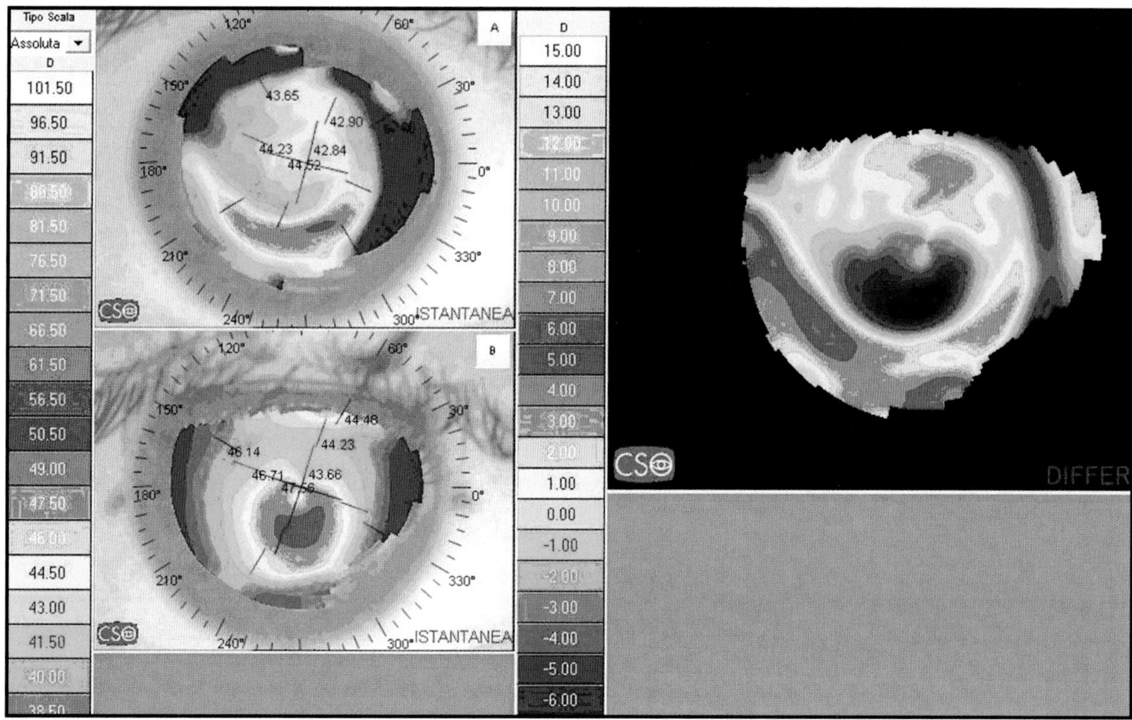

FIGURE 9-11: A typical expected outcome after Ferrara ring implantation. Flattening is observed on the topographic difference map (right) for an eye with phase I keratoconus that is 4 years after surgery. Postoperative astigmatism is less than 1.00 D.

In study of 400 eyes with mean follow-up of 10 months, mean reduction in keratometry values was 4.18 D and spherical equivalent was reduced by 4.65 D on average.[21] Mean UCVA improved from <20/150 to 20/100 and mean BCVA changed from 20/100 to 20/50 postoperatively. This is the largest study published to date evaluating the Ferrara ring.

Safety

We evaluated the incidence of clinically significant complications directly related to the ring segments. In doing so, we excluded cases where complications were surgical in origin, the most frequent of which was shallow implantation that can lead to early segment extrusion or poor patient selection that involved segment placement in corneas that were too thin or where keratoconus was too advanced for Ferrara rings. There were 11 eyes (1.8%) that experienced complications related to Ferrara rings.

- Two eyes developed delayed infective keratitis (about 0.3%), one was bacterial in origin and the other was fungal in etiology, which was associated with use of soft contact lenses, that led to severe tissue loss that required penetrating keratoplasty that uneventfully healed with a good outcome.
- Three eyes had extrusions (about 0.5%) that occurred at four, six and seven months postoperatively, despite adequate depth of implantation. Significant stromal melting prevented reimplantation, which is typically a feasible option when superficial segments extrude. Eye rubbing was suspected as the being responsible for extrusion in these cases. In two cases, lamellar keratoplasty was performed without complication. There was no need to remove segments prior to the transplant procedure, since they are far away from the trephination areas. Segments may help with centration of the procedure.

Similarly to Intacs® lamellar channel deposit, whitish intralamellar channel deposits around both segments' sides were noted. These deposits were more evident at the superior edge of the inferior segments. They are commonly observed three months after surgery and can increase in density for up to one year postoperatively before becoming stable. Although their origin and nature have not been conclusively established,[22] these deposits do not seem to adversely affect visual performance. They remain confined to the intrastromal channels and do not extend centrally or peripherally toward the limbus. They can disappear after segment removal. No chronic ocular itching, no neovascularization, and no epithelial ingrowth of the stromal channels were observed.

Pellucid Marginal Degeneration

We have implanted 47 eyes with pellucid marginal degeneration (PMD). After some cases of severe keratoectasia after LASIK, an unrecognized "subclinical" PMD was described.[23] It is now recognized that PMD is a contraindication to LASIK. Ferrara ring surgery outcomes are particularly good with PMD, PMD is one of the best indications for intrastromal implant surgery as long as the peripheral thinning is not severe enough to risk corneal segment perforation.

Case Report

A patient with PMD had Ferrara ring **(Figure 9-12)**. Preoperatively, the BSCVA was 20/80 with –9.00 –11.00 × 105° and14 months postoperatively, BSCVA improved to 20/30 with –8.25 –2.75 × 98°. Based on residual refractive error, a toric Visian ICL was implanted with the goal of plano. Postoperative UCVA was an impressive 20/20 for this case.

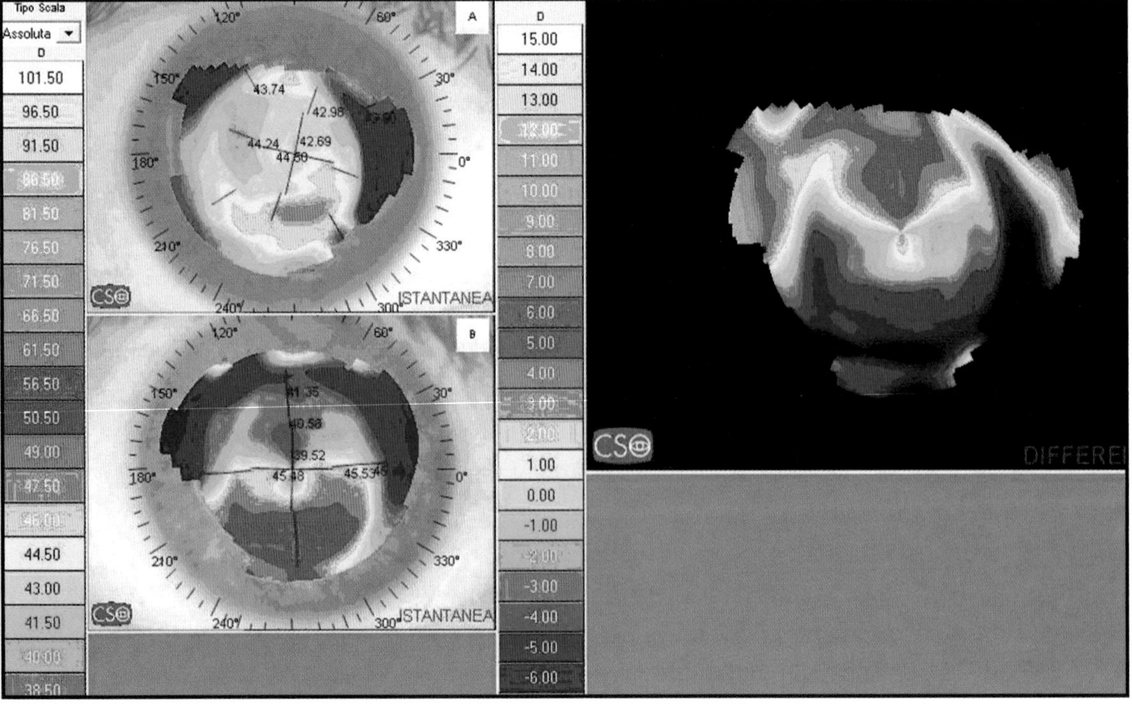

FIGURE 9-12: Topographic outcome shown by difference map of a single 210° Ferrara ring segment implanted in the lower cornea in a patient with pellucid marginal degeneration. Note the marked improvement in corneal symmetry.

Radial Keratotomy and Astigmatic Keratotomy Ectasia

Ferrara ring implantation may help in restoring a physiological shape of the anterior corneal surface.[24,25] Patients who had radial keratotomy (RK) and astigmatic keratotomy (AK) in the past may experience similar types of corneal ectasia. We have used Ferrara rings for 19 eyes that experienced complications after RK. When a post-RK keratoectasia shows develops, before proceeding with a transplant surgery, we believe it is worth treating these cases with one or two, symmetrical (same thickness) or asymmetrical (different thickness) Ferrara ring segments. The rationale of segment's choice is still controversial and mainly left to the each surgeon's experience.

Case Report

A patient underwent RK and AK. Preoperative topography was unremarkable and BSCVA was 20/20 with –6.00 –3.00 × 180°. Post-RK and AK surgery, BSCVA was reduced to 20/40 with –2.75 –3.75 × 90° **(Figure 9-13)**. A symmetrical pair of 250 μm Ferrara ring segments were implanted through a temporal incision two years after the complicated RK and AK surgery. Three years after Ferrara ring surgery and two single 10-0 nylon sutures of the inferior transverse incisions, clinical appearance and refraction are stable, with an uncorrected visual acuity of 20/30, a BSCVA of 20/20 with –1.50 × 90°.

Despite several theoretical advantages of Ferrara rings for RK ectasia, it is prudent to acknowledge the increased risk of incision dehiscence during channel dissections or segment positioning. Similar to what has been described during penetrating keratoplasty,[26] when the dissector passes through the RK incision, even though no particular resistance is encountered, the dissector always creates torque that can separate and eventually may open the old RK incisions **(Figure 9-14)**. RK incision dehiscence requires tight closure with 10-0 nylon sutures that are placed perpendicular to the incision; Ferrara ring segments should not be implanted in this situation. Even if tunnel dissection does not open an RK incision at the time of surgery, it may not be safe in the long-term. Considering the space-occupying effects of the segments which put RK incisions under constant strain and tension, a potential risk is the delayed postoperative opening and wound melt.[3]

Keratoectasia

We have performed Ferrara ring surgery in 63 eyes that underwent previous LASIK or PRK. Most cases had excimer laser surgery before it was recognized that forme fruste keratoconus (FFKC) or PMD were risk factors for keratoectasia.[27,28] Excluding those cases, 12 eyes can be considered "true" iatrogenic corneal ectasia without identifiable preoperative risk factors, which makes future keratoectasia a very rare disorder. There is a distinction between "LASIK on keratoconus" vs. "true" iatrogenic keratoectasia in which LASIK was performed on a completely normal cornea that developed keratoectasia. "LASIK on keratoconus" will lead to almost immediate progression of ectasia postoperatively that can involve a large area of corneal topography. On the other hand, "true" iatrogenic keratoectasia will often have good, stable results until 5 to 6 years after surgery. At which time a localized area of steepening can become apparent inducing more spherical and higher order aberrations than coma, and without a progressive thinning of the stroma. It is not clear if these patients were pre-destined to develop keratoconus or if the laser vision procedure was a cause in the delayed development of the ectasia. Ferrara ring outcomes are less predictable for keratoectasia than for naturally occurring keratoconus and PMD but case still be of benefit.

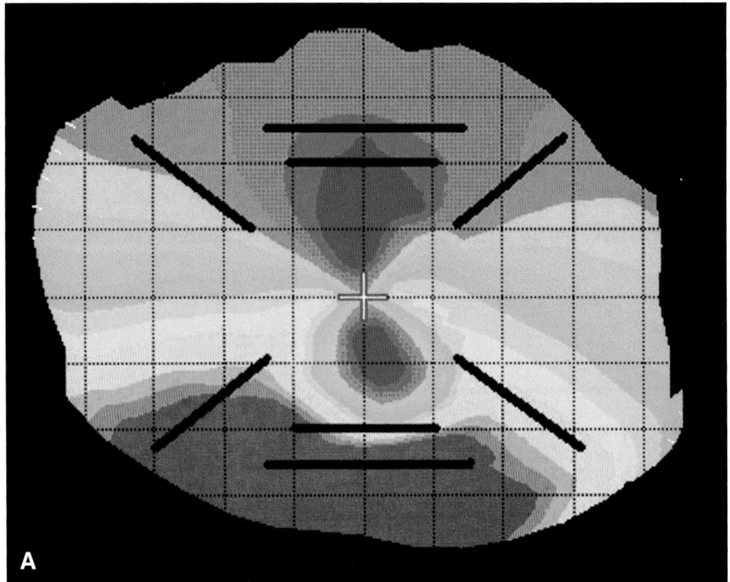

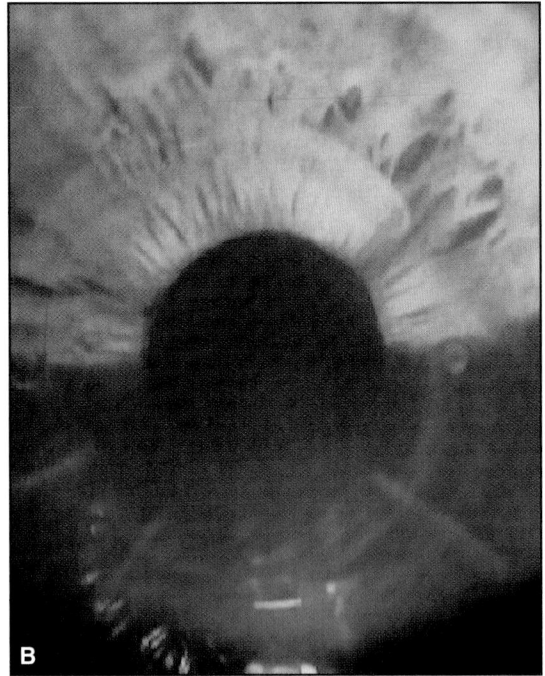

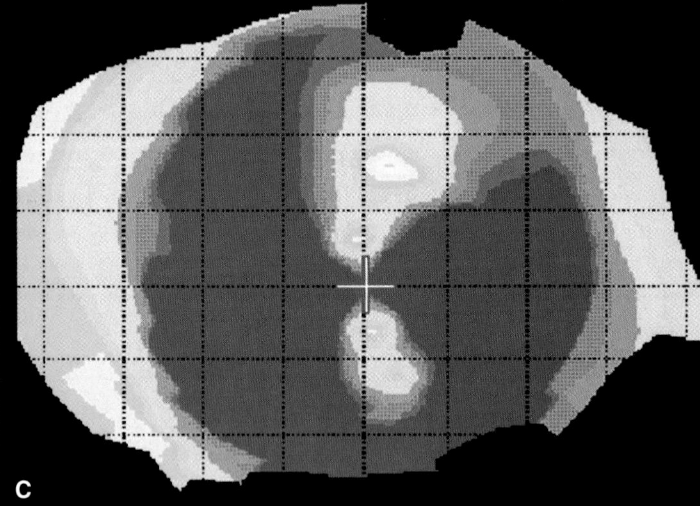

FIGURE 9-13: Ferrara ring for RK and AK. Post-RK and AK corneal topography shows the astigmatic overcorrection and the keratoectasia of the inferior radial and astigmatic transverse incisions (A) along with locaton of the RK and AK incisions (black lines). Ferrara rings were placed through the RK incisions (B). The topography difference map (C) shows the coupling effect: flattening on the temporal incision meridian and vertical steepening of the meridian peripendicular to the entry incision.

Case Report

'True' iatrogenic corneal ectasia was detected 6 years after uneventful LASIK for –9.75 sphere. Preoperative Orbscan (not shown) was normal and postoperative course was uneventful. The 160-head Hansatome flap thickness, measured with VHF ultrasound (Artemis 2), ranged from 149 to 122 microns. Keratoectasia is shown **(Figure 9-15)**. The patient underwent Ferrara ring surgery with one single 200 μm segment inserted through incision on the coma axis. Seventeen months later, UCVA was 20/40 and BSCVA is 20/20– with plano –1.25 × 85°.

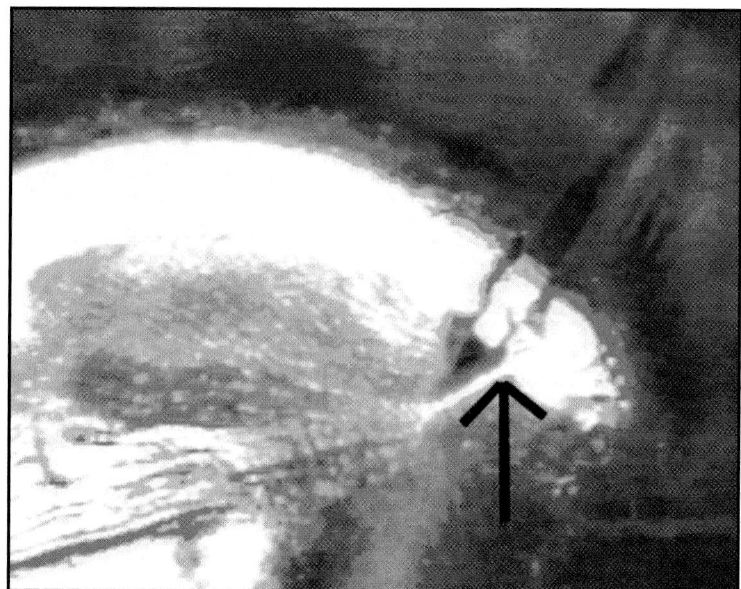

FIGURE 9-14: Intraoperative dehiscence and reopening of an old RK incision during Ferrara ring segment implantation.

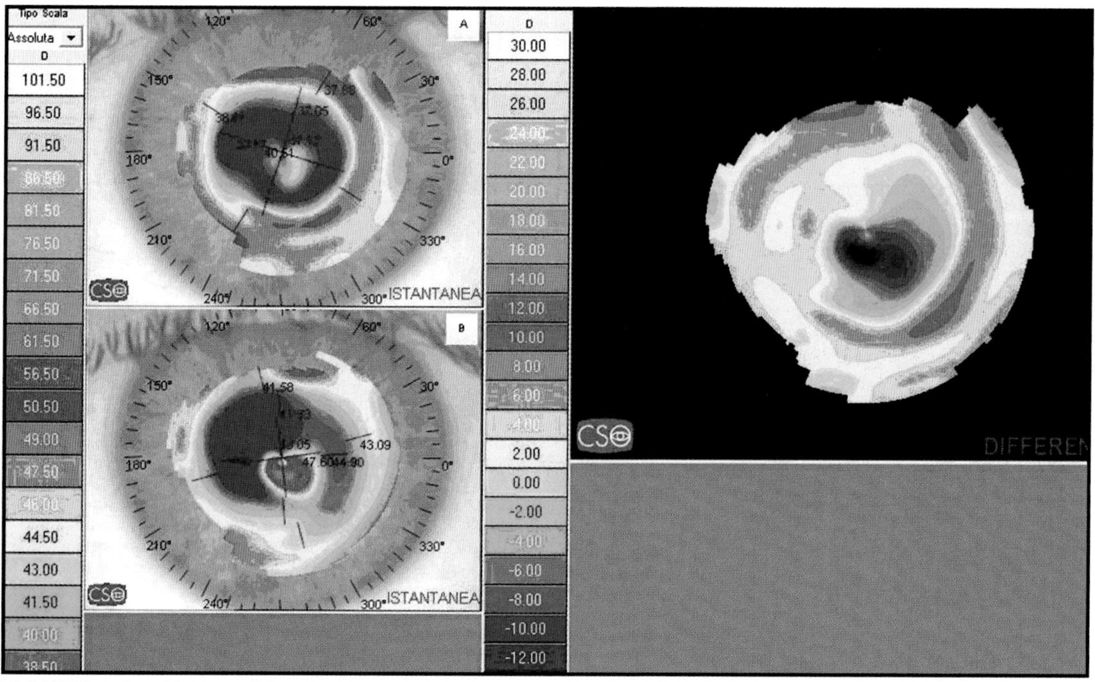

FIGURE 9-15: Ferrara Ring for iatrogenic keratoectasia. Inferior steepening is evident (lower left) and post-Ferrara ring flattening is shown (upper left). The difference map (right) shows significant flattening.

Case Report

A patient with FFKC underwent LASIK and development keratoectasia (**Figure 9-16**). A single 250 μm Ferrara ring segment was inferiorly implanted and yielded UCVA of 20/25 with a BSCVA of 20/40 with –1.75 – 3.00 × 48°.[29]

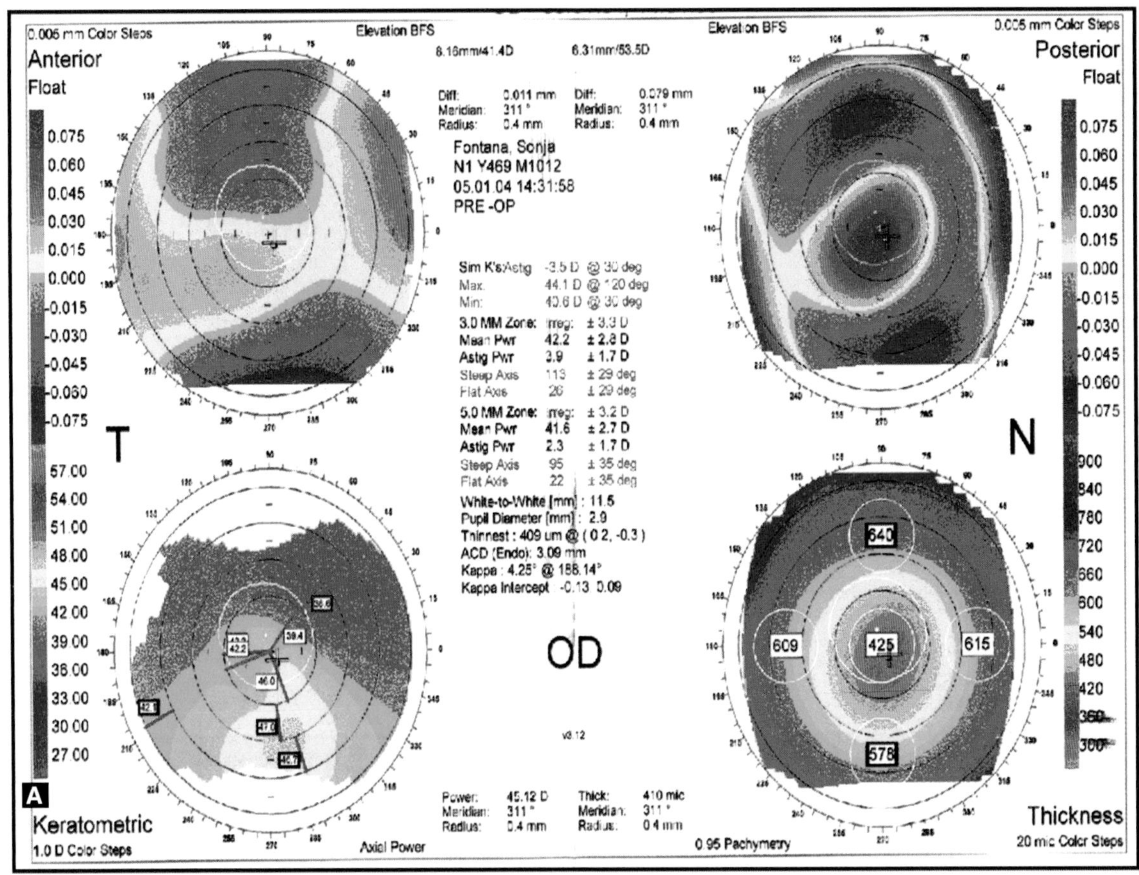

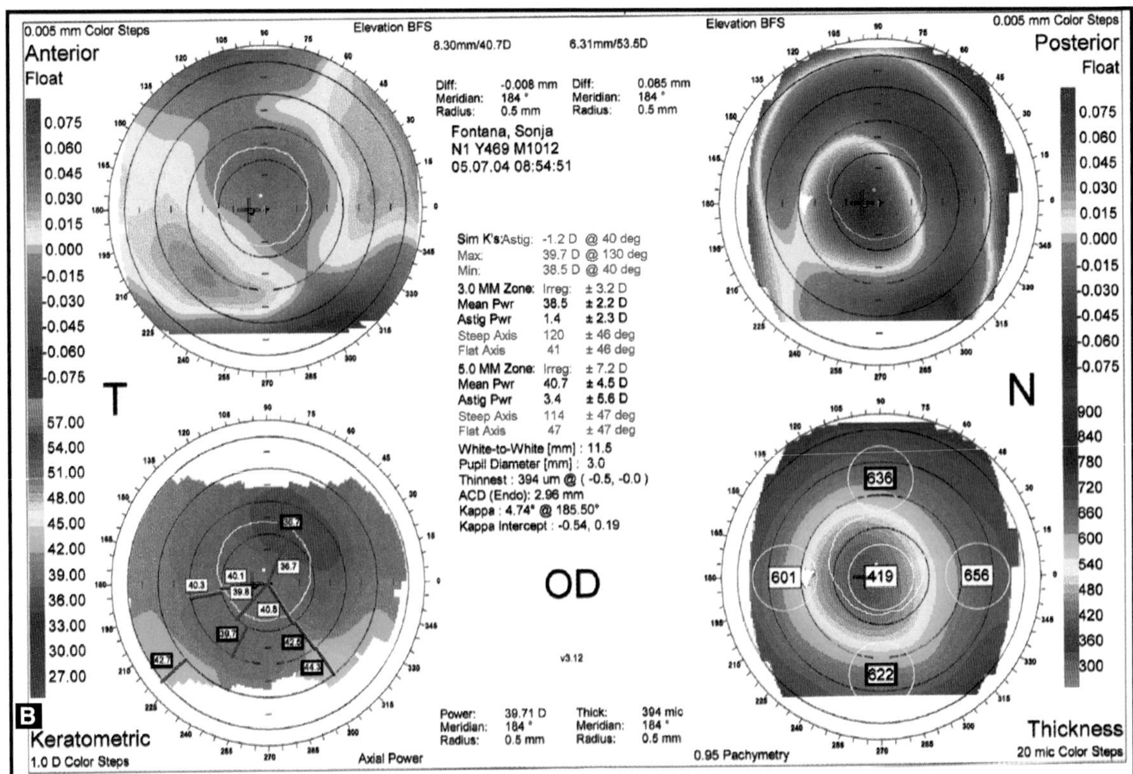

FIGURE 9-16: Ferrara ring after "LASIK on FFKC". Preoperative Orbscan has with inferior steepening (lower left) (A). Post-Ferrara ring Orbscan (B) shows flattening on topography (lower left).

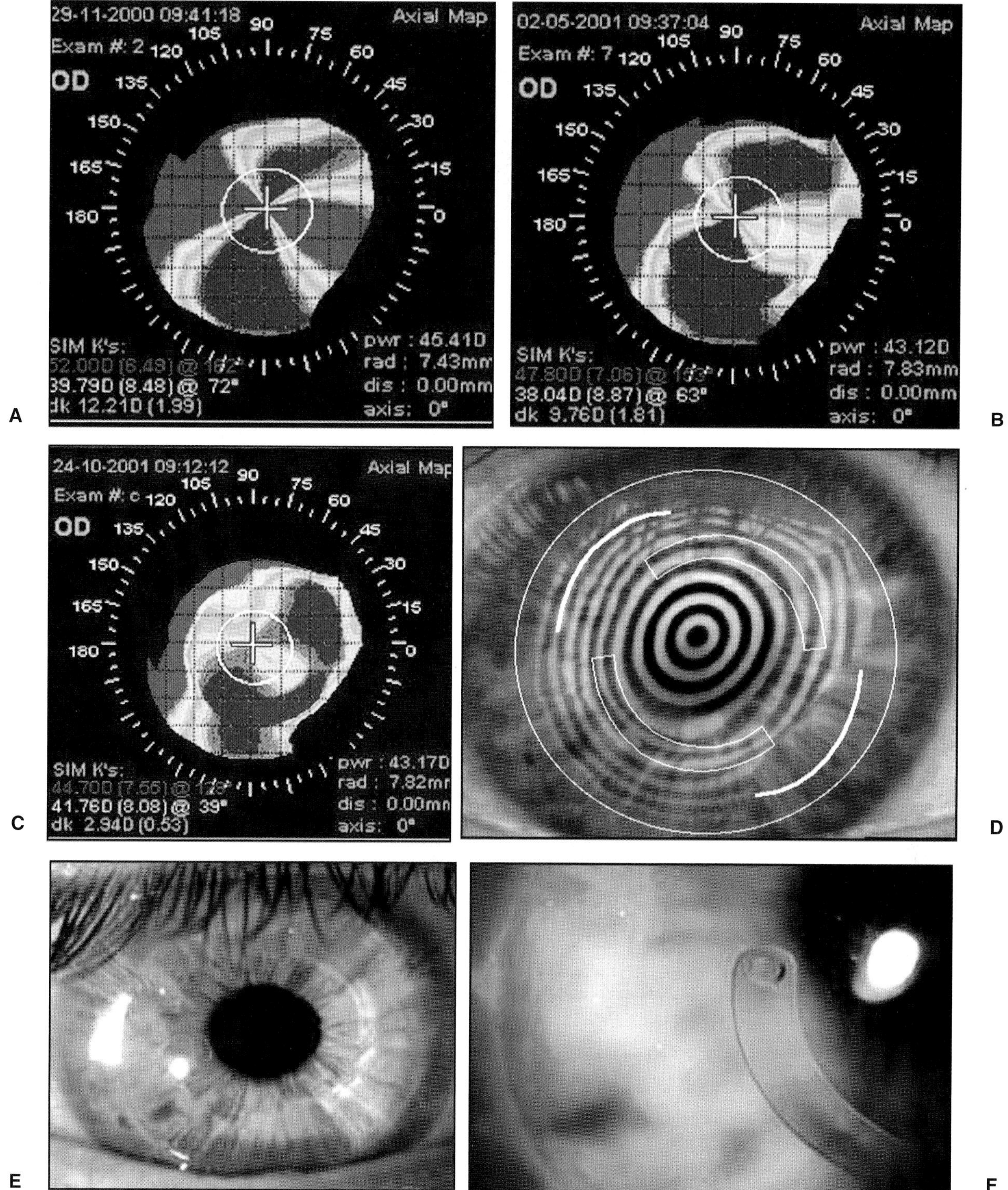

FIGURE 9-17: A case of Ferrara rings after PKP. Six months after PKP sutures were removed, a high amount of regular, post-PKP astigmatism was present (A). Three months after Ferrara ring surgery (B), corneal astigmatism was reduced, but relatively high. AK was performed outside the graft, on the steep axis. Four months after AK incisions, astigmatism was significantly reduced (C). Segments were implanted with incision on the steep axis and placed inside the graft as shown by white diagram outlines of segments. White curved lines show location of paired AK incisions made on the steep axis (D). Slit lamp photograph shows segments within the graft (E and F).

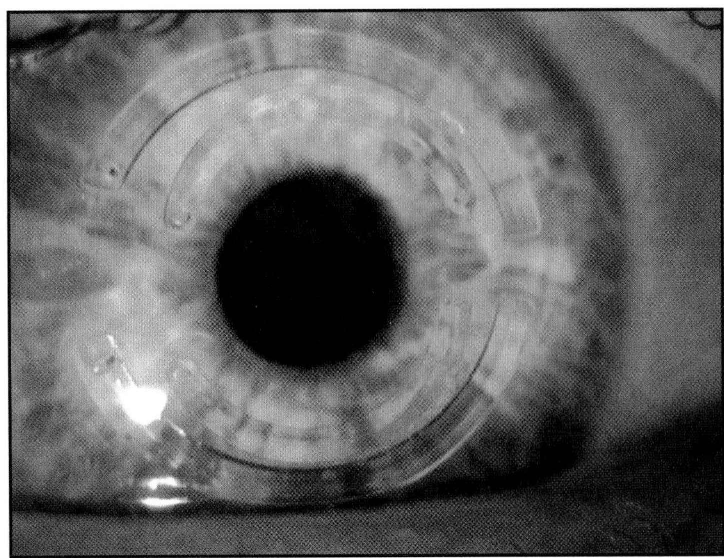

FIGURE 9-18: Slit lamp photograph showing two Intacs segments placed in the periphery and two Ferrara ring segments located within the borders of the Intacs.

Corneal Transplantation

We performed Ferrara ring surgery on 24 eyes that had prior corneal transplantation (23 penetrating keratoplasty, 1 lamellar keratoplasty) to treat their high irregular astigmatism. In 8 eyes, we combined AK with Ferrara rings **(Figure 9-17)**. In other 6 eyes, we performed topography-linked custom PRK for the residual lower and higher order aberrations with excellent outcomes.

Combined Intacs and Ferrara Rings

Case Report

This 'LASIK-on-keratoconus' eye received four ring segments, a pair of 450 μm Intacs and a pair of 250 μm Ferrara ring.[8] Five years after surgery, the patient maintained UCVA of 20/80 and a BSCVA of 20/50 **(Figure 9-18)**.

Conclusion

We have gained considerable knowledge of the long-term outcomes in eyes with keratoconus whether left to their natural course or surgically influenced by intrastromal synthetic implants. . We believe that this procedure will move from a niche procedure to one that is routinely performed as we gain greater understanding of corneal physiopathology and biomechanics, in pharmacological control of inflammation.

References

1. Ferrara de Cunha P. Tecnica cirurgica para correcao de myopia com implante de anel corneano intraestromal. II Congresso Internacional da Sociedade Brasileira de Cirurgia Refractiva, Sao Paulo, 1994.
2. Ferrara de Cunha P. Intrastromal ring in myopia. Revista Brasileira de Oftalmologia 1995;54(8):19-30.
3. Lovisolo CF, Fleming JF, Pesando PM. Intrastromal corneal ring segments. Fabiano Editore Canelli Italy 2002.
4. Barraquer JI. Modification of refraction by means of intracorneal inclusion. Int Ophth Clin 1966; 6:53.
5. Kwitko S, Severo NS. Ferrara intracorneal ring segments for keratoconus. J Cataract Refract Surg 2004;30(4):812-20.

6. Siganos D, Ferrara P, Chatzinikolas K., et al. Ferrara intrastromal corneal rings for the correction of keratoconus. J Cataract Refract Surg. 2002;28(11):1947-51.
7. Shabayek MH, Alio JL. Intrastromal corneal ring segment implantation by femtosecond laser for keratoconus correction. Ophthalmology, 2007.
8. Lovisolo CF, Fleming JF. Intracorneal ring segments for iatrogenic keratectasia after laser in situ keratomileusis or photorefractive keratectomy. J Refract Surg 2002;18:535-41.
9. Akaishi L, Tzelikis PF, Raber IM. Ferrara intracorneal ring implantation and cataract surgery for the correction of pellucid marginal corneal degeneration. J Cataract Refract Surg 2004;30:2427-30.
10. Reinstein DZ, Srivannaboon S, Holland SP. Epithelial and stromal changes induced by intrastromal corneal ring segments examined by three-dimensional very high-frequency digital ultrasound. J Refract Surg 2001;17:310-8.
11. Colin J, Simonpoli S. Keratoconus: current surgical options. J Fr Ophtalmol 2005;28:205-17.
12. Miranda D, Sartori M, Francesconi C, et al. Ferrara intrastromal corneal ring segments for severe keratoconus. J Refract Surg 2003;19:645-53.
13. Chalita MR, Krueger RR. Wavefront aberrations associated with the Ferrara intrastromal corneal ring in a keratoconic eye. J Refract Surg 2004;20:823-30.
14. Ertan A, Bahadir M. Intrastromal ring segment insertion using a femtosecond laser to correct pellucid marginal corneal degeneration. J Cataract Refract Surg 2006;32:1710-6.
15. Bisantis C. Intrastromal perioptic implants for the correction of high myopia. Invest Ophthalm Vis Sci 1997; 38:s538.
16. Amsler M. Keratocone classique et keratocone fruste. Arguments Unitaires Ophthalmologica 1946;111:96-101.
17. Alio JL, Artola A, Hassanein A, et al. One or 2 Intacs segments for the correction of keratoconus. J Cataract Refract Surg 2005;31:943-53.
18. Sharma M, Boxer Wachler BS. Comparison of single-segment and double-segment Intacs for keratoconus and post-LASIK ectasia. Am J Ophthalmol 2006;141:891-5.
19. Andreassen TT, Simonsen AH, Oxlund H. Biomechanical properties of keratoconus and normal corneas. Exp Eye Res Oct 1980; 31:435-41
20. Avitabile T, Marano F, Uva MG, et al. Evaluation of central and peripheral corneal thickness with ultrasound biomicroscopy in normal and keratoconic eyes. Cornea 1997; 16:639-44.
21. Cunha PFA, Alves EAF, Silva FBD, Cunha GHA. Study of the ocular changes after stromal Ferrara ring implantation in patients with keratoconus. [Estudo das modificaçöes oculares induzidas pelo implante estromal do anel de Ferrara em portadores de ceratocone]. Arq Bras Oftalmol 2003;66:417-22.
22. Rodrigues MM, Mc Carey BE, Waring GO II. Lipid deposits posterior to impermeable intracorneal lenses in Rhesus monkeys: clinical, histochemical, and ultrastructural studies. Refract Corneal Surg 1990;6:32-37.
23. Ambrosio JrR, Klyce SD, Smolek MK, et al. Recognizing pellucid marginal degeneration: preoperative clues that make the diagnosis. Review Refract Surg 2001 Nov;39-41.
24. Fleming JF, Lovisolo CF. Intrastromal corneal ring segments in a patient with previous laser in situ keratomileusis. J Refract Surg 2000;16:365-7.
25. Lovisolo CF, Calossi A, Fleming JF. Corneal bioptics. Improving success and managing complications of refractive surgery. In Lovisolo CF, Fleming JF, Pesando PM (Eds): Intrastromal Corneal Ring Segments Fabiano (Canelli) Chapter 7, 2002;171-204.
26. Rashid ER, Waring GO 3rd. Complications of radial and transverse keratotomy. Surv Ophthalmol 1989;34:73-10.
27. Bilgihan K, Ozdek SC, Konuk O, et al. Results of phothorefractive keratectomy in keratoconus. J Refract Corneal Surg 1994; 10:368-72.
28. Bowman CB, Thompson KP, Stulting RD. Refractive keratotomy in keratoconus suspects. J Refract Surg 1995; 11:202-6.
29. Lovisolo CF. La tomografia altitudinale nella cheratectasia post-laser ad eccimeri e nel trattamento con segmenti corneali intrastromali Ferrara Ring in: Mularoni A., Tassinari G. La topografia altitudinale. Fabiano Ed. Canelli 2005;402-31.

***Brian S Boxer Wachler,* MD, *Shawn Jalali,* MD**

10 Conductive Keratoplasty

Introduction

Using heat to alter the corneal curvature was first introduced by Gayat[1] in 1876 however, the new era of thermal keratoplasty first began in 1984 when Svyatoslav Fyodorov[2,3] inserted a hot probe (nickel-chromium probe) in the peripheral cornea to induce shrinkage. Modern conductive keratoplasty (CK) was later developed by Mendez[4] for correction of hyperopia. His results were published in 1997. CK is a surgical technique aimed to alter the corneal curvature. CK uses a low-energy, radiofrequency (350 kHz) current to heat the peripheral cornea. This results in shrinkage of the peripheral stromal collagen, and therefore, flattening the peripheral cornea, and steepening of the central cornea.[5-10]

In 2002, CK using the Viewpoint system (Refractec, Inc, Irvine, Ca) received Food and Drug Administration approval for temporary treatment of mild to moderate hyperopia (+0.75 to +3.0 D) with astigmatism of –0.75 D or less. In 2004, CK was FDA approved for treatment of presbyopia in the non-dominant eye of presbyopic patients with a target of –1.0 to –2.0 D.

CK is painless and is performed with a hand-held probe at the end of which is a disposable stainless steel tip **(Figure 10-1)** that penetrates about 450 microns into the corneal stroma. The eyelid speculum is attached to the probe to allow for the electrical return path. In CK, a controlled release of radiofrequency energy is delivered intrastromally via a probe tip. Impedance of the corneal tissue results in local heat contraction of tissue that induces the shape change. Thermal profile is homogeneous to approximately 80% of the depth of the cornea. The CK footprint has an average width of 405 microns and an average depth of 509 microns. Its major advantage is the greater stability of the refractive effect compared to other forms of thermal keratoplasty. CK allows the surgeon to customize the astigmatism correction for each patient.

It is a novel concept to apply selective CK spots to the cornea for keratoconus in order to reduce astigmatism.[11] This chapter will discuss CK for astigmatism in keratoconus. It is important to note that to reduce likelihood of complete regression, CK should be performed with C3-R® on the same day or on a cornea previously treated with C3-R®. Using CK in a cornea without C3-R® has a high rate of regression of the astigmatism effect.

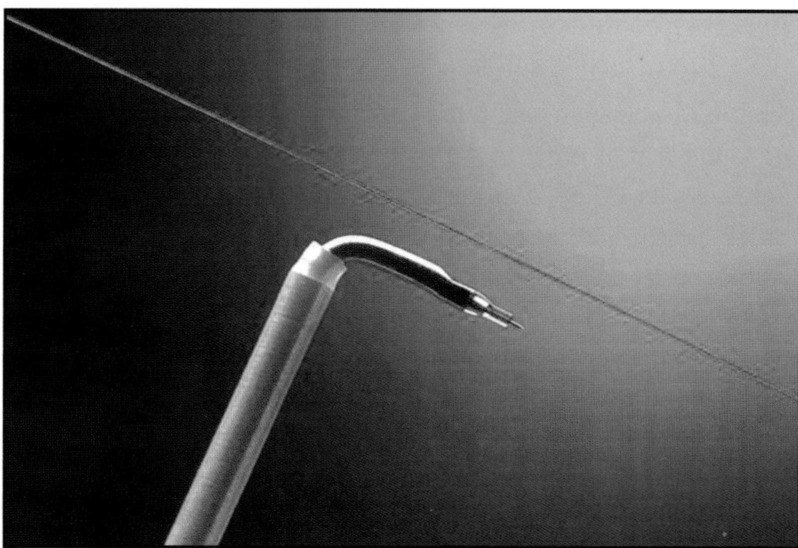

FIGURE 10-1: The disposable CK tip.

Surgical Technique

CK for Hyperopia

After topical anesthetics are applied and the CK speculum is inserted, the surgeon first marks the cornea in a set circular pattern for either 8 or 16 spots according to the surgical plan and nomogram. Using Light Touch technique, the tip is placed into the stroma and released so there is a minimal dimple **(Figure 10-2)**. The footswitch is depressed and the CK unit delivers a set power for 0.6 seconds. Additional spots are applied to complete a circular pattern. The number and location of spots determines the amount of refractive changes; an increasing number of spots and rings are used for higher amount of hyperopia. The CK procedure typically takes less than 5 minutes.

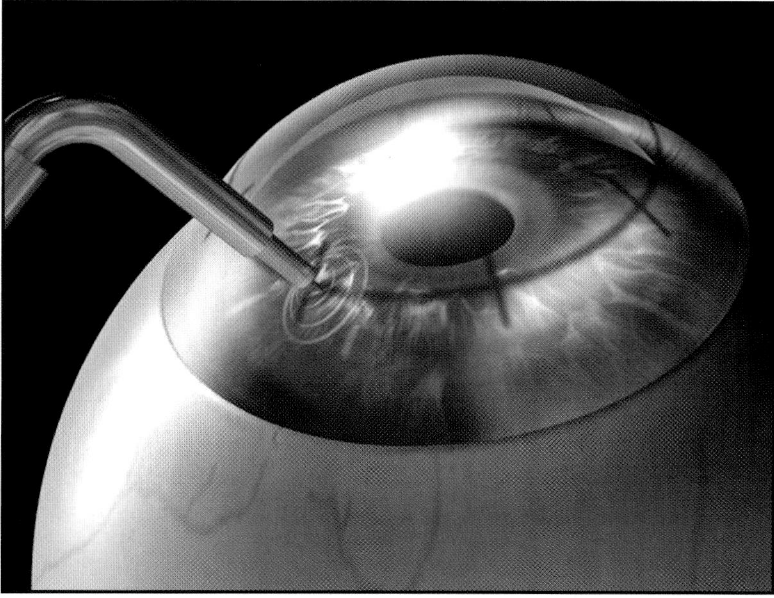

FIGURE 10-2: The CK probe placed in the cornea and the concentric waves of radiofrequency energy during the treatment.

CK for Astigmatism in Keratoconus

We use CK to reduce moderate to high astigmatism (4 D to 15 D). We frequently use CK in our keratoconus and keratoectasia patients in combination with Intacs or after Intacs if they were previously placed. It is worth repeating that we have found that in order to achieve a long-lasting effect, CK should be performed on a cornea that has been treated with C3-R®. We found that CK for astigmatism without C3-R® results in near complete regression of the benefit initially achieved. We use CK in patients who:

1. Had C3-R® in the past, or
2. Have C3-R® immediately after CK on the same day.

Presumably, the collagen crosslinking makes the cornea resistant to regression that would otherwise occur without C3-R® treatment. Therefore, we do not recommend using CK for astigmatism for keratoconus without prior crosslinking therapy or without crosslinking therapy on the same day as CK.

CK spots cause selective corneal steepening via collagen contraction. Therefore, CK spots are placed in the flat axis of the manifest refraction to help "pull" against the astigmatism 90 degrees away from it. This can reduce astigmatism. Often the topography flat axis will be close to manifest refraction axis. If there is a discrepancy between the axes, we treat based on the manifest refraction axis.

1. Depending on the degree of astigmatism, one or two CK spots are initially applied in the flat axis at a 7 mm optical zone (OZ).
2. Walk the patient out of the procedure room and obtain corneal topography to assess the induced astigmatism effect. For most cases, our target is 2 to 3 D of overcorrection of topography astigmatism as there will be some expected regression in the first 2 to 3 weeks. Topography astigmatism is typically different than refractive astigmatism. We will subtract refractive astigmatism from that of topography and add overcorrection amount desired.
3. If our desired topographic astigmatism overcorrection is not achieved, we return to the procedure room. We apply additional 1 to 2 spots at either a 6 mm optical zone (if we desire greater effect than initial spots at 7 mm OZ) or apply 1 to 2 spots at 8 mm OZ (if we desire less effect than initially achieved at 7 mm OZ).
4. We bring the patient out for repeat topography and reassess change. Additional CK spots may be applied again in the sequence described above until we are content with our final topography end point.
5. On occasion, the last application of CK spots will yield a larger, unexpected overcorrection of astigmatism than desired. Our experience is that with time postoperatively, the regression will be greater and it would be rare for a patient to remain overcorrected after 3 months. We have also used 2 to 4 weeks of topical steroids drops to facilitate regression of overcorrection. For this reason, it is prudent to apply CK spots in a conservative fashion.
6. After end-point is reached, we use a dry surgical sponge to wipe off the opacified epithelium overlying the CK spots **(Figure 10-3)**. This facilitates comfort postoperatively as the eyelid is not moving over roughened epithelium.

Nuance to Note

1. If patient's UCVA is relatively good (e.g. 20/40), but refraction shows more astigmatism than expected for given level of UCVA, it is prudent to be cautious and conservative with amount of CK applied. Significant overcorrection of astigmatism and worse UCVA postoperatively could occur initially. Even with expected regression, the patient may remain with significantly overcorrected astigmatism and worse final UCVA. After

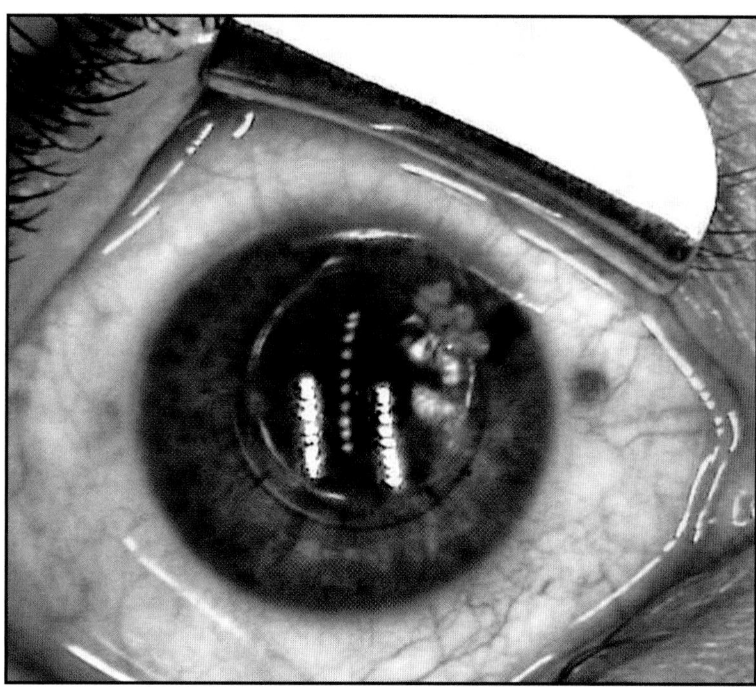

FIGURE 10-3: Three CK spots at 7 mm and 3 additional spots at 8 mm. Note the opacified epithelium overlying the CK spots which will then be removed with a dry surgical sponge to maximize patient comfort postoperatively.

1 week assessment, if there is still high induced astigmatism and UCVA is reduced from pre-CK, use of steroid eyedrops tapering down over 2 to 4 weeks to facilitate regression is an option.

2. If treating keratectasia after LASIK or PRK, CK can yield a greater than expected effect. Having a prior flap with laser ablation or ablation makes the cornea biomechanically more sensitive to CK. Therefore, proceed very conservatively with CK spots to avoid significant overcorrection surprises.

Postoperatively, fourth generation fluoroquinolone antibiotic (e.g. Vigamox) is used TID for 1 week. We do not routinely use steroids postoperatively as they may facilitate regression. Postoperative visits are typically 1 day, 3 months, and 1 year, which include UCVA, manifest refraction, BCVA, and corneal topography. New glasses or contact lenses can be dispensed as soon as 2 weeks, but the cornea and hence refraction will be more stable if patient can wait 1 month. There may be further changes as the cornea heals after 1 month which may necessitate a prescription update.

If we are planning Intacs, CK, and C3-R® for a patient on the same day, our sequence is first the perform Intacs. For beginner surgeons, we recommend obtaining topography to assess change. CK is applied at 7 mm OZ and titrated as described above. Then walk the patient to another room where we perform C3-R®. The patient is instructed to rest as home with eyes closed for the remainder of the day and the patient will be seen the following day for first postoperative examination.

Clinical Case Reports

Case 1

A 53-year-old male keratoconus patient with high myopia and irregular astigmatism.
Preoperative manifest refraction (MRx) in right eye was –8.75 –14.75 × 075 producing 20/50. Uncorrected visual acuity (UCVA) was count fingers. Preoperative topography showed 13.35 D of astigmatism at axis 071 **(Figure 10-4)**.

Treatment

1. Single segment inferior Intacs (0.35 mm); care is taken when marking center of cornea with Sinskey hook to not indent epithelium as indentation may affect accuracy of subsequent topography for CK titration.
2. CK at 075 degrees axis to reduce the astigmatism.
   Three CK spots were placed at 8 mm OZ in 075 degrees axis. The patient was taken out of room for repeat topography which showed astigmatism reduced to only 11.34 D **(Figure 10-5)**. As this cornea was resistant to CK, 3 additional superior spots were added at 7 mm OZ which reduced astigmatism to 3.09 D **(Figure 10-6)**. 3 additional CK spots were applied at 9 mm OZ, which has less effect as it is a larger OZ to give a small overcorrection of the astigmatism.
3. C3-R® was then used to stabilize CK effect.
4. On the first postoperative day, there is dramatic improvement in astigmatism **(Figure 10-7)**.
5. 3-month results **(Figure 10-8)**.
   MRx was: –6.75 –5.75 × 105 which produced 20/30.

Case 2

A 37-year-old male keratoconus patient with high irregular astigmatism. Preoperative MRx in the left eye was –0.25 –12.25 × 120 with 20/25. UCVA was count fingers. Preoperative topography showed 12.84 D of astigmatism at axis 120 **(Figure 10-9)**.

Treatment

1. Single segment inferior Intacs (0.35 mm) with incision in 030 degrees axis.
2. CK at 120 degrees to reduce the astigmatism.
   2 upper CK spots were placed at 7 mm OZ in 120 degrees axis. The patient was taken out of room for repeat topography which showed astigmatism reduced to 3.74 D, and no additional CK spots were needed. **(Figure 10-10)**.
3. C3-R® was then used to stabilize CK effect
4. At the 1 day postoperative visit, corneal topography showed only 3.44 D of astigmatism remaining **(Figure 10-11)**.

Case 3

A 22-year-old patient with keratoconus, high myopia, and irregular astigmatism
Preoperative MRx in the left eye was –7.50 –8.75 × 157 giving 20/40–1 and UCVA was 20/200. Preoperative topography showed 7.08 D of astigmatism at axis 168 **(Figure 10-12)**.

Treatment

1. Single segment temporal Intacs (0.35 mm) with incision in 067 degrees axis.
2. CK at 157 degrees axis to reduce the astigmatism
   2 upper CK spots were placed at 7 mm OZ in 157 degrees axis. The patient was taken out of room for repeat topography which showed astigmatism reduced to 1.72 D at axis 168 **(Figure 10-13)**.

Contd....

Contd....

3. C3-R® was then used to stabilize CK effect.
4. 1 day postoperative results **(Figure 10-14)**
5. 3-month postoperative result MRx: OS: –4.50 –2.50 × 120 yielding 20/40. UCVA was 20/100. Topography shows marked improvement in astigmatism **(Figure 10-15)**

Case 4

A 43-year-old female patient with keratoectasia in the left eye after LASIK. She later had multiple CK treatments between 2001 and 2004 with another surgeon with complete regression of effect as C3-R® was not performed. In 2005, single segment Intacs were placed inferiorly as ectasia was progressing. She was referred to us for evaluation and further treatment. **(Figure 10-16).**

Our testing showed MRx in the left eye was plano –5.00 × 85 with 20/20-1 and UCVA was 20/100.

Treatment

1. CK at 85 degrees axis to reduce astigmatism.
   2 superior CK spots were place at 7 mm OZ in 85 degrees axis. The patient was taken out of the operating room for repeat topography which showed astigmatism reduced to 2.93 D in 80 degrees, representing a flip in the axis from against-the-rule to with-the-rule **(Figure 10-17)**.
   One additional CK spot was added at the conservative 8 mm OZ **(Figure 10-18)**.
   Since the astigmatism axis was flipped, no more CK spots were applied. The patient was moved to another room where C3-R® was performed to stabilize the CK effects.
2. 1 day postoperative results
   UCVA was 20/40. Corneal topography showed reduced astigmatism of 1.62 D **(Figure 10-19)**.
3. 1 week postoperative results, MRx was +0.25 –0.75 × 180 yielding 20/25 and UCVA was 20/30. Topography was not available.

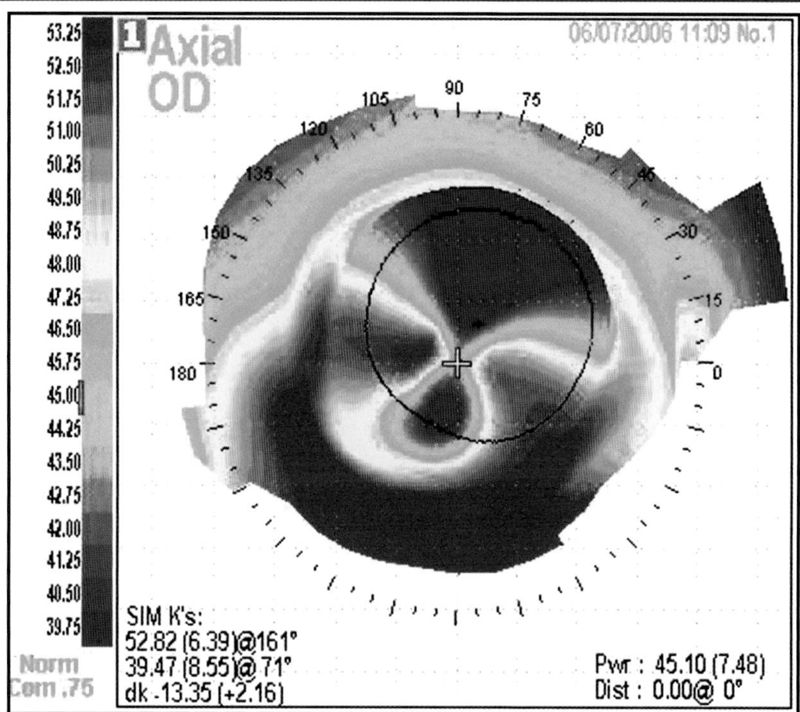

FIGURE 10-4: Preoperative corneal topography. Note the inferior cone and the high irregular astigmatism of 13.35 D.

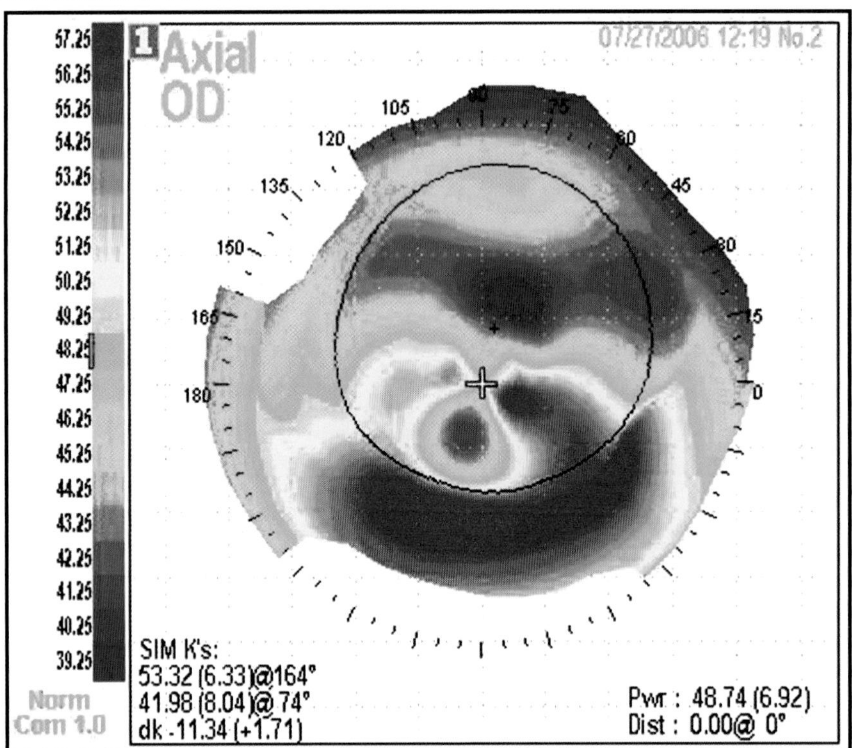

FIGURE 10-5: Corneal topography after superior 3 CK spots were applied at 8 mm OZ.

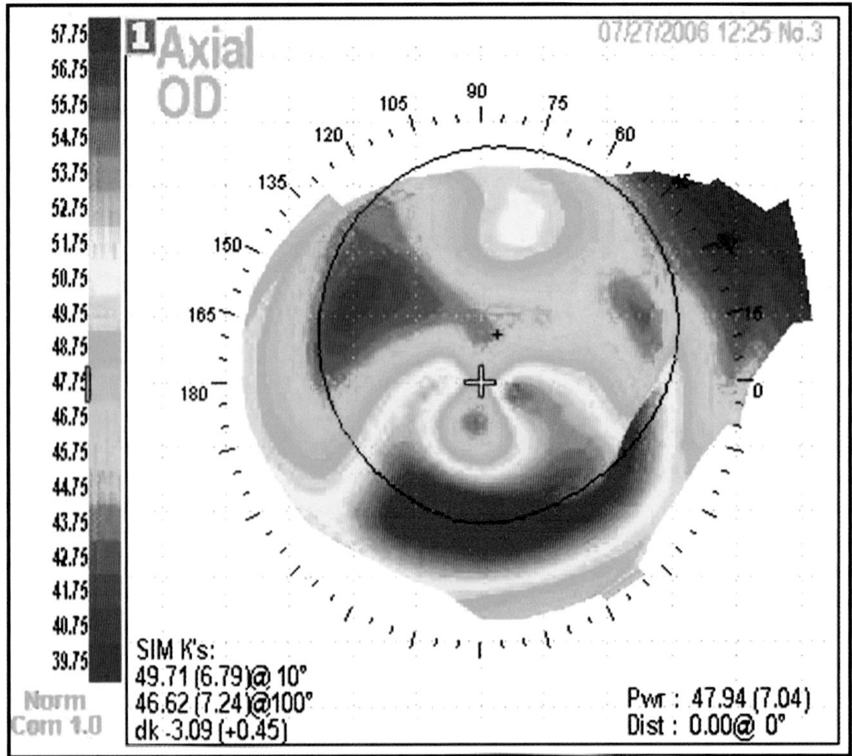

FIGURE 10-6: Corneal topography after 3 additional superior spots were applied at 7 mm OZ.

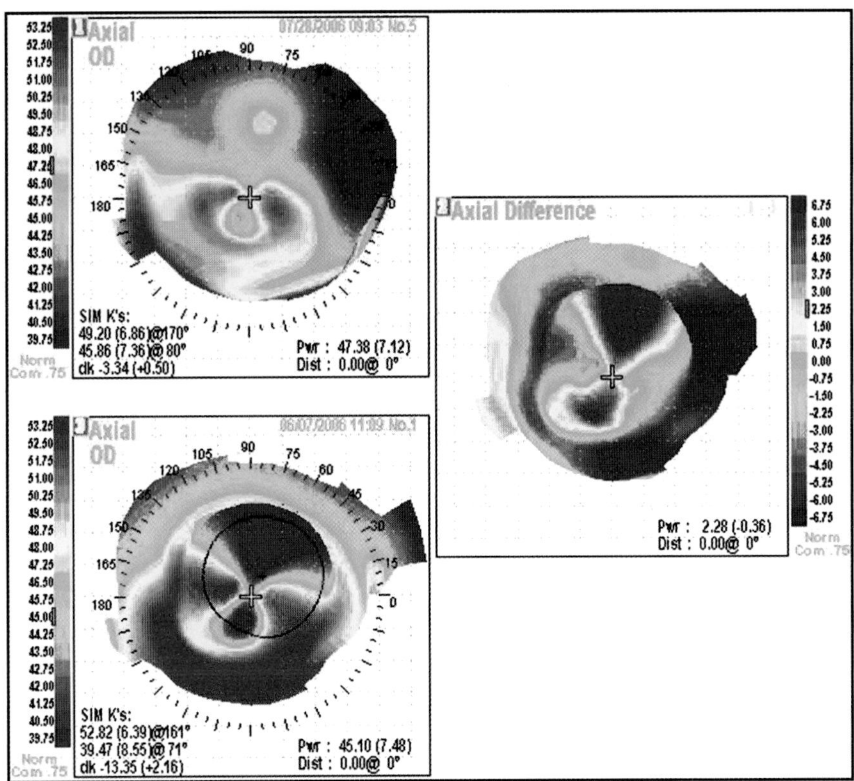

FIGURE 10-7: Preoperative corneal topography (lower left) and 1 day postoperative topography (upper left) with 10 D of astigmatism correction and difference map (right).

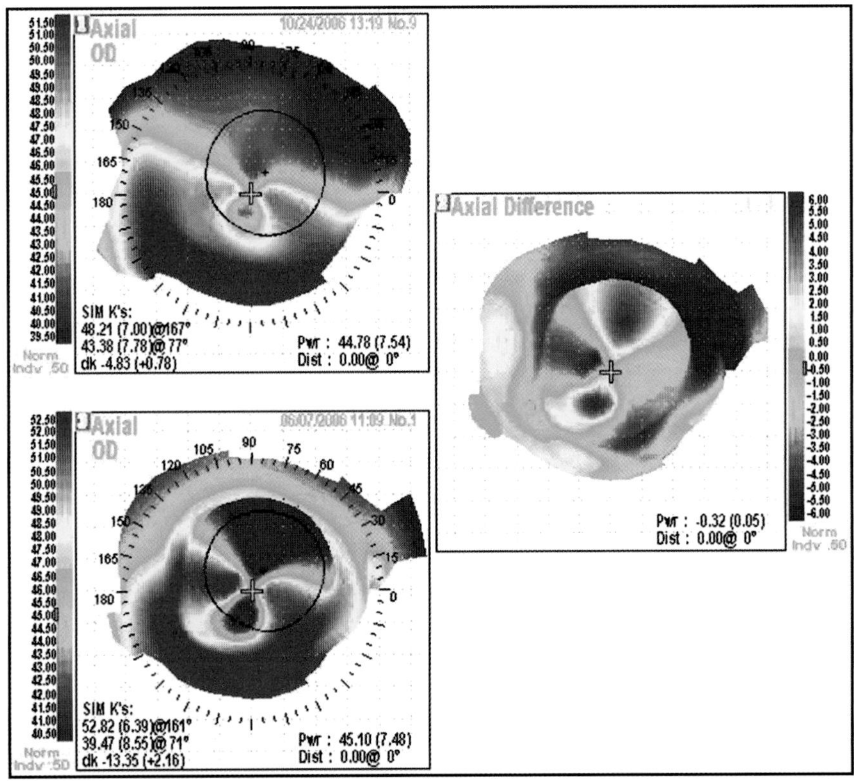

FIGURE 10-8: Preoperative corneal topography (lower left) and 3 month postoperative topography (upper left) with over 8 D of astigmatism correction and difference map (right).

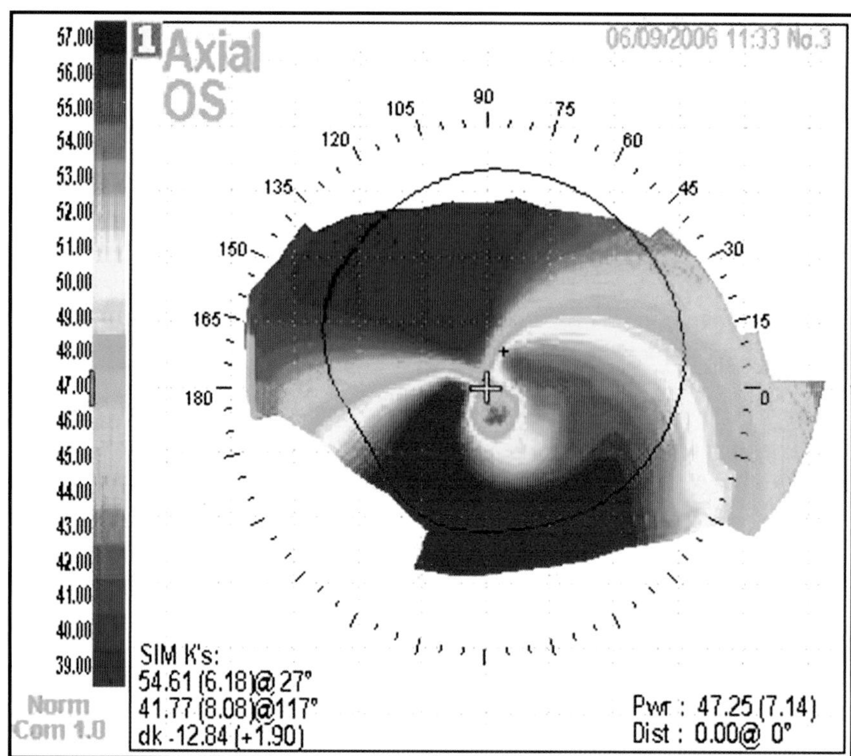

FIGURE 10-9: Preoperative corneal topography of a keratoconic eye. Note the inferior cone and the high irregular astigmatism of 12.85.

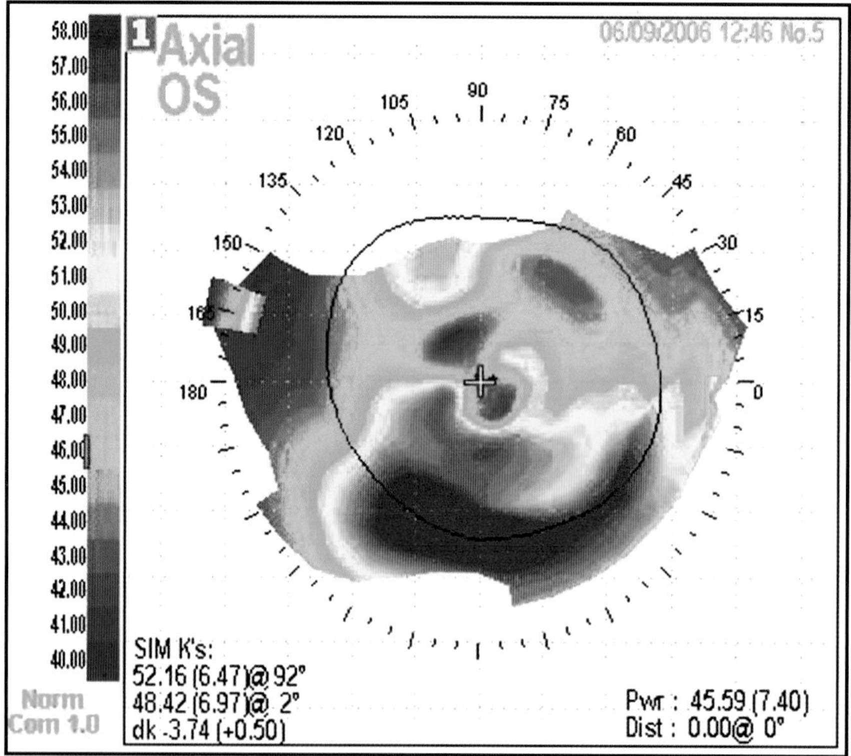

FIGURE 10-10: Corneal topography of the same patient after 2 CK spots were applied.

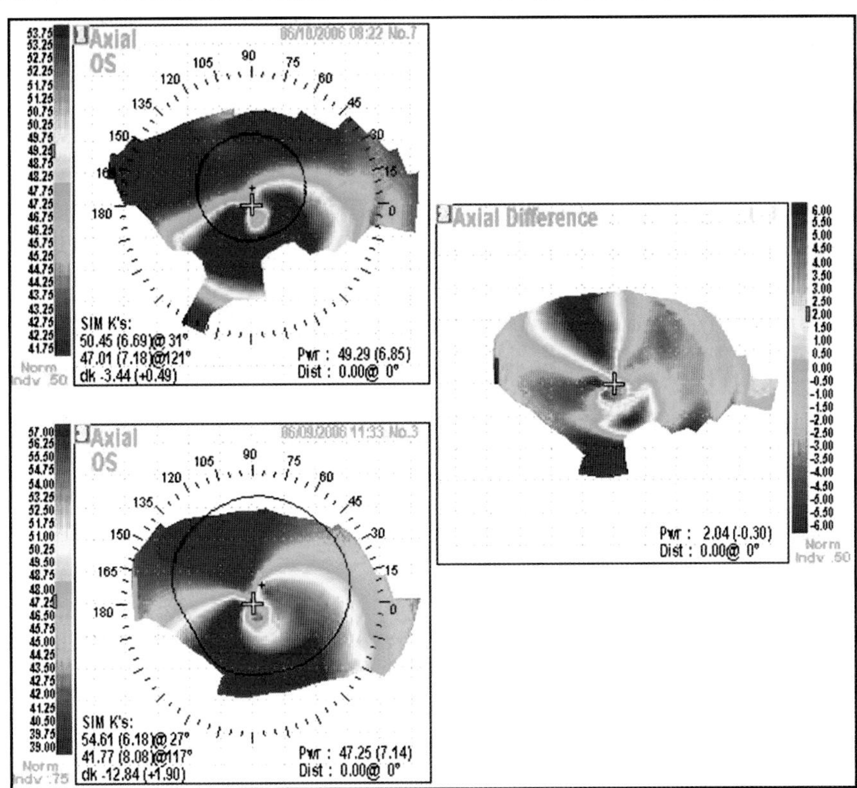

FIGURE 10-11: Preoperative corneal topography (lower left) and 1 day postoperative topography (upper left) with over 9.0 D of astigmatism correction and difference map (right).

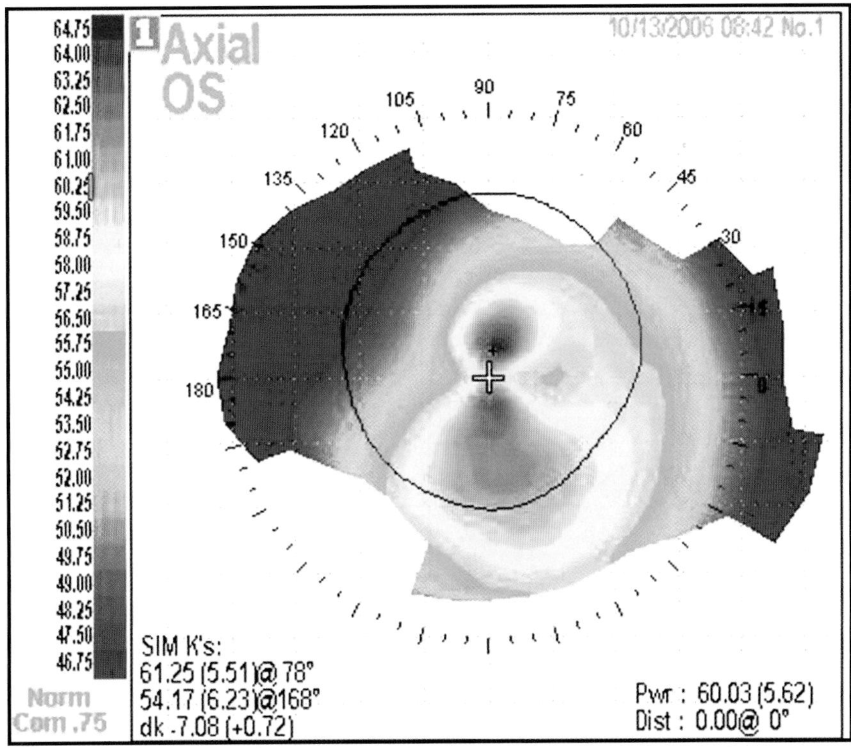

FIGURE 10-12: Preoperative corneal topography with the temporal cone and the high irregular astigmatism of 7.08 D.

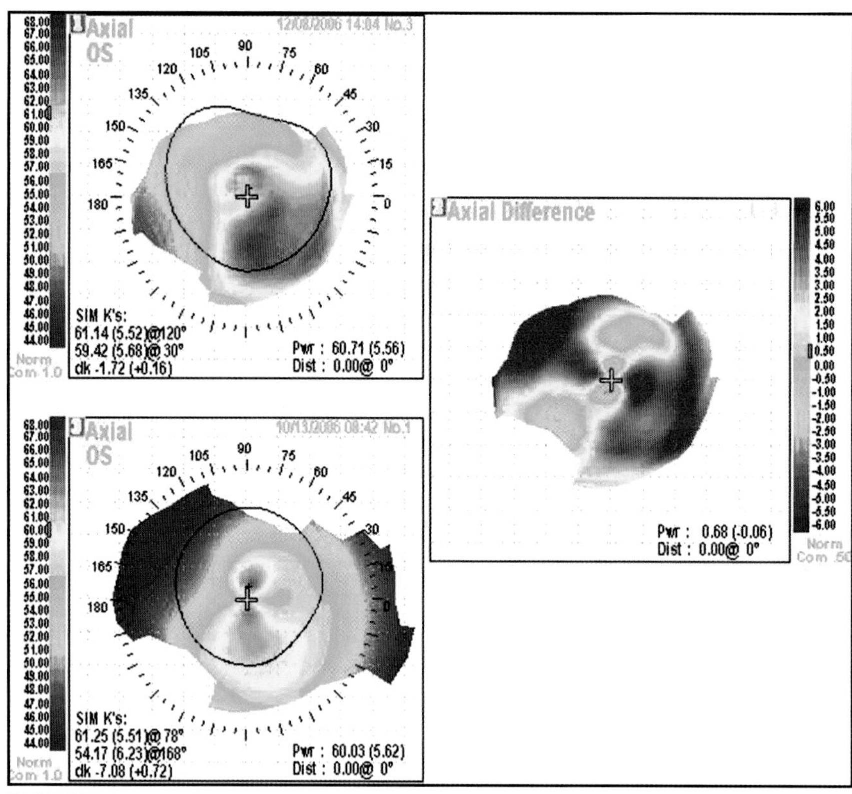

FIGURE 10-13: Preoperative corneal topography (lower left) and immediate topography on same day of surgery after 2 CK spots were applied with less than 2 D of astigmatism (upper left) and difference map (right).

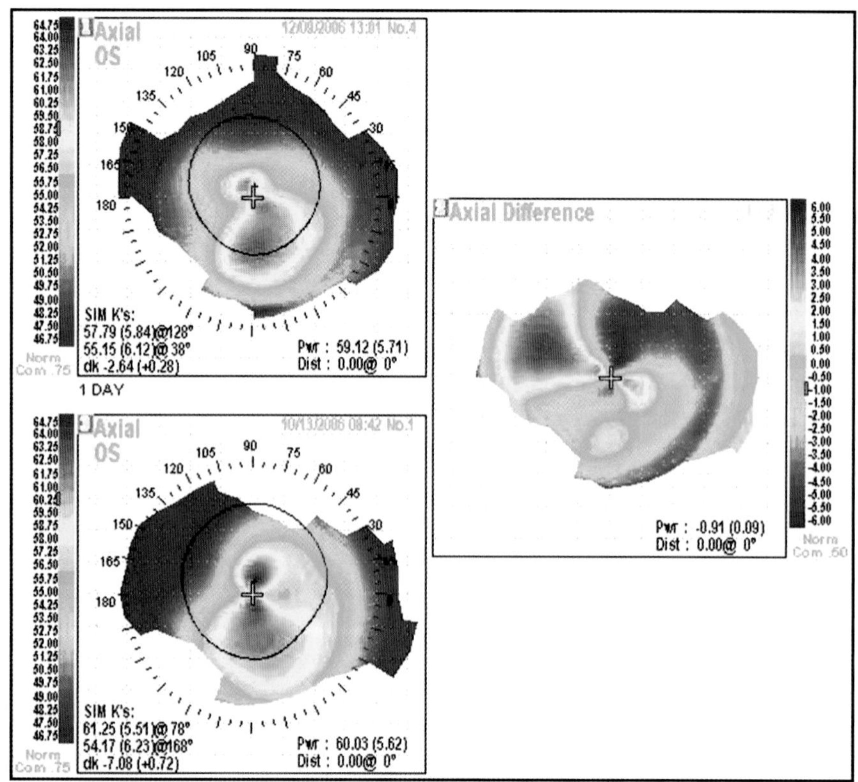

FIGURE 10-14: Preoperative corneal topography (lower left) and 1 day postoperative topography (upper left) and difference map (right).

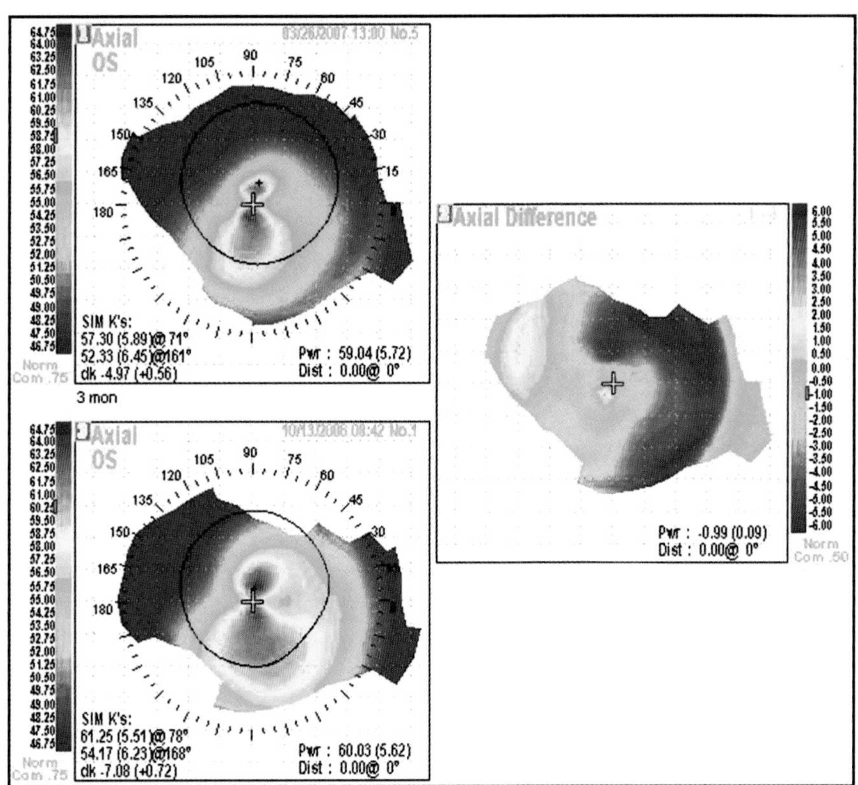

FIGURE 10-15: Preoperative corneal topography (lower left) and 3 months postoperative topography (upper left) and difference map (right). The 3 months topography shows slight regression from 1 day topography (Figure 10-14). MRx astigmatism was only 2.50 D.

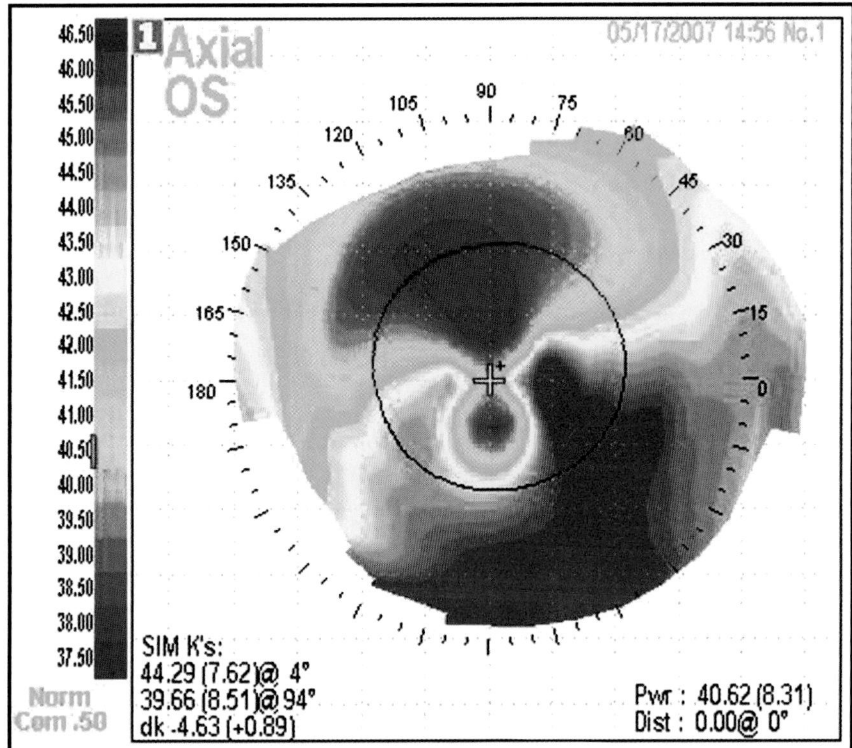

FIGURE 10-16: Preoperative corneal topography of a patient with keratoectasia after LASIK and high irregular astigmatism. Inferior Intacs (pink) was placed by another surgeon 2 years earlier.

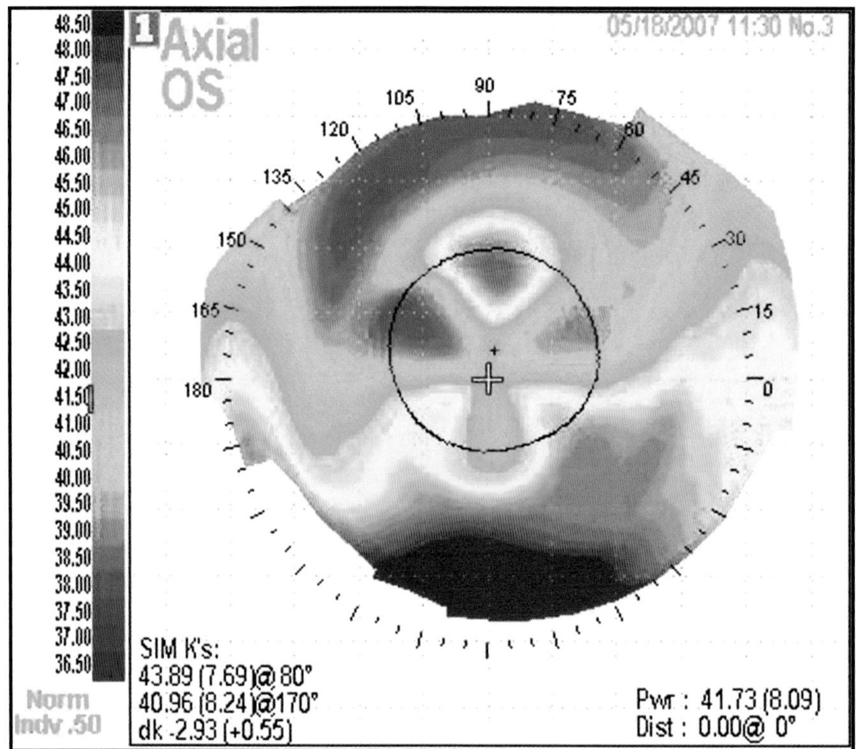

FIGURE 10-17: Corneal topography of the same patient after 2 CK spots were applied. Astigmatism is reduced. The decision was made to apply additional CK for more effect.

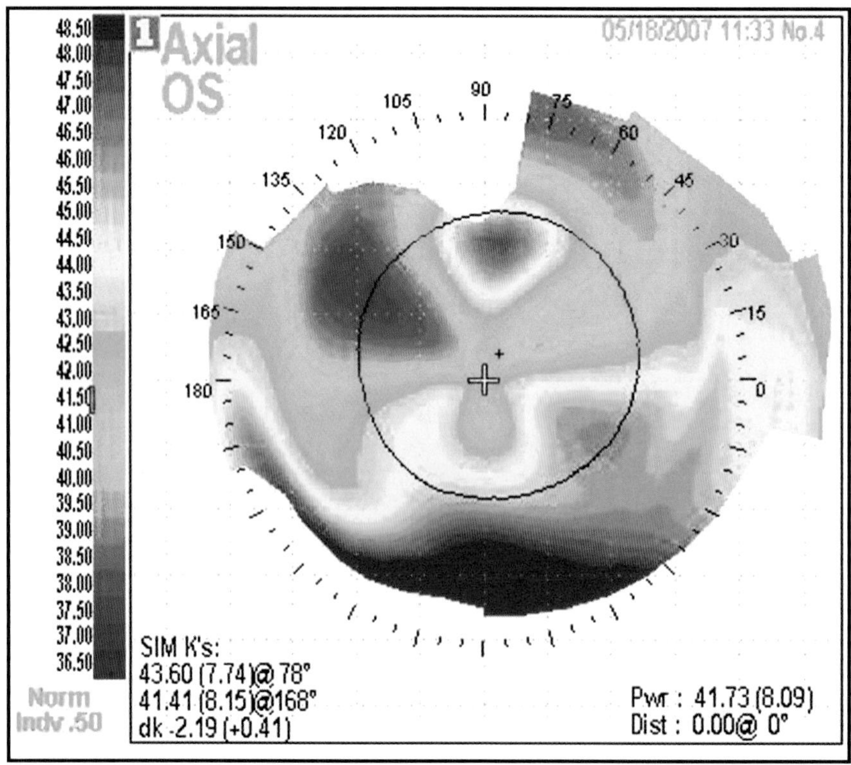

FIGURE 10-18: Shows the corneal topography after 1 additional CK spot was applied and astigmatism was further reduced to 2.19 D.

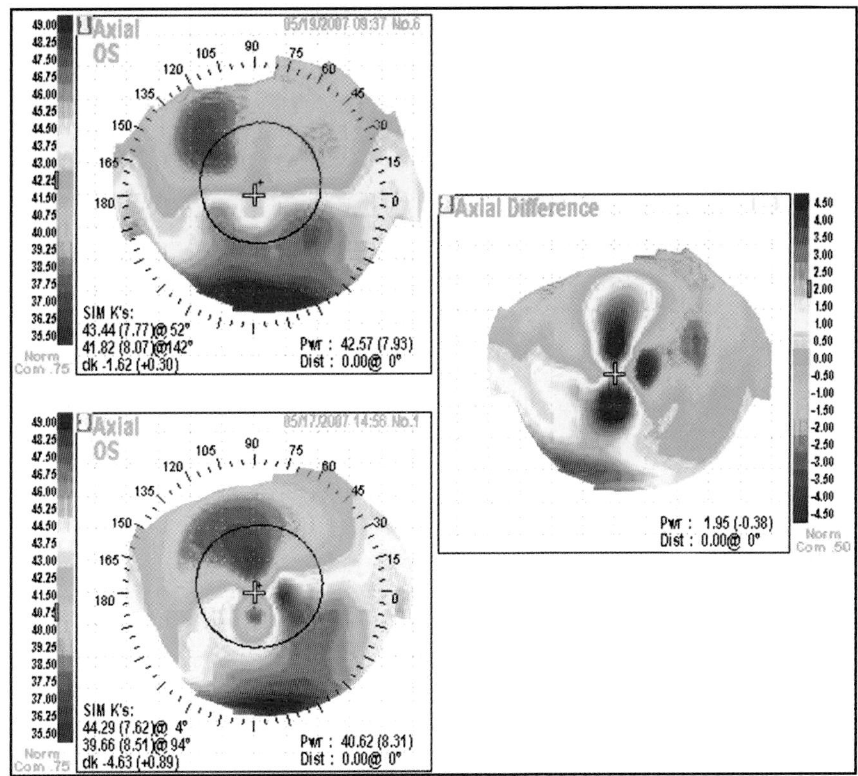

FIGURE 10-19: Preoperative corneal topography (lower left) and 1 day postoperative topography (upper left) and difference map (right) shows astigmatism effect. The 1 day topography shows astigmatism reduced to 1.62 D. MRx astigmatism was only 2.50 D.

Conclusion

CK provides an important tool for surgeons to manage astigmatism in patients with keratoconus and keratoectasia. CK can be combined with Intacs to enhance results achieved with Intacs alone in patients with high astigmatism. We describe our technique, however, each cornea can respond differently which makes using CK for keratoconus both science and art. It is prudent to combine CK with C3-R® to provide long-lasting benefits of CK for astigmatism.

References

1. Gayat J. Ulcerazione grave della cornea cagionata dai vapori della radice. Annali di ottalmologia 1876 ott. Volume 5. Fascicolo 4.
2. Fyodorov S, Danders DR. Radial thermokeratoplasty for correction of hyperopia. J of Ophthalmology 1981;88:755-60.
3. Caster AI. The Fyodorov technique of hyperopia correction by termal coagulation: a preliminary report. J Refract Surg 1988;4:105.
4. Mendez A. Conductive keratoplasty for the correcion of hyperopia. J Cataract Refract Surg 1997;23:480-7.
5. Naoumidi TL, Kounis GA, Astyrakakis NI, Tsatsaronis DN, Pallikaris IG. Two-year follow-up of conductive keratoplasty for the treatment of hyperopic astigmatism. J Cataract Refract Surg 2006;32:732-41.
6. Alió JL, Claramonte PJ, Cáliz A, Ramzy MI. Corneal modeling of keratoconus by conductive keratoplasty. J Cataract Refract Surg 2005;31:190-7.
7. Alió J, Claramonte P, Ramsey R. Conductive keratoplasty in the correction of residual hyperopia following LASIK. J Refract Surg 2005 Nov-Dec;21(6):698-704.

8. McDonald MB, Davidorf J, Maloney RK, et al. Conductive keratoplasty for the correction of low to moderate hyperopia; 1-year results on the first 54 eyes. Ophthalmology. 2002;109:637–49 discussion by CL Blanton, 649–650; correction, 1583.
9. McDonald MB, Hersh PS, Manche EE, et al. Conductive keratoplasty for the correction of low to moderate hyperopia: US clinical trial 1-year results on 355 eyes; the Conductive Keratoplasty United States Investigators Group. Ophthalmology 2002; 109:1978-89 discussion by DD Koch, 1989-1990.
10. Lin DY, Manche EE. Two-year results of conductive keratoplasty for the correction of low to moderate hyperopia. J Cataract Refract Surg 2003; 29:2339-50.
11. Sekundo W, Stevens JD. Surgical treatment of keratoconus at the turn of the 20th century: a historical overview. In Alió J, Belda JI (Edn): Treating Irregular Astigmatism and Keratoconus. Panama: Highlights of Ophthalmology International; 2004;235.

Brian S Boxer Wachler, *MD*

11 Lowering Intraocular Pressure for Keratoectasia

Introduction

Keratoectasia is a known iatrogenic complication following LASIK.[1-15] Chapter 2 discusses the findings and risk factors in detail. In some cases, the steepening associated with keratoectasia may be improved or even reversed by lowering intraocular pressure (IOP) with eyedrops. We have had success in such patients if two criteria are met:

1. If ectasia occurred within several months after LASIK was performed and
2. If ectasia was treated with IOP lowering drops within 1 to 2 months after diagnosis.

Our experience in using IOP lowering for ectasia that occurred several years after LASIK has met with limited or no success. We also have limited or no success if ectasia occurred within several months after LASIK, but IOP lowering was begun years later.

Below is a case that describes a success of using IOP lowering in a patient who developed ectasia shortly after LASIK and was promptly treated.[16]

Case Report

A 40-year-old Caucasian female presented in January 2003 to inquire about LASIK surgery. The patient was out of her soft contact lenses for 10 days prior to preoperative testing. Preoperative manifest refractions were –7.75 –0.75 × 020 in the right eye and –7.50 –1.50 × 165 in the left eye. Marco 3 D system (Marco Technologies, Jacksonville, FL) standard topographies were normal with regular, symmetrical astigmatism in both eyes. Corneal pachymetries (Pachette 2; DGH Technology, Inc; Exton, PA) were normal in both eyes (531 microns (μ) right, 548 μ left). IOPs (Applanation Tonometer; Tono-Pen XL; Medtronic; Jacksonville, FL) were high-normal at 22 mm Hg in each eye. We used a tonopen to measure IOP since it is not subject to the post-LASIK adjustments that applanation tonometry requires. Infrared-tested pupil size was 7.0 mm and 7.2 mm in right and left eye respectively (Pupilscan II, Keeler, Broomall, Pa).

LASIK was performed without complication in each eye with targets of –1.25 D residual myopia in the right eye and plano in the left eye. The Moria M2 microkeratome (Moria, Doylestown, PA) with

Contd....

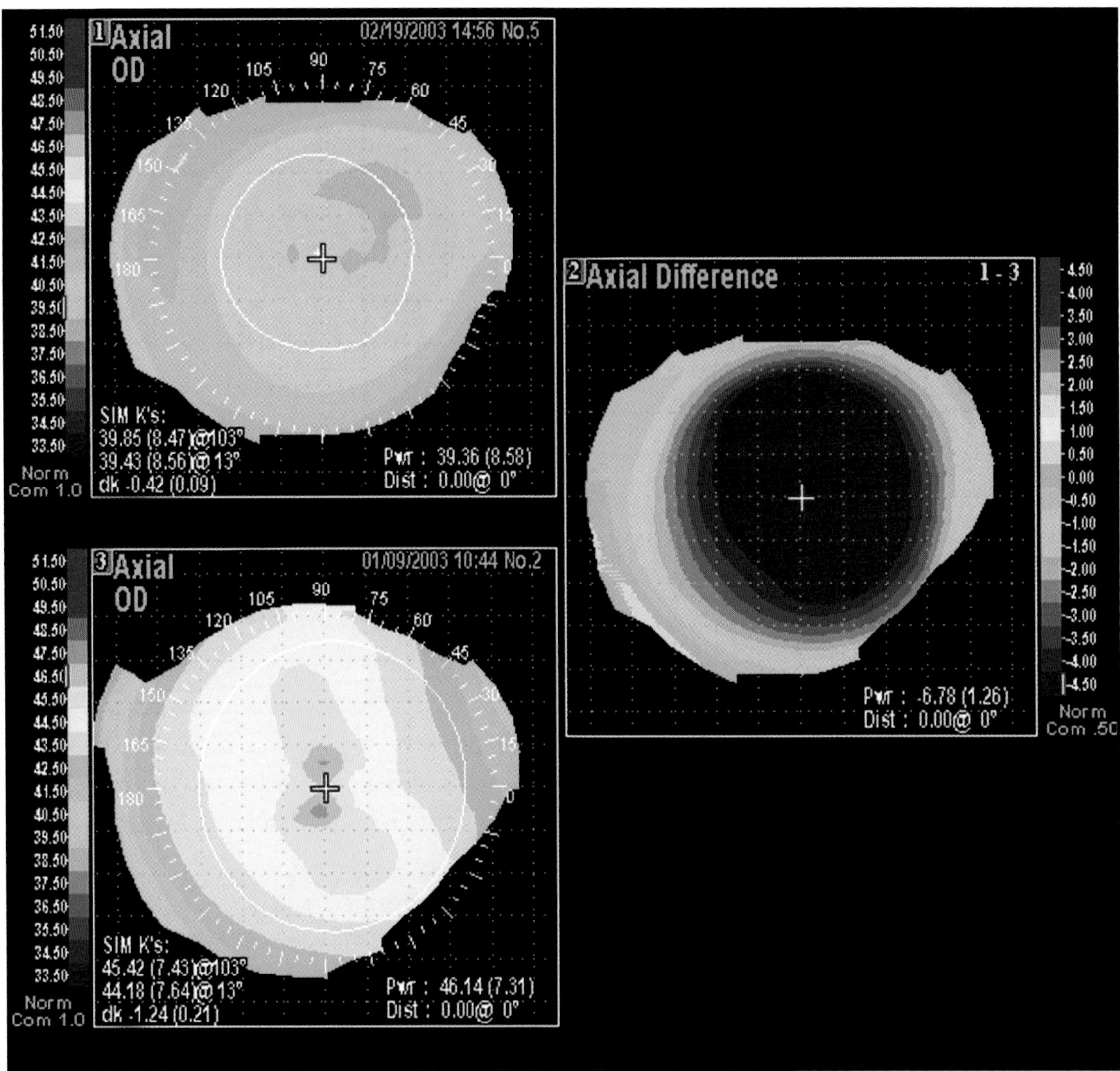

FIGURE 11-1: The patient's preoperative topography (lower left) and 1 month postoperative topography (upper left) is shown. Difference map (right) illustrates effects of LASIK surgery on the corneal shape. On the difference map, green denotes no net change in curvature (see scale to the left of the map); blue denotes net flattening. The white cross in the middle of each figure represents the patient's visual axis. From the difference map, one can deduce the net effect of the LASIK surgery on the cornea. Difference map shows a well-centered myopic correction without inferior steepening.

....Contd

a 110 μ head was used to create the LASIK flap in both eyes. An estimated flap thickness of 150 μ (standard deviation in our experience was 18 microns) was used for residual stromal bed thickness calculations; this estimated thickness was based on an average previous flap thickness using this specific microkeratome. The LADARVision 4000 excimer laser (Alcon, Fort Worth, TX) was used. Ablation depth with a 7.0 mm laser optical zone was 115 μ in the right and 138 μ in the left. A large 7.0 optical zone was used because of the combination of high myopia and large pupils to reduce the risk of symptomatic spherical aberrations postoperatively. A smaller optical zone with the LADARVision or other lasers could have been used, but the risk of symptomatic spherical aberrations is increased. Postoperative residual corneal stromal bed thickness was calculated to be 266 μ on the right and 260 μ on the left.

Contd....

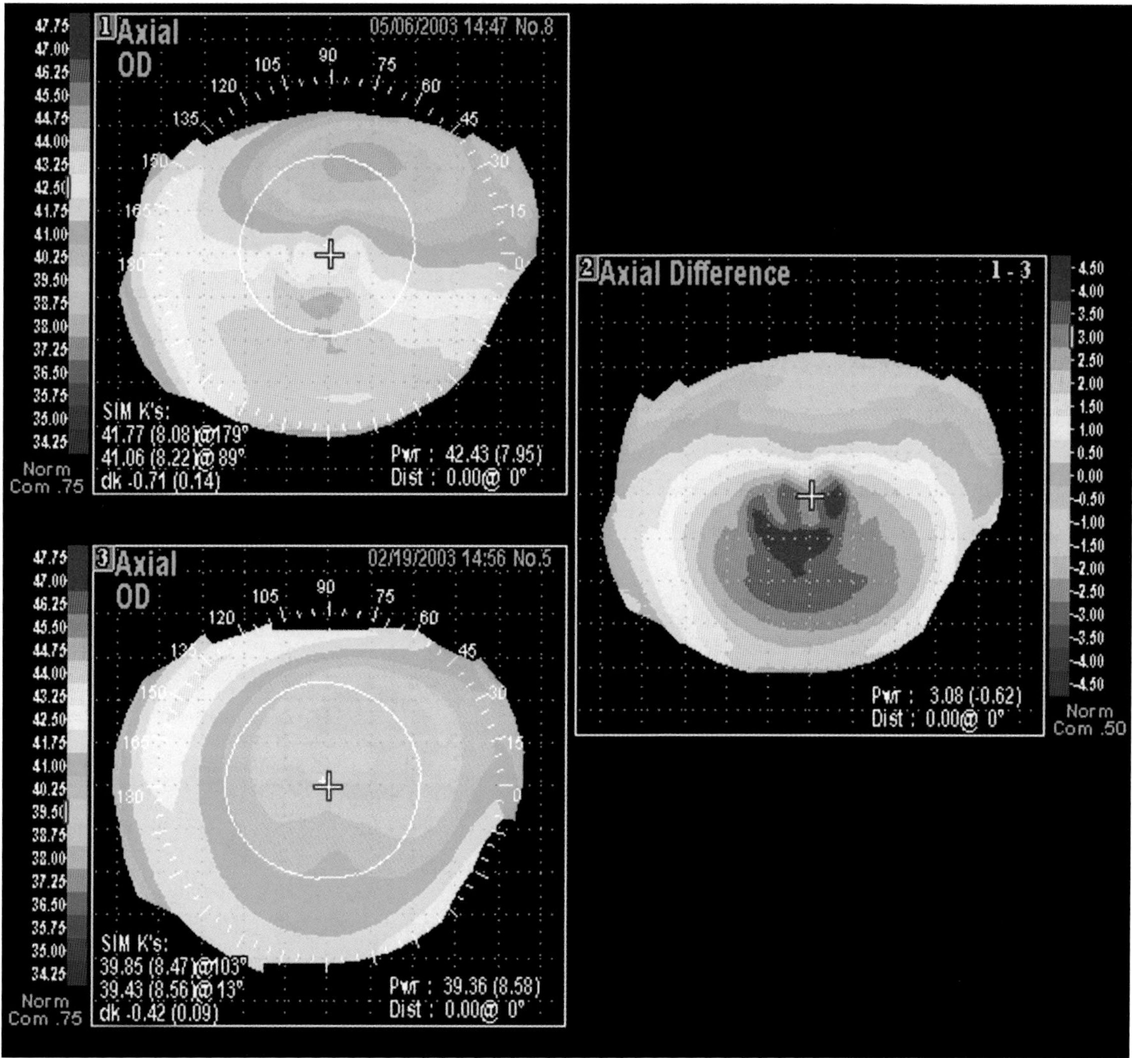

FIGURE 11-2: The 1 month postoperative topography (lower left) and 4-month postoperative topography (upper left) show new development of inferior steepening (red). Difference map (right) makes the diagnosis of ectasia easy.

....Contd

Follow-up best spectacle-corrected Snellen visual acuity (BSCVA) was 20/20, and topographies were normal at 1 day, 1 month, and 3 months postoperatively in both eyes. Flap thickness in the right eye was subjectively estimated to be significantly thicker than normal, based on observations of interface depth relative to that typically seen with the microkeratome used. Slit lamp examinations were otherwise normal **(Figure 11-1)**.

At 4 postoperative months, the patient presented with a report of decreased visual acuity in the right eye. BSCVA was found to have decreased to 20/40-2, and corneal topography was noted to have significant asymmetric inferior steepening in the right eye **(Figure 11-2)**. Intraocular pressure was 19 mm Hg in both eyes. There was no change in the left eye. Corneal ectasia of the right eye was diagnosed, and the patient was prescribed Timoptic XE to be taken once per day in the right eye. The rationale for this prescription was that lowering IOP relieves biomechanical strain on the cornea, just as deflating a car tire relieves pressure from the inner tire wall.

Contd....

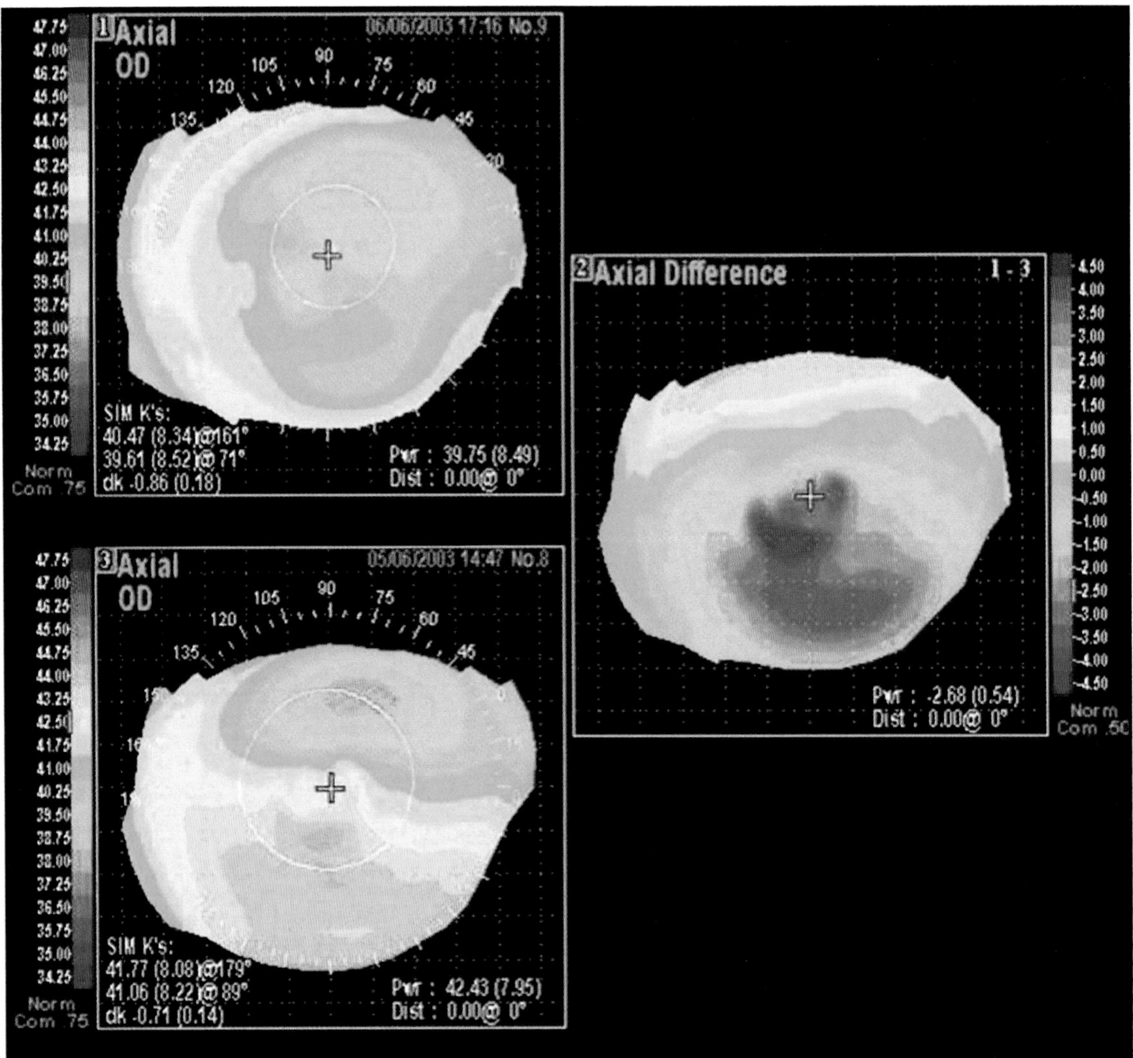

FIGURE 11-3: The 4-month topography (lower left) and 5-month topography show near complete ectasia reversal. Difference map (right) indicates flattening (blue) after starting the IOP-lowering topical medication.

....Contd

At month 5, the patient's IOP had decreased to 14 mm Hg, BSCVA was 20/30, and corneal topography had improved significantly **(Figure 11-3)**, with mild evidence of asymmetric, predominantly inferior, astigmatism in the right eye **(Figure 11-3)**. At month 11, the patient's BSCVA in the right eye returned to 20/20, and corneal topography remained normal without any topographic inferior steepening. The patient's cornea was believed at this time to have stabilized, so she was taken off Timoptic. At month 14, the patient returned with a BSCVA of 20/30 and recurrence of inferior steepening on topography. She was again placed on topical Timoptic. **Figure 11-4** shows mean keratometry changes over the course of 14 months postoperatively.

This case demonstrated that ectasia that developed early followed by treatment can be reversed. Intraocular pressure can influence corneal shape and that its reduction can improve early ectasia. The cornea has two opposing forces acting upon it: IOP inside the eye which pushes against the back of the cornea and atmospheric pressure (ATM) outside the eye which pushes against the front of the cornea

Contd....

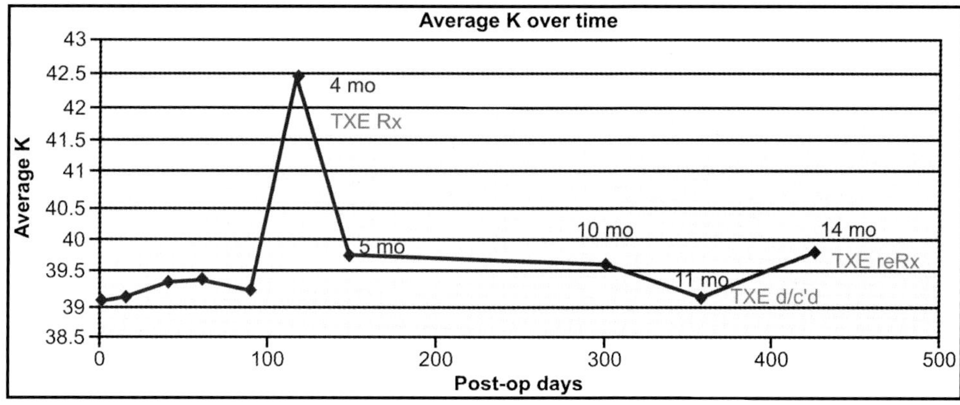

FIGURE 11-4: Shows a linear graphical representation of mean keratometry over time postoperatively. The axis represents time (days); the Y axis is mean keratometry (D). The peak steepening was at 4 months at which time Timoptic was started (TXE Rx). Flattening while on IOP-lowering medication from 4 to 11 months is illustrated. Recurrent steepening after Timoptic was stopped (TXE dc'd) at 11 months is evident.

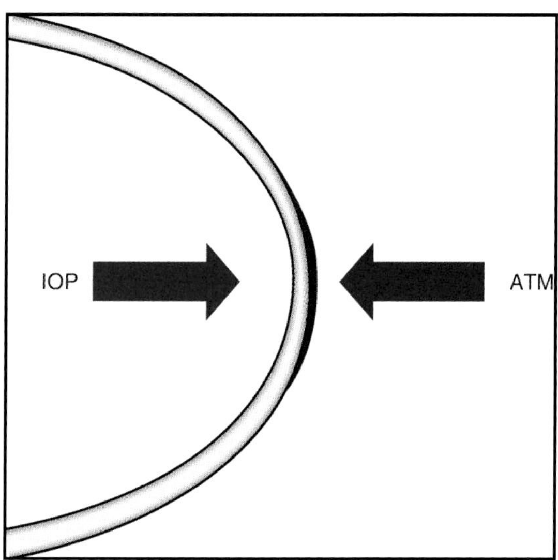

FIGURE 11-5: The cornea is constantly under the influence of two types of pressure: IOP pushing on the back of the cornea and ATM pushing on the front of the cornea.

....Contd

(Figure 11-5). In an uncompromised cornea, the biomechanical strength of the cornea makes it resistant to shape change if one pressure force exceeds the other. In a surgically compromised cornea, the collagen fibers are not strong enough to hold the corneal shape. The result is bulging forward due to intraocular pressure that effectively pushes the cornea out. A delicate balance may exist that can be more easily influenced by intra-and extraocular pressure differences.

Even though we used one specific medication for IOP reduction, we believe the potential benefit would be for other IOP lowering medications, although that has yet to be evaluated. We believe that there is a window of opportunity to reverse ectasia with simple IOP lowering. We have attempted such IOP treatment in patients with long-standing ectasia without success. We hypothesize that the cornea may be malleable during early and active ectasia and amenable to flattening from IOP reduction.

Conclusion

It appears that for ectasia that develops early after LASIK, prompt reduction in IOP has the ability to reverse ectasia. Such cases may benefit from C3-R® to 'lock in" the normal shape. Use of IOP lowering on late occurring ectasia and/or late diagnosed ectasia appears to be of little benefit.

References

1. Randleman JB, Russell B, Ward MA, Thompson KP, Stulting RD. Risk factors and prognosis for corneal ectasia after LASIK. Ophthalmol 2003;110: 267-75.
2. Clair-Florent M, Schmitt-Bernard C, Lesage C, Arnaud B. Keratectasia induced by laser in situ keratomileusis in keratoconus. J Refract Surg 2000;16:368-70.
3. Seiler T, Quurke AW. Iatrogenic keratectasia after LASIK in a case of forme fruste keratoconus. J Cataract Refract Surg 1998; 24:1007-10.
4. McLeod S, Kisla T, Caro N, McMahon T. Iatrogenic keratoconus: corneal ectasia following laser in situ keratomileusis for myopia. Arch Ophthalmol 2000;118:282-4.
5. Lafond G, Bazin R, Lajoie C. Bilateral severe keratoconus after laser in situ keratomileusis in a patient with forme fruste keratoconus. J Cataract Refract Surg 2001;27:1115-8.
6. Argento C, Cosentino MJ, Tytiun A, Rapetti G, Zarate J. Corneal ectasia after laser in situ keratomileusis. J Cataract Refract Surg 2001;1438-48.
7. Jabbur NS, Stark WJ, Green WR. Corneal ectasia after laser-assisted in situ keratomileusis. Arch Ophthalmol 2001;119: 1714-6.
8. Seiler T, Koufala K, Richter G. Iatrogenic keratectasia after laser in situ keratomileusis. J Refract Surg 1998;14:312-7.
9. Joo CK, Kim TG. Corneal ectasia detected after laser in situ keratomileusis for correction of less than -12 diopters of myopia. J Cataract Refract Surg 2000;26:292-5.
10. Amoils SP, Deist MB, Gous P, Amoils PM. Iatrogenic keratectasia after laser in situ keratomileusis for less than -4.0 to –7.0 diopters of myopia. J Cataract Refract Surg 2000;26:967-77.
11. Geggel HS, Talley AR. Delayed onset keratectasia following laser in situ keratomileusis. J Cataract Refract Surg 1999; 25:582-6.
12. Haw WW, Manche EE. Iatrogenic keratectasia after a deep primary keratotomy during laser in situ keratomileusis. Am J Ophthalmol 2001;132: 920-1.
13. Pallikaris IG, Kymionis GD, Astyrakakis NI. Corneal ectasia induced by laser in situ keratomileusis. J Cataract Refract Surg 2001: 27: 1794-802.
14. Rao SN, Epstein RJ. Early onset ectasia following laser in situ keratomileusis: case report and literature review. J Refract Surg 2002;18:177-84.
15. Wang JC, Hufnagel TJ, Buxton DF. Bilateral keratectasia after unilateral laser in situ keratomileusis: a retrospective diagnosis of ectatic corneal disorder. J Cataract Refract Surg 2003;29:2015-8.
16. Hiatt JA, Boxer Wachler BS, Grant CN. Reversal of laser in situ keratomileusis-induced ectasia with intraocular pressure reduction. J Cataract Refract Surg 2005;31:1652-5.

Section 4

Cornea Replacement Treatments

Jes Mortensen, *MD*

12 Lamellar Keratoplasty

Introduction

In 1891 Arthur von Hippel introduced the motorized, clockwork-driven trephine to aid in lamellar keratoplasty (LK) which proved to enhance the safety of the procedure.[1] The automated LK technique became the preferred technique in corneal transplantation for many years. In 1906 Edward Zirm reported the first successful penetrating keratoplasty (PKP)[2] and later in 1919 Anton Elschnig reported on 100 PKPs with a success rate of 10%.[3] Lack of thin sutures was a significant obstacle that hindered the success of PKP until the 1960s at which time 10:0 nylon and prolene sutures were developed along with improved needle designs. In the 1970s PKP began to replace LK even though LK was a less invasive and safer procedure. The reason for the transition to PKP was the safety of the surgical procedure improved with the development of more accurate trephines and with the introduction of viscoelastic. Another reason for the shift away from LK was the optical quality of the hand-dissected lamellar graft was not as high as that of a full thickness graft used for PKP. In South America, LK remained a prevalent procedure due the automated microkeratome developed by Jose Barraquer, which was the foundation of his "refractive lamellar technique".[4-6] The microkeratome system produced a lamellar dissection with host and donor lamellar surface quality that was superior to that of hand-dissection. Additionally, the thickness of tissue produced by the microkeratome was significantly more uniform and predictable compared to hand-dissection technique.[7] In the early 1980s, PKP became a refined surgical procedure that largely replaced LK throughout the world. During this time, a small number of epikeratophakia operations (suturing a lamellar graft onto Bowman's layer after corneal epithelium was removed) were performed[8] along with tectonic LKs.

In keratoconus, LK can enhance vision by replacing the anterior portion of the cornea with a thicker, structurally intact anterior corneal donor graft. Because the posterior portion of the patient's cornea is not disrupted, the healing time is faster than PKP. Once healed, patients will often need some of contact lens or glasses for full vision correction.

Immunology of the Eye

It is impressive how a corneal graft can be transplanted from one individual to another individual and survives for a sustained time. The unique immunology of the eye accounts for this ability as the cornea is considered to be an "immune privileged site"[9-11] like the brain, testes and placenta. The historical definition of an immune privileged site was an anatomical site where a transplanted allograft survives for an extended period of time in an immunocompetent host. Immune privilege is a dynamic process that is actively acquired and continued by immunological regulatory systems that represent a type of immunological tolerance. For more information read Chapter 13 on Penetrating Keratoplasty (PKP).

Reintroduction of Lamellar Keratoplasty

The author worked extensively with PKP for over 15 years, but was not satisfied with the results, which was the motivation to work with LK. When the author began as a corneal specialist in a university hospital, more complicated cornea patients were referred to us which increased PKP risk and led to discouraging results. The problems with PKP were: rejection of the graft,[12] high astigmatism, slow healing, irregularity of the surface of the graft, and the risk of developing secondary glaucoma that could lead to severe vision loss. The detailed risks of PKP are covered in Chapter 13. Because the risk of PKP is spread over the patients' life, we transitioned PKP for keratoconus in younger patients to those patients in their forties or older. There have been several younger patients with severe loss of vision in one or both eyes due to PKP problems early in the postoperative period that required repeat corneal transplant only to be followed by recurrent episodes of rejection that eventually led to glaucomatous loss of vision.

Sweden was reintroduced to LK through the generosity of Professor Massimo Busin of Italy. In January 2003, Professor Busin treated the first patient in Sweden. The patient was a 29-year-old woman who, at the age of 17, had a PKP due to keratoconus **(Figure 12-1)**. The transplanted eye experienced profound vision loss from glaucoma caused by repeated graft rejection episodes. As a result, she was not comfortable with proceeding with PKP in her fellow eye. She was comfortable with LK and underwent a successful LK. She has done very well for over four years later without any side effects.

Lamellar Keratoplasty

We perform LK on primary eyes with advanced to severe keratoconus. We used the Moria ALT-K system **(Figures 12-2 and 12-3)**. Keratoconic eyes that had a PKP are also candidates for LK. In the latter cases, patients

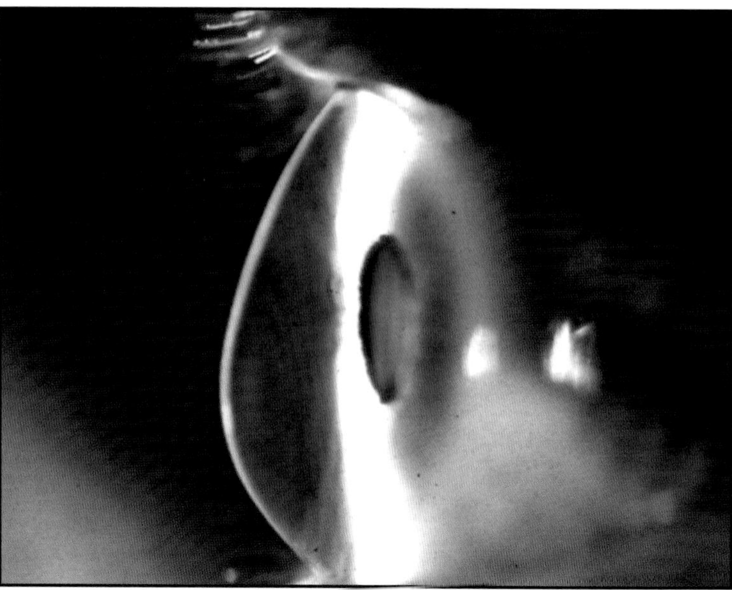

FIGURE 12-1: Advanced keratoconus.

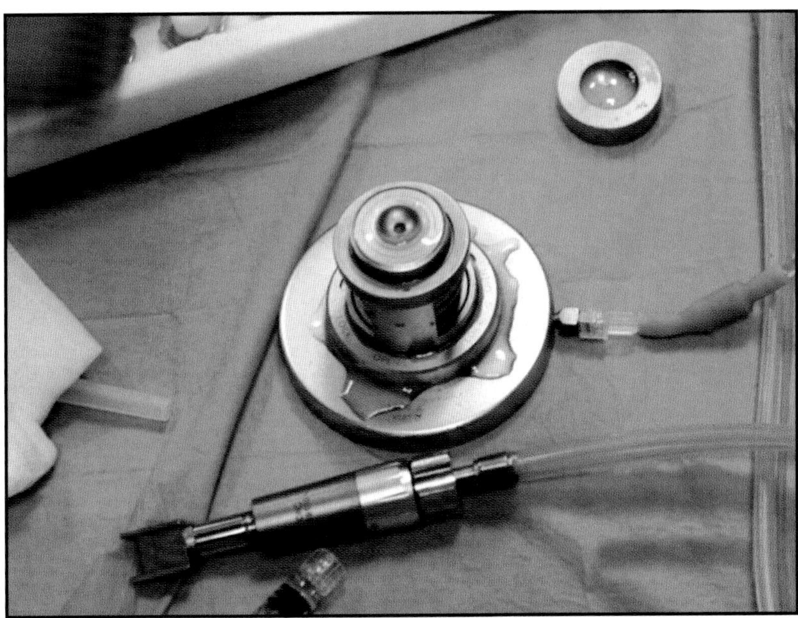

FIGURE 12-2: The Moria ALT-K system and artificial anterior chamber (upper) and LSK microkeratome (lower).

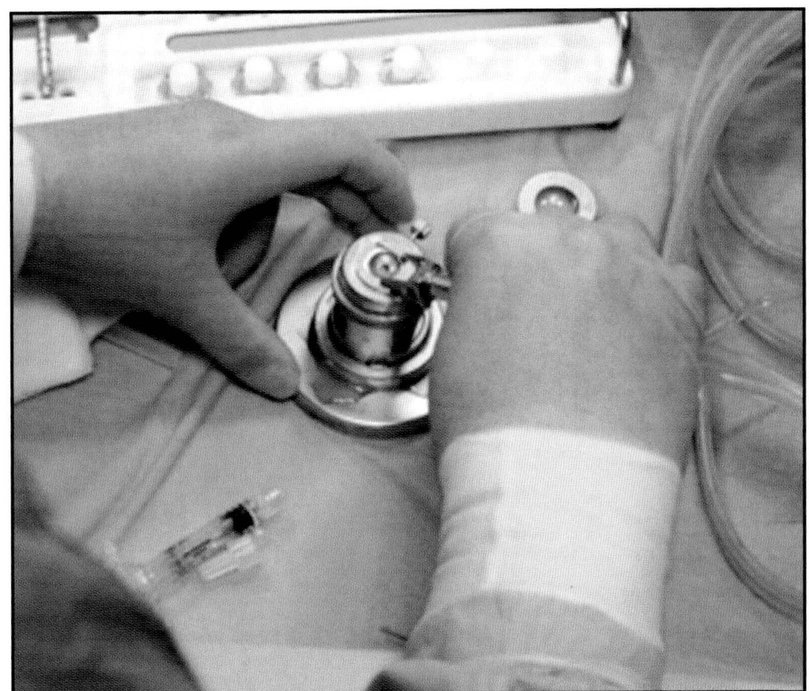

FIGURE 12-3: Harvesting of donor lamellar graft using microkeratome. The donor cornea is secured in the artificial anterior chamber.

after PKP experienced high astigmatism and/or irregularity of the surface of the transplant. Helena Sonne, MD, and the author have until now performed LK on more than 150 eyes. Last year, we presented the postoperative results of our first 63 cases. In our series, 100 eyes were operated on for different diagnoses: keratoconus, post-PKP, anterior corneal dystrophy, and post-trauma. We had follow-up for 63 eyes. Of these eyes, 26 had keratoconus and 3 eyes experienced keratoectasia after LASIK. Of these 26 eyes, 19 eyes were primary LK and 7 had prior PKP.

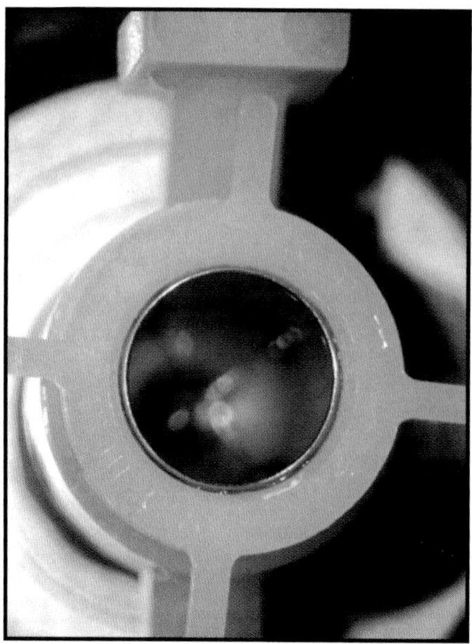

FIGURE 12-4: Hessburg-Baron trephine that is used to incise the patient's cornea in preparation for the lamellar graft to be placed on Bowman's layer.

Keratoconus

We have evaluated 26 eyes treated with LK using two different methods were used for advanced keratoconus as catagorized by the thin cornea group and thick cornea group.

The thin cornea group (group 1) had 15 eyes with pachymetry was less than 300 microns pachymetry as measured by Orbscan or Sonogage if Orbscan was not possible due to irregularity of the cornea. We used the Hessburg-Baron vacuum trephine **(Figure 12-4)** to make a circular partial penetration of about 180 microns. In the outer edge of this circular incision, a 0.5 mm pocket was created to allow the donor lamella to be tucked into the pocket minimizing the risk of epithelial ingrowth. The donor lamellar graft was cut with a microkeratome using a 130 microns head using the Moria ALT-K system. As these patients' corneas were less than 300 micons, a lamellar resection was not performed. In these cases the corneal epithelium was removed and the graft was placed on Bowman's layer. The edges were tucked into the peripheral cornea after a circular incision was made. This is different than epikeratophakia as the lamellar graft tissue was not frozen, but living tissue for LK. Tisseel tissue glue has proven useful to prevent epithelial ingrowth evidenced by only one case of occurrence since we began using it. We put a thin layer of Tisseel glue on the corneal bed and posterior side of the graft and waited two minutes before the graft was sutured. We secured the graft with 8 interrupted sutures and one running suture.

Thick cornea group (group 2) had 11 eyes with pachymetry greater than 300 microns. The lamellar graft was cut from the patient's cornea with the 130 microkeratome head **(Figure 12-5)**. The lamellar graft was cut with a microkeratome using a 250 microns head. The lamella was placed with glue and sutured with the same technique as above mentioned. A silicone contact lens was inserted after operation in both groups.

Analyzing the results of both groups as a whole (26 eyes), the mean best spectacle corrected visual acuity (BSCVA) before surgery was 20/160 (range 20/2000 to 20/30). Mean BSCVA postoperatively was 20/40 (range 20/200 to 20/20) **(Figure 12-6)**. The mean follow up time was 12 months (range 1 to 33 months). The mean spherical correction was +0.80 (range +5.5 to –4.0 D), mean cylinder was –3.8 D (range 0 to –12.0 D). Ten eyes were fitted with a gas permeable contact lens to optimize BCVA.

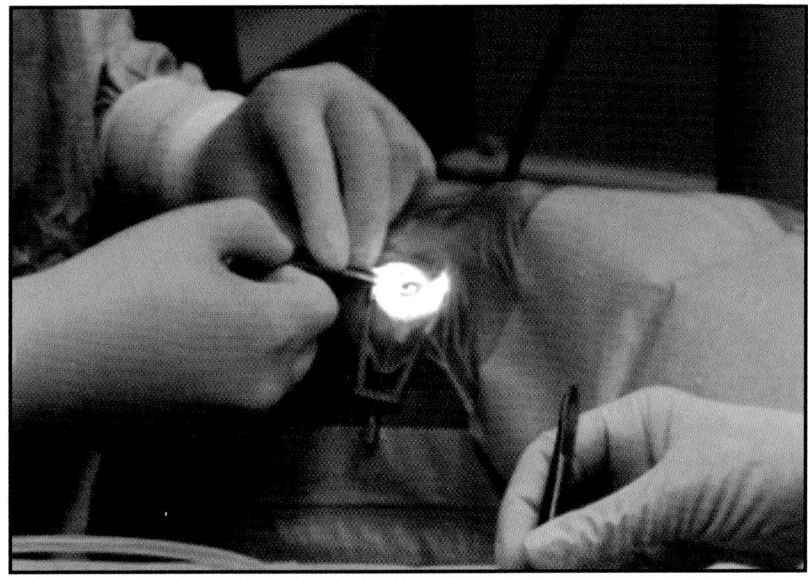

FIGURE 12-5: The microkeratome is used to remove lamellar dissection of patient's cornea if pachymetry is greater than 300 microns.

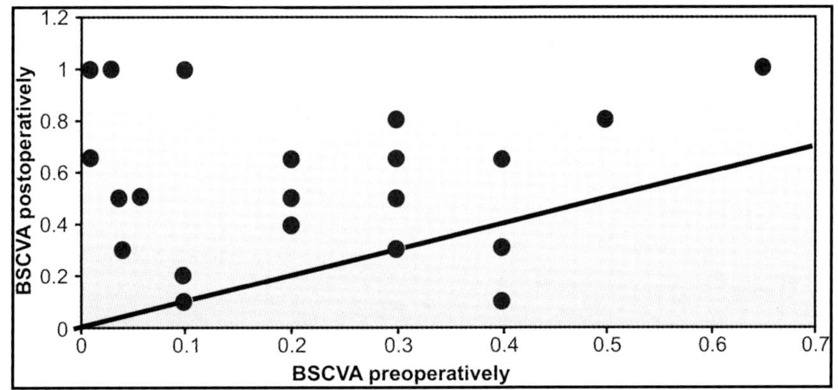

FIGURE 12-6: A diagram showing BSCVA before and after lamellar keratoplasty for keratoconus in 26 eyes. Note that most eyes are above the line which indicates improvement in BSCVA postoperatively.

Group 1 (only the adding the lamellar graft to corneal surface) had mean BSCVA before surgery of 20/160 (20/2000 – 20/30). Group 2 had mean BSCVA of 20/160 (20/2000–20/40). In group 1, mean BSCVA after surgery was 20/40 (20/200–20/20) and in group 2 was 20/40 (20/200 – 20/25). In group 1, the postoperative sphere was +0.70 D (range +2.0 to –4.0 D) and the mean cylinder was – 3.82 D (range 0 to –12.0 D). In group 2, the mean postoperative sphere was +0.93 (range –1.0 to +5.5 D), and mean cylinder was –3.88 D (range 0 to –9.0 D). Three eyes were operated for LASIK-induced ectasia. The eyes were treated with the same protocol as the keratoconus eyes in group 2 above. Mean visual acuity was 20/125 before operation and 20/40 after operation. Follow-up time was 6 months (range 1 to 9 months). **Figure 12-7** shows the results for groups 1 and 2.

Postoperative Care

Patients can expect to feel very little discomfort the day after operation and can typically return to work in one to two weeks. Corticosteroid eyedrops are prescribed times 4 times a day, tapering that dose with one

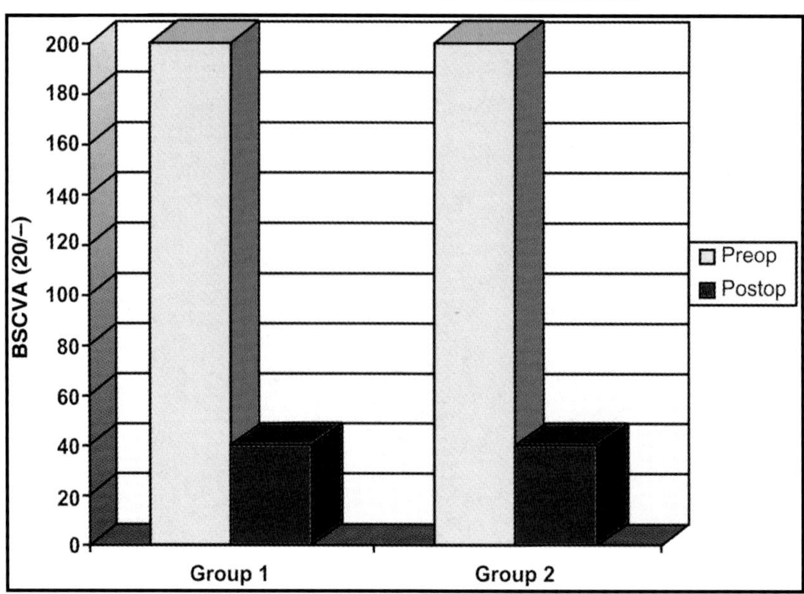

FIGURE 12-7: BSCVA Results for groups 1 and 2.

drop every second month thereafter. The patient is seen the day after operation and again after 5 days for removal of the contact lens when complete epithelialization has occurred. The sutures are removed after 3 months, but may be earlier if the sutures loosen which may cause minor discomfort. Loose sutures are not uncommon in keratoconic eyes since the corneal strength is less than in the normal cornea. The technique using 8 interrupted sutures and one running suture has reduced the incidence of loose sutures before 3 months. Once sutures are removed, the corneas are typically very clear, even in eyes with LK after previous PKP for keratoconus **(Figure 12-8)**.

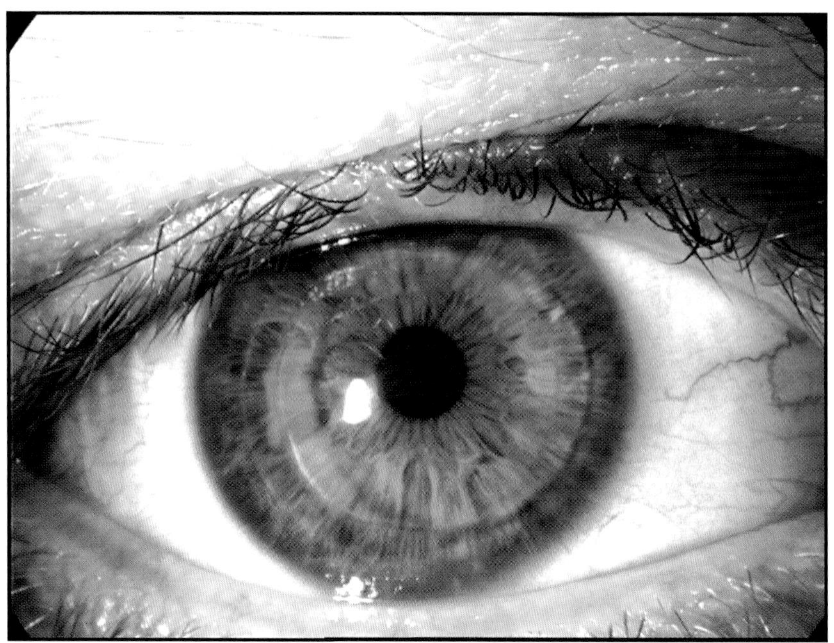

FIGURE 12-8: Well-healed LK. This 40-year-old woman had PKP several years ago, but was unable to use glasses and contact lenses. Six months after LK, vision was 20/20 with a contact lens.

Contact Lens Fitting

The optometrist plays an important role in the postoperative visual rehabilitation. To optimize the results, it is essential to have a relationship with a skilled optometrist to achieve the best visual results. Our optometrist, Lars Carlsson, has many years of experience fitting soft and hard contact lenses and has worked with many patients with keratoconus, PKP, LK and even normal contact lens users. He states: "Lamellar keratoplasty has proven to give a very smooth and even convex surface often giving a very good possibility to attain an excellent comfort and good quality of vision for the contact lens patient."

There are many benefits of LK over PKP. Patients after LK appear to tolerate contact lenses better (less discomfort) compared post-PKP. High induced astigmatism occurs less frequently after LK compared to PKP. The patients after LK often do not experience double vision or aberration disturbances which are often seen after PKP. LK seems to provide better quality of vision than PKP. High quality of daytime and nighttime vision after LK, even with a BSCVA 20/40 or 20/30, leads to very satisfied patients. The refraction is stable even after the sutures are removed. Vision in both LK and PKP improves over 2 years postoperatively.

Complications

Very few complications have been seen with LK. Even though all patients in our study were operated on under general (universal) anesthesia, three male patients complained of severe pain after the operation for several days. Once we began adding subTenons' local anesthetia, we have not observed this occurrence.

Initially, we had a few highly irregular lamellar dissections as we were not experienced with the Moria ALTK keratome system. Pushing the keratome with too high speed will cause the soft corneal tissue in a keratoconic cornea to be pressed up in front of the blade causing deep irregular cuts. Using a slow keratome translational speed avoids deep irregular cuts and yields uniform smooth surface.

We had one case of a prior PKP dehiscence during the lamellar cut in a patient with Downs syndrome. The patient required cataract surgery. Immediately following the procedure, we performed LK during the same session. Subepithelial ingrowth occurred which led to graft dehiscence. The lesson learned here is that it is not recommended to suture a lamellar graft on a soft eye.

Gluing the lamellar graft with Tisseel tissue glue has virtually eliminated epithelial ingrowth. Rejection of the graft occurred in one eye operated with a deep lamellar graft for keratoconus. This was one epithelial rejection that occurred after 6 months and was successfully treated with corticosteroid drops. There were no stromal rejection episodes in our LK series. The risk of any form of rejection after PKP was 16% in the Swedish Corneal Register following up study over 5 years. In our series of 26 eyes with LK for keratoconus, the risk of any type of rejection was approximately 3.8%, which is significantly lower than 16% rejection rate for PKP. We now have performed LK on over 50 eyes and still have only seen one epithelial rejection which is a very favorable 2% rejection rate.

Conclusion

The future of LK for keratoconus is bright. We expect that modern lamellar techniques will replace old PKP techniques as the risk of rejection is much less and visual recovery and vision quality is better with LK. An artificial cornea is underdevelopment and is approaching clinical tests in human eyes in Sweden and Canada (personal communication by professor Per Fagerholm, Linkoping, Sweden). The femtosecond laser is perhaps the most promising advanced in LK as the precise cutting of the recipient cornea and the donor cornea is expected to induce less astigmatism and less irregularity of the surface after transplantation. Even very thin corneas can be cut without risk of perforation.

References

1. von Hippel A. Ein neue methode der hornhauttransplantation. Albrecht v Graefes. Arch Ophthalmol 1888;34:108-30.
2. Zirm E. Eine erfolgreiche totall keratoplastik. Albrecht Von Graefes Arch Ophthalmol 1906;64:580.
3. Elschnig A. Keratoplasty. Arch Ophthalmol 1930;4:165.
4. Barraquer JI. Safety technique in penetrating keratoplasty. Transactions of the Ophthalmol Soc of the UK 1949;69:77.
5. King JH Jr. Variations in technique in lamellar keratoplasty. An Inst Barraquer 1966; 7:365-85.
6. Barraquer JI. Lamellar keratoplasty (Special Techniques). Annals of Ophthalmol 1972;4:437-69.
7. Haimovici R, Culbertson WW. Optical lamellar keratoplasty using the Barraquer microkeratome. Refract Corneal Surg 1991;7:42-5.
8. Werblin TR Kaufman HE. Epikeratophakia: the surgical correction of aphakia II. Primary results in a non-human primate model. Current Eye Res 1981;1:131-7.
9. Niederkorn, Jerry Y. The immune privilege of corneal allografts [overviews] transplantation 1999;67;1503-8.
10. Niederkorn JY, Peeler JS, Mellon J. Phagocytosis of particulate antigens by corneal epithelial cells stimulates interleukin-1 secretion and migration of Langerhans cells into the central cornea. Reg Immunol 1989; 2:83.
11. Kenji Inoue, et al. Risk factors for corneal graft failure and rejection in penetrating keratoplasty. Acta Ophthalmol Scand 2001:79;251-5.
12. Vail ASM, Gore BA, Bradley DL, CA Rogers. Corneal transplant follow-up study. Invest. Ophthalmol Vis Sci 1993;34:1366.

Jes Mortensen, *MD*

13 *Penetrating Keratoplasty*

Introduction

Penetrating keratoplasty (PKP) or full-thickness corneal transplantation is the oldest and still the most successful transplantation in humans. In 1824 Franz Reisinger reported on experimental corneal transplantations in rabbits. All the corneal transplants opacified, but they healed into the recipient cornea. These results encouraged the belief that this kind of transplantation might be feasible. Kissam performed the first human corneal transplantation in 1838. A pig cornea was transplanted to a human eye without anesthesia and without success.[1] In 1905 Edward Zirm carried out a successful corneal allograft (cornea from another human) to a 45-year-old patient who had been blind in both eyes from lye burns. Bilateral PKP was performed and one transplant remained clear. [2] In the subsequent decade, PKPs became more popular and in 1919 Elschnig reported on 100 PKPs with a success rate of 10%.[3]

In Sweden, renowned professor Henrik Sjögren **(Figure 13-1)** was one of the pioneers in corneal grafting. He was born 1899 in a little town, Koping and received his medical degree from The University of Stockholm. His thesis: "Zur Kenntnis der Keratoconjunctivitis Sicca" made him world-famous when it was translated to English in the late 1940s.[4] He was founding director of The Eye Clinic in Jonkoping and remained as director for 31 years at which time he retired in 1967. His clinic in Jonkoping became the leading center for PKPs. He invented a special punch **(Figure 13-2)** which functioned like a ticket punch. The operation started with a cataract incision, one of the arms of this punch was introduced into the anterior chamber and the cornea was punched **(Figure 13-3)**. The same procedure was performed on the donor eye to achieve a similar size corneal donor button. This technique, however, likely led to damage to the donor endothelium as the importance of the endothelium was not understood until the 1970s. In the 1950s, the only sutures available were 4:0 and 5:0 silk **(Figure 13-4)**. In an article from 1961 on lamellar keratoplasty, Professor Mauno Vannas related that they started to use fibers from rat tails, which caused no irritation to the corneal tissue.[5] In the 1960s, 10:0 nylon and polypropylene sutures became available.

The goal of PKP is to replace the full-thickness keratoconic portion of the cornea. This differs from lamellar keratoplasty, which replaces the anterior section of the cornea. After patients heal, they often will need to use some form of contact lenses or glasses to realize full vision potential.

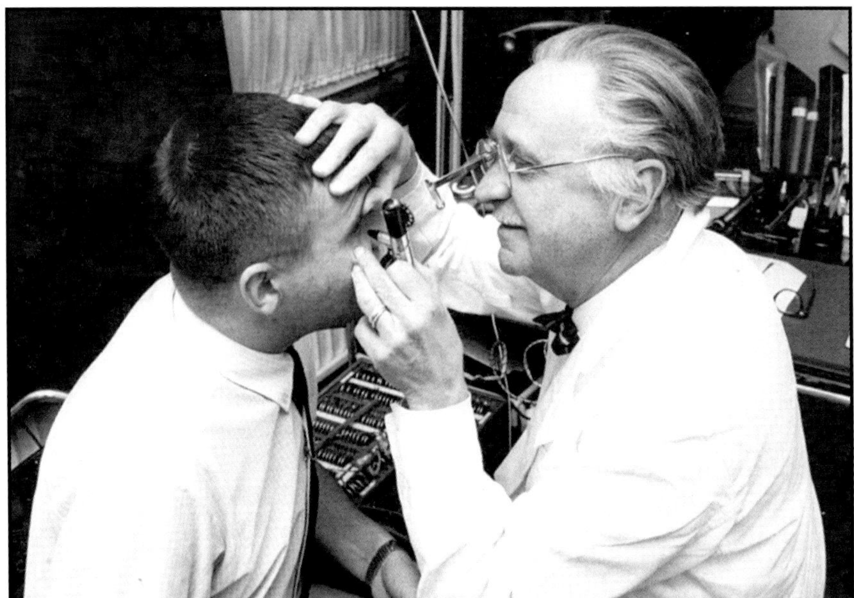

FIGURE 13-1: Professor Henrik Sjögren investigating one of his patients using his own designed ophthalmoscope (Picture from 1967).

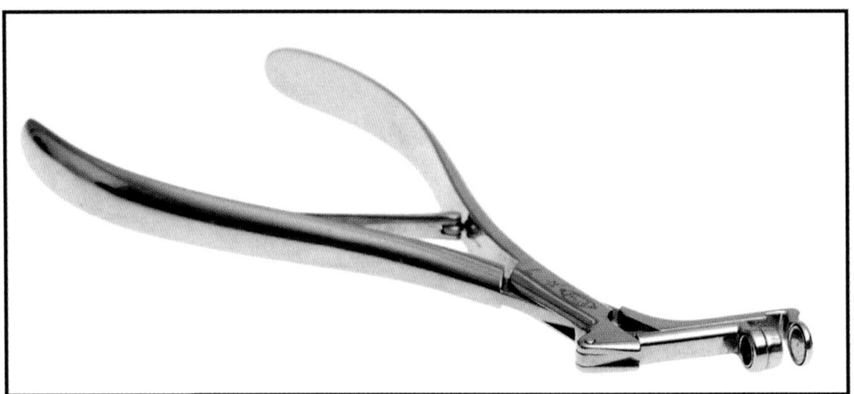

FIGURE 13-2: Forceps designed by Professor Henrik Sjögren for punching the recipient and donor cornea.

Immunology Role

It is prudent to understand the reason that a corneal allograft can be transplanted from one individual to another individual and survive for a sustained time. The immunology of the eye is the unique reason that allows this feat to occur. The eye is considered to be an immune privileged site like the brain, testes and placenta. The historical definition of an immune privileged site was an anatomical site where a transplanted allograft survives for an extended period of time in an immunocompetent host. Immune privilege is a dynamic process and is actively acquired and sustained by immunological regulatory systems that represent a type of immunological tolerance. We have gained a deep understanding into the immune privilege of the eye.[6]

The "neural reflex arc" **(Figure 13-5)** is considered an important sequence to aid in understanding the immune cycle. An afferent stimulus is sent to the spinal cord and processed, causing an efferent response sent to the effector organ as a reflex. The immune system can be described in the same manner—an afferent lymphatic limb, a central processing organ (lymph node), an efferent lymphatic limb. Corneal transplantation evokes an "immune reflex arc" that is analogous to the neural reflex arc. In the immune arc, a stimulus (alloantigen-

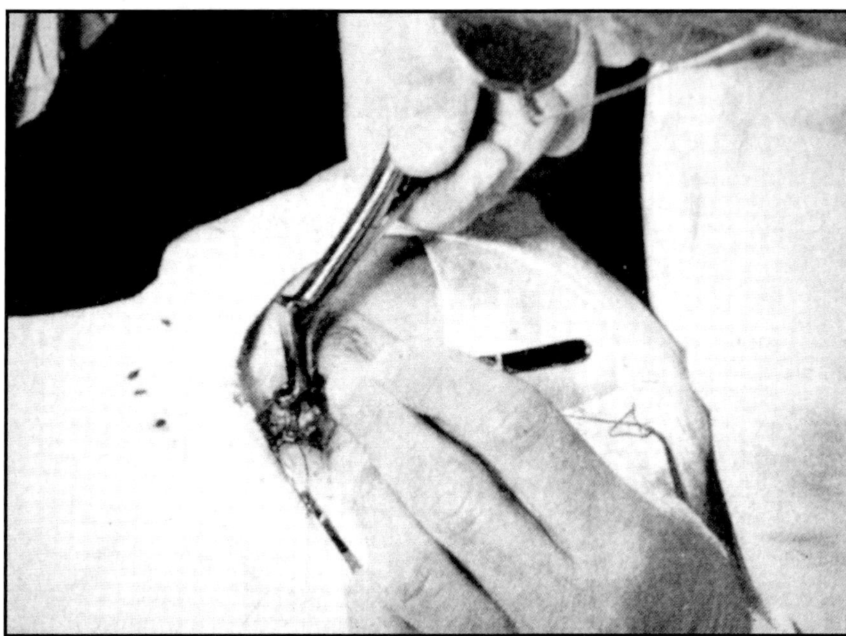

FIGURE 13-3: Professor Henrik Sjögren using his special forceps punching the recipient cornea through a cataract incision (Picture from a Swedish family journal 1956).

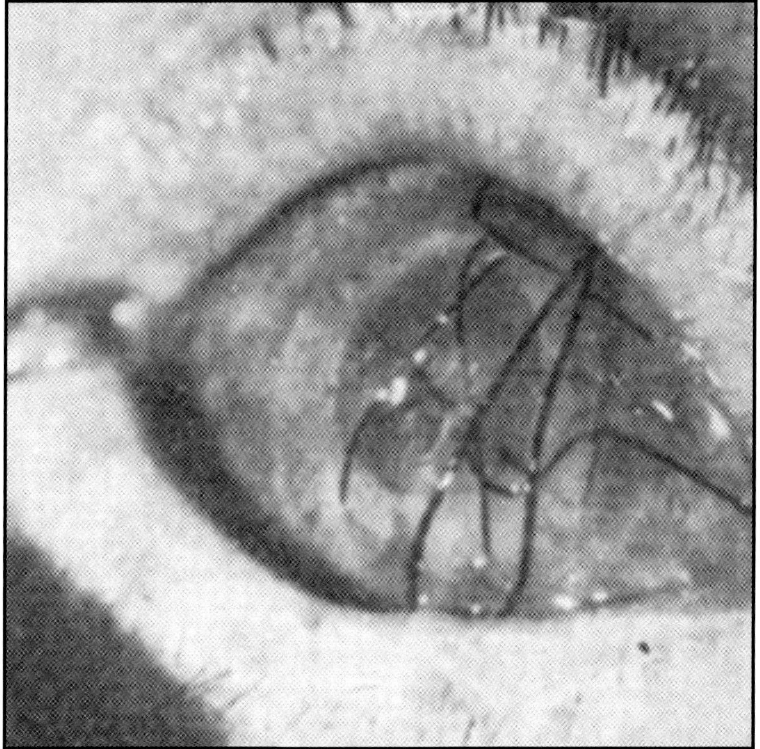

FIGURE 13-4: The sutures are visible immediately after a PKP was performed by Professor Henrik Sjögren (Picture from a Swedish family journal 1956).

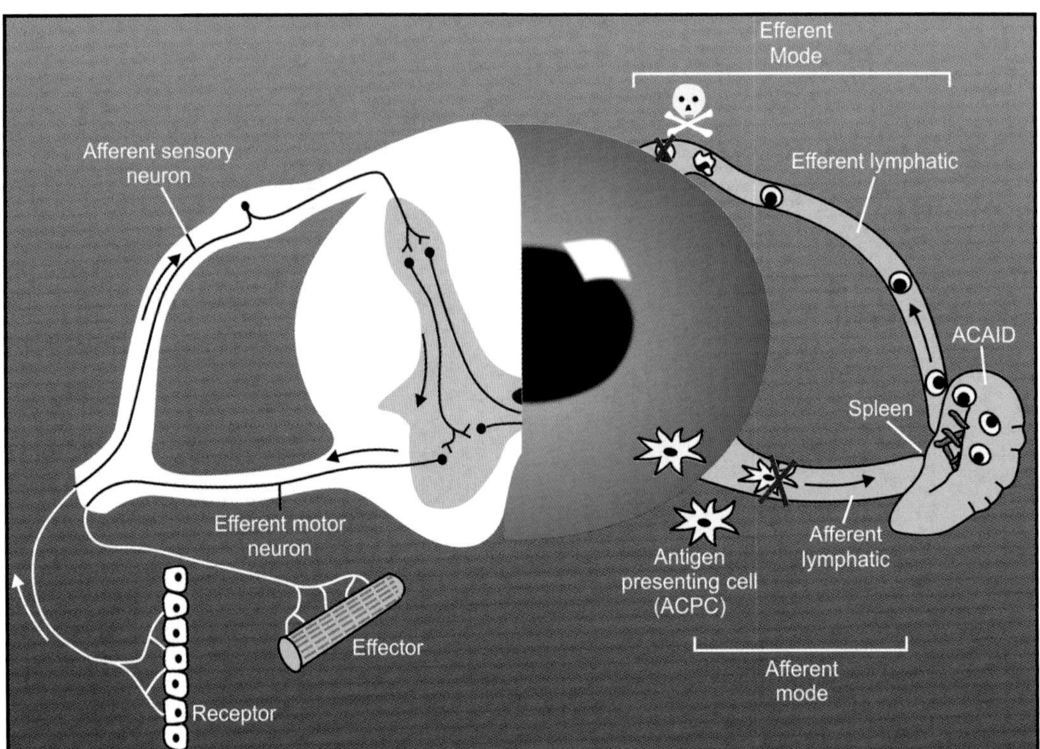

FIGURE 13-5: Disruption of the immune reflex arc promotes immune privilege of corneal allograft. The absence of donor-derived passenger antigen-presenting cells (APC) in the corneal graft blocks the afferent arm of the immune reflex arc. Corneal alloantigens shed from the allograft enter the anterior chamber and are transported via the blood vasculature to the spleen, where they deviate the systemic immune response away from a Th1 phenotype to a Th2 phenotype. Immune effector cells (if generated by extraocular immunization) undergo apoptosis when they encounter FasL that is expressed on the epithelial and endothelial cells of the corneal allograft (Courtesy: The author and Lippincott Williams & Wilkins).

presenting cell) is transmitted via an afferent pathway to a central processing component (lymph node), and an effector component (e.g. effector TH1 cells, cytotoxic antibody, cytotoxic T lymphocyte) is transmitted via an efferent pathway. Interruption of any of these three components of the immune reflex arc will shelter the immune privilege of the corneal graft.

Historically, it was postulated that the corneal privileged status was due to three special qualities:

1. Corneal cells did not have histocompatibility antigens from the donor.[7,8]
2. Donor cells in the corneal graft were replaced in a very short period, and
3. Corneal bed is devoid of lymphatics and blood vessels and the afferent and efferent arms of the immune reflex arc are blocked.

All components of the cornea do have MHC class I antigens and even minor histocompatibity antigens. Animal studies using sex chromatin markers have revealed that donor cells stay in the transplant for a long period.[9] Maumenee demonstrated that orthoptic corneal allografts placed into avascular beds failed to sensitize the hosts to donor alloantigens as the host later rejected skin grafts from the donor strain in a first-set tempo.[10] The afferent limb hypothesis was supported by observations that corneal grafts transplanted into vascular beds were always rejected. This rejection is now thought to be caused by small lymphatic vessels following the blood vessels that recreate the afferent immune limb.

Jerry Niederkorn, PhD concludes that the immune privilege of corneal allografts is a product of at least three unique qualities:

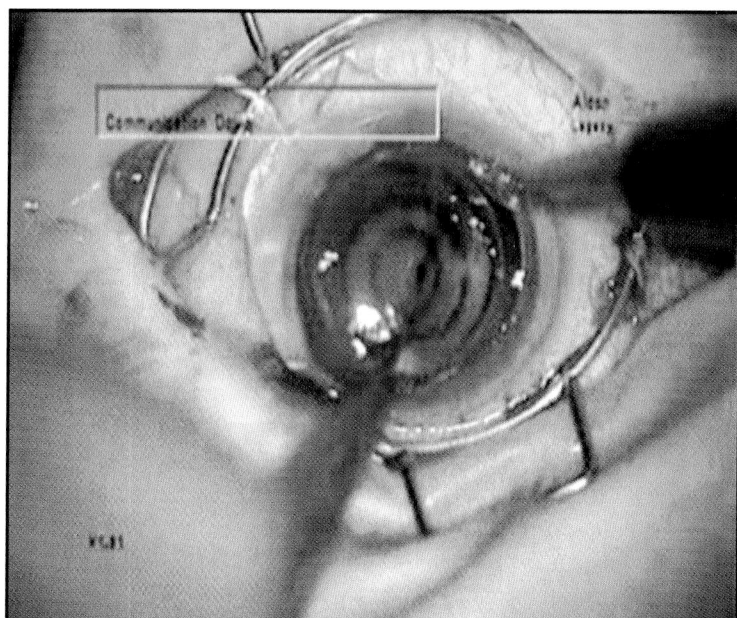

FIGURE 13-6: The McNeill-Goldman ring blepharostat is being used. The corneal cap is trephined and then removed with a diamond knife.

a. Absence of donor-derived, antigen-presenting passenger Langerhans' cells in the corneal graft.[11]
b. Expression of Fas ligand on the epithelium and endothelium of the corneal allograft,[12] and
c. Capacity of the corneal allograft to induce immune deviation of the systemic immune response.[13-16]

Present Status

In the United States more than 40,000 corneal transplantations are performed each year. In Sweden 500 to 600 transplantations are performed annually. During the1990s iatrogenic endothelial damage after phacoemulsification was one of the most frequent etiologies, with the modern phacomachines that incidence has fortunately remarkably diminished. Today keratoconus is the leading reason for PKP in Sweden. Over the past four years in our clinic we have transitioned from PKP to lamellar keratoplasty (LK). Other clinics in Sweden have followed the same trend, so PKPs will become less frequently performed. The PKP technique has not changed significantly since the 1980s when viscoelastic was introduced which greatly aided success rates of PKP.

Current Technique

If the patient is young, general anesthesia is recommended, while with older patients, subtenon's anesthesia is appropriate. We use the McNeill-Goldman ring blepharostat **(Figure 13-6)** to fixate the eye. In most cases four symmetric sutures are placed to minimize any force against the sclera which aids in corneal trephination of the patient's cornea as well as suturing the corneal button. Excessive scleral force increases the risk of high astigmatism postoperatively.

The center of the cornea is marked and the size of the corneal trephination area determined. The size in most cases is 7 to 8 mm. Before the actual trephination, a corneal button 0.25 to 0.50 mm larger is punched from the donor cornea. We use the Barron Markin corneal punch **(Figure 13-7)**, and cut the graft from the posterior surface. Punching from the anterior surface is possible with an anterior chamber maintainer and may provide more precise donor-recipient edge matching.

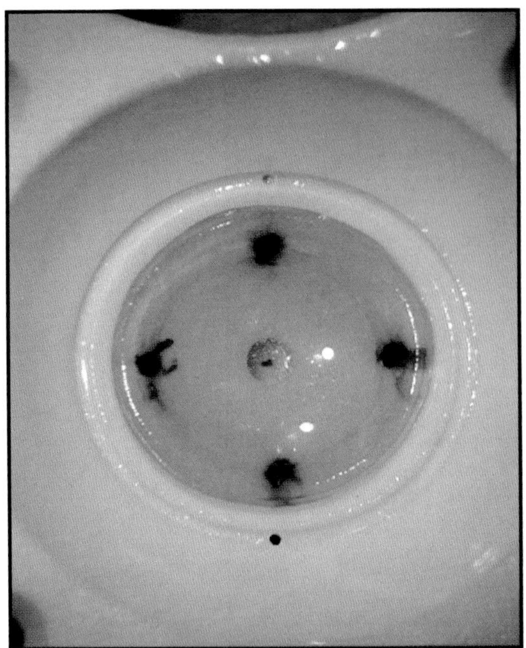

FIGURE 13-7: The Barron Markin corneal punch. The donor remains in the well before being suture to recipient.

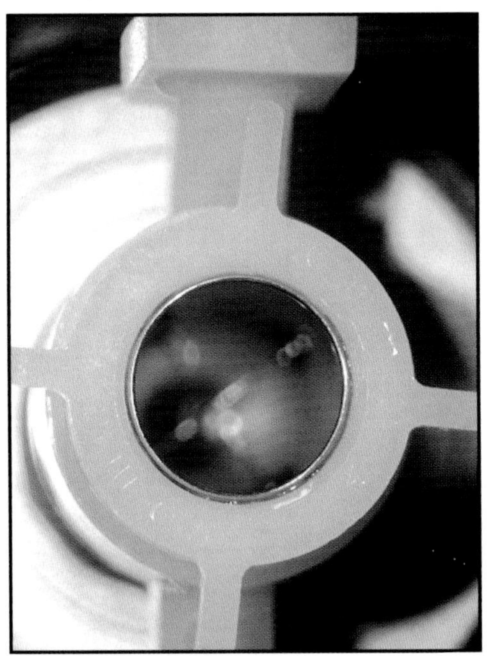

FIGURE 13-8: The Hessburg-Barron vacuum trephine (single use).

Then we prepare for trephination of the recipient cornea. Miochol is injected into the anterior chamber to minimize the risk of producing a dilated, non-reactive pupil. The cornea center is marked with a Sinkey hook. The periphery is marked with a radial keratotomy marker for the desired number of sutures to be placed. A variety of trephines have been developed—we use the Hessburg-Barron vacuum trephine which is a single use device **(Figure 13-8)**. This trephine can be used for partial penetration to allow for precise, partial penetration of the cornea. The trephine consists of a spring-loaded syringe connected by a plastic tube to a cylinder chamber. The circular blade is a cylinder connected to a screw assembly running in the cylinder chamber. The syringe is depressed in and held in position. The metal cylinder chamber is then placed on the cornea and the plunger released. The vacuum created in the chamber fixates the trephine to cornea. There is a view of the cornea through the cylinder of the trephine. A fixation cross located within the cylinder aids in centering the trephine on the premarked center of the cornea. For each quarter clockwise rotation the blade will cut 60 microns.

If a penetration is intended, the rotation continues until the quick "rush" of aqueous humor is evident within the cylinder, then the syringe is depressed in and the vacuum is released. The anterior chamber is filled with viscoelastic and the corneal cap is removed with corneal scissors or a diamond knife.

The donor button is removed from the well with a Paton spatula and placed on the cornea supported by the Healon. Using 10-0 nylon suture, the first cardinal interrupted suture is placed at twelve or six o'clock and the second interrupted cardinal suture is placed exactly 180 degrees opposite. The third and fourth cardinal interrupted sutures are placed 90 degrees from the two first sutures, a regular "baseball" diamond (square) figure is seen on the donor button due to compression of the four cardinal sutures. A running suture is placed with a 10:0 nylon suture, four bites per quadrant, 0.75 mm from each side of the wound down to Descemet´s membrane. When the running suture is tightened the four cardinal sutures are removed. Viscoelastic is generally removed with bimanual irrigation. In complicated cases after trauma or retransplantation, 16 single sutures are placed as some sutures may become loose. In complicated cases, single sutures are easier to replace compared to one loose running suture might endanger the whole transplant.

In eyes with dense cataracts, cataract surgery can be combined with PKP. After the trephination and removal of the recipient cornea, a capsulorhexis is performed. The nucleus is gently luxated out of the capsular bag and the cortex is removed with an irrigation and aspiration instrument. A foldable lens is placed in the bag and miochol is injected and the donor button is placed and sutured as already described. In most cataracts, we choose to perform the cataract operation at another day postoperatively. This staging provides an opportunity to correct refractive error induced by the PKP.

If the eye is aphakic, scleral fixation of the IOL is an option, but it is difficult to predict the end refraction which may result in significant anisometropia that can only be resolved by a contact lens. It might be prudent to wait and perform a secondary scleral fixation of the lens after one year.

In complicated eyes with invasive blood vessels, we either pretreat the cornea with a sutured amniotic membrane patch graft over the cornea or suture the amniotic membrane graft at the same time as the transplantation. This has significantly reduced the risk of an early rejection or delayed healing of the graft.

Postoperative Care

We have our patients stay overnight in the hospital, although elsewhere PKP is consider outpatient surgery and patients return home the same day. The day after the operation, biomicroscopy is performed and the IOP is measured. In complicated cases, i.e. after trauma, a contact lens is placed to reduce the risk of wound leakage; leaving the viscoelastic in the anterior chamber will also help to maintain a normal anterior chamber.

The patient is seen in one week to check the IOP and the sutures to assess that no wound leakage is seen using fluoroscein in the tear film. Steroid eyedrops are administered 6 times a day along with the addition of antibiotic eyedrops until full epithelialization of the graft occurs.

The next visit is one month where the visual acuity may still be poor, but the transplant is often totally clear and no reaction is seen in the eye. Steroid eyedrops are reduced to four times a day and the intraocular pressure (IOP) is measured. In eyes with glaucoma, IOP assessment is highly recommended as there is increased risk that the eye will respond with higher IOP from prolonged use of steroid eyedrops compared to eyes without glaucoma. In such cases, IOP should be checked regularly. The patient with an uncomplicated eye will have the next visit at three months. At that time, streroid drops can be reduced to three times a day. The next visit will be at 6 months and then 9 months at which time steroid drops can be reduced to twice a day. After one year we usually discontinue steroid drops in uncomplicated cases. A Swedish study of all PKPs performed in Sweden over a 5-year-period showed a rejection rate of 16% which is rather high. We now continue steroid drops for a longer period. After one year, some surgeons recommend one steroid drop every Monday, Wednesday, and Friday for the patients' life to reduce the risk of rejection. The sutures are removed after 18 months and glasses or a contact lens can be prescribed in many cases.

Complications

Postoperative complications are rarely seen today. Tissue banks now use advanced preservation techniques and media which has led to improved preservation of endothelial cell counts and has improved the survival of grafts to almost 100% in uncomplicated cases.

The most serious complication is rejection of the graft. The rejection rate is 10 to 16% in most countries. This might be due to the fact that steroid drops were discontinued after one year. With a second (repeat) PKP in the same eye, the rejection risk increases to 35% and after the third graft the risk is greater than 65%. The risk of rejection always exists as the immune tolerance is a dynamic process. If rejection cannot be controlled, there is a higher risk of developing secondary glaucoma—if this occurs early in life, there is a high risk of severe visual disability later in life. Infection of the graft is very rarely seen.[17]

Keratoconus Expectations

In 1997, Professor Claus Dohlman of Massachusetts Eye and Ear Infirmary at Harvard Medical School stated that 50% of patients will not experience better vision after PKP. At first, this statement appears counter intuitive since a diseased cornea is being replaced with a healthy cornea. Our experience confirmed that of Professor Dohlman: PKP even in uncomplicated keratoconus eyes does not always lead to better vision. This is largely due to high astigmatism and irregularity of the corneal surface that frequently occurs after PKP. A hard contact lens cannot always achieve functional vision in these extreme cases as it may be difficult to use a contact lens.

We have attempted to correct many eyes with high astigmatism with corneal relaxing incisions with and with a "LASIK-type flap". In some cases we performed an excimer laser ablation as well. The immediate results are often good but the cornea is often unstable and the problems of high astigmatism may recur. Four years ago we started to treat those eyes that had a clear transplant but an irregular surface and high astigmatism with LK. A 150-micron lamella is cut on the recipient cornea and 250-micron lamella is taken from the donor cornea and sutured in the corneal bed. That procedure will in most cases result in an eye that can tolerate a contact lens or even produce acceptable vision with glasses. In cases of irregularity, the surface of the lamella can be smoothed with the excimer laser and also reduce anisometropia.

Conclusion

The rate of penetrating keratoplasty is decreasing. It appears that modern lamellar techniques are on track to replace the old penetrating technique as the risk for rejection is much less with the former. We have performed more than 150 LK procedures with the follow-up of almost 4 years. We have seen only one epithelial rejection.[18] The recovery of LK is fast, the sutures are removed after three months, and in most cases glasses or contact lenses can be prescribed shortly thereafter. Artificial corneas are being used after repeat PKP failures. Alphacor (Addition Technology, Des Plaines, IL, USA) is approved by the Food and Drug Administration in the United States. The femtosecond laser is perhaps the most promising new technique for PKP as the precise cutting of the recipient cornea and the donor cornea may induce less astigmatism. The cutting may even be modified to give the transplant a wide base with a top-hat-shaped incision. In that way more endothelium may be placed and at the same time achieve a stronger, more stabile wound.

References

1. Kissam RS. Ceratoplastice in man. NY J Med 1844;2:281.
2. Zirm E. Eine erfolgreiche totall keratoplastik. Albrecht Von Graefes Arch Ophthalmol 1906;64:580.
3. Elschnig A. Keratoplasty. ARCH Ophthalmol 1930;4:165.
4. Henrik Sjögren. Zur Kenntnis der Keratoconjunctivitis sicca (Keratitis filiformis bei Hypofunktion der Tränendrüsen). Acta Ophthalmologica, Copenhagen, 1933; supplement II:1-151.
5. Henrik Sjögren. Lamellar keratoplasty. Acta Ophthalmologica 1961;Vol 39.
6. Niederkorn, JY. The immune privilege of corneal allografts. [Overviews] Transplantation: 1999;67(12):1503-8.
7. Whitsett CF, Stulting RD. The distribution of HLA antigens on human corneal tissue. Invest Ophthalmol Vis Sci 1984;25: 519.
8. Baudouin C, Fredj-Reygrobellet D, Gastaud P, Lapalus P. HLA DR and DQ distribution in normal human ocular structures. Curr Eye Res 1988;7:903.
9. Basu PK, Miller I, Ormsby HL. Sex chromatin as a biologic cell marker in the study of the fate of corneal transplants. Am J Ophthalmol 1960;49:513.

10. Maumenee AE. The influence of donor-recipient sensitization on corneal grafts. Am J Ophthalmol 1951;34:142.
11. Niederkorn JY, Peeler JS, Mellon J. Phagocytosis of particulate antigens by corneal epithelial cells stimulates interleukin-1 secretion and migration of Langerhans cells into the central cornea. Reg Immunol 1989;2:83.
12. Griffith TS, Brunner T, Fletcher SM, Green DR, Ferguson TA. Fas ligand-induced apoptosis as a mechanism of immune privilege. Science 1995;270:1189.
13. Li X-Y, D'Orazio T, Niederkorn JY. Role of Th1 and Th2 cells in anterior chamber-associated immune deviation. Immunology 1996;89:34.
14. Sonoda Y, Streilein JW. Impaired cell-mediated immunity in mice bearing healthy orthotopic corneal allografts. J Immunol 1993;150:1727.
15. She S-C, Steahly LP, Moticka EJ. Intracameral injection of allogeneic lymphocytes enhances corneal graft survival. Invest Ophthalmol Vis Sci 1990;31:1950.
16. Niederkorn JY, Mellon J. Anterior chamber-associated immune deviation promotes corneal allograft survival. Invest Ophthalmol Vis Sci 1996;37:2700.
17. Kenji Inoue, et al. Risk factors for corneal graft failure and rejection in penetrating keratoplasty. Acta Ophthalmol. Scand. 2001:79:251–5.
18. Stephanie L, Watson, Stephen J, Tuft, John K.G Dart. Patterns of rejection after deep lamellar keratoplasty. Ophthalmology 2006;113:556-60.

Section 5

Contact Lenses

Robert Joyce, OD

14 Contact Lens Fitting Overview

Introduction

When a patient has lost vision to keratoconus or keratoectasia, achieving a proper contact lens fit and restoring vision can be life changing for the patient. However, fitting keratoconic corneas can also be one of the greatest challenges in a contact lens practice. As the cornea is irregularly shaped in keratoconus, each cornea needs to be individually treated. In addition, each cornea belongs to a patient who has unique needs. There are many aspects of the patient, unrelated to the cornea itself which need to be considered when selecting the lens of choice.

After corneal rehabilitation procedures, patients may further benefit from glasses or contact lenses. Intacs, C3-R®, CK, LK, or PKP often enable further improvement in the quality of vision with contact lenses. The goal of Intacs, C3-R®, and/or CK is often to maximize vision with contact lenses or glasses. Depending on the degree of keratoconus before the procedures, some patients may be preoperatively counseled to expect being able to transition from rigid gas permeable contact lenses to soft toric contacts. Other patients may expect the procedures to allow them to wear glasses instead of contacts. For mild keratoconus, the procedures may improve vision without the need of any corrective lenses.

The type of contact lens and care system for keratoconus patients with or without prior Intacs, C3-R®, CK is also a function of the degree of acceptable vision based on patients' needs. An understanding of lifestyle, including career, hobbies and personality, need to be considered in the decision tree **(Figure 14-1)** when choosing a contact lens modality. For example, a student who frequently travels and spends most of the free time engaged in ocean sports may be required to trade some visual acuity for a convenient lens and care system. On the other hand, a very detailed-oriented person who is a "perfectionist" may be more inclined to wear glasses in combination with a complicated contact lens and care system to achieve as perfect vision as possible. It is helpful to know the expectations of each patient in order to be able to manage expectations with treatments.

Patient History

Patient history is a vital part of the fitting process. At the beginning of the initial contact lens fit, it is prudent to obtain the history through discussions with the patient, or, at the very least, to review a pre-examination

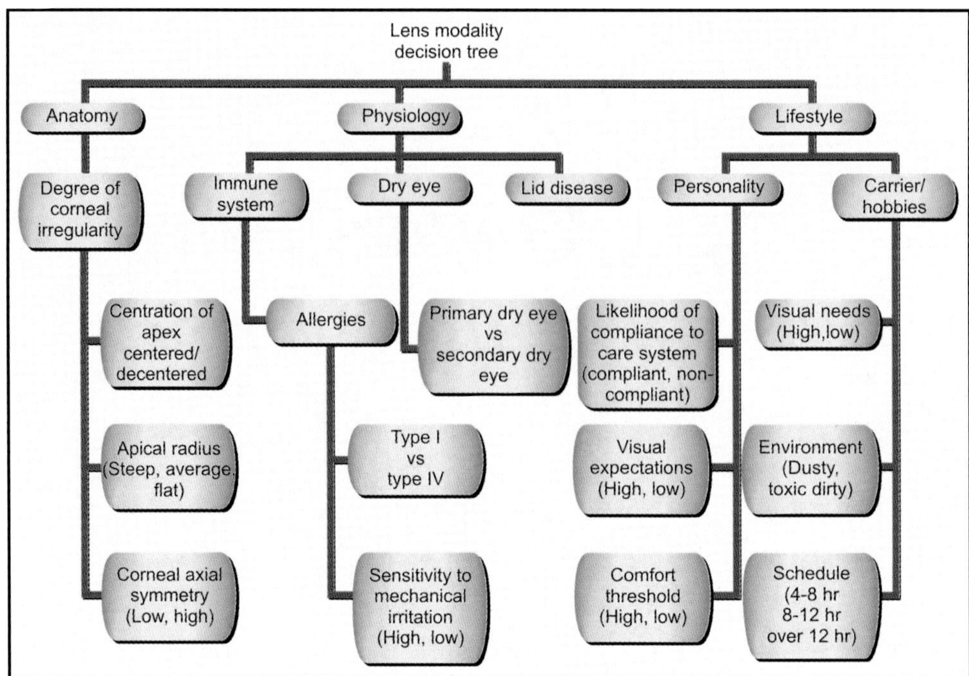

Figure 14-1: Decision tree for helping select type of contact lens.

history worksheet. The history taking, as with any examination, needs to paint a picture of the patient's past and present medical and physiological condition, along with inquiries about lifestyle. There should be a clear understanding of the patient's expectations at the end of the history taking process.

Anatomy

Corneal geometry has typically been the primary determining factor in the decision of type of lens that is fitted for keratoconus. Wavefront technology which directs the prescribing of higher order aberration corrections could prove in the future to diminish the importance of the understanding of corneal geometry.[1] Soft contact lenses with custom aberration controlled optics may compete with the optics that once only rigid gas permeable lenses could provide. New materials and developments with hybrids currently challenge soft lens comfort and provide rigid optics. Even though anatomy is an important consideration in the decision of what lens to use, it is becoming secondary.

Physiology

Considering the eye's physiology is very important to a successful fit, as eyes often react very differently to the same environment. Sometimes even two eyes of the same patient react differently from each other. The individual eye's immune response to the normal environment can be an indicator to how the eye will respond to wearing a contact lens for 14 to 16 hours a day. Patients who have eyelid disease (e.g. blepharitis) or dry eye syndrome need to be treated for their conditions to optimize results. Educating the patient on the need to manage these conditions for better success will also help manage patient expectations. Care products and systems can determine the success or failure of a fit. For example, hybrid lenses can trap solution or metabolic waste products under them and cause physiological problems that may not exist when the same solution is used with a soft lens or good adherence to digital cleaning with a fingertip is followed. Lubrications may be required to provide better comfort or a cushion to ease mechanical irritation. Some eyes are very sensitive to mechanical irritation and the slightest apical touch causes corneal staining in seconds; other eyes do not seem to be bothered to even heavy apical bearing. Good cleaning techniques are required to remove any pellicle that may build up on the ocular surface. This is especially important in large vaulting rigid or hybrid lenses. Large diameter rigid and hybrid lenses which vault the cornea are prone to trapping solution under them and some eyes will have reactions to the metabolic changes under the lens.

Since there is an exhaustive list of lenses to choose from, it is unreasonable to think a typical practitioner can become an expert or even familiar with all of them. It is advisable that the practitioner be familiar with a few modalities within the various lens groups. A well-formed decision tree that considers the anatomy, physiology and lifestyle needs of the patient is part of efficiently determining the most appropriate modality for the patient **(Figure 14-1)**. It is appropriate to choose the least complex system first and add complexity as needed.

Lifestyle

Career/Hobbies

Visual acuity is not the only consideration in managing expectations. The practitioner should consider the amount of time the patient spends at various visual tasks and diverse working environments, coupled with considerations and complications in contact lens care. For example, a firefighter will have very different needs than an accountant.

Personality

It is prudent to determine the likelihood that the patient will be compliant to prescribed treatments. Some patients want to be involved with the decisions about their care modality, while other do not. Some patients may come in with prior education on the different modalities and appreciate being further enlightened and involved in the decision about what lens modality is prescribed, while others have no prior knowledge of lenses. In either case, the prescribing professional is responsibile for the decision making and consultative prescribing.

Potential Side Effects

When fitting contact lenses, it is important to be aware that they are not without some degree of risk. Below is a summary of potential complications from contact lenses and solutions.[2]

- Irritation
- Dry eyes
- Corneal abrasion
- Bacteria/debris accumulation on lens
- Corneal edema (swelling)
- Corneal neovascularization
- Giant papillary conjunctivitis
- Sterile subepithelial infiltrates from allergic reaction
- Infectious corneal ulcers
- Corneal scars from infectious ulcers (some of which require corneal transplant).

Conclusion

There are many options to help improve vision in patients with keratoconus and keratoectasia. Understanding the patients and their needs greatly aids in contact lens fitting and ultimately success. It is prudent to consider patient history, anatomy, physiology, and lifestyle. There is no panacea for contact lens fittings of corneas with keratoconus and keratoectasia. Being able to match lens geometry to the cornea regardless of the modality is important, but considering the patient's needs and expectations is paramount to fitting success. Many patients with irregular corneas do not function well without their lenses and expectedly often over-wear them. This is the reason when fitting compromised corneas, regular office follow-up examinations are essential. To best manage patient expectations and make fitting irregular corneas a success in practice, a practitioner can select a lens from each of the various types of lenses available, become familiar with the various consultants of each of the lens manufacturers, treat the whole patient with a well-formed decision tree, and most of all, enjoy the results of helping restore better vision to these patients who suffer from keratoconus and keratoectasia.

References

1. Charman, WN. Cont Lens Anterior Eye. 2005;28(2):75-92. Epub 2005 Apr 26.
2. St Louis, MO. American Optometric Association. Optometric Clinical Practice Guidelines Care of the Contact Lens Patient. 2nd ed. 2006.

Robert Joyce, *OD,* **Carl Garbus,** *OD, FAAO*

15 Soft Contact Lenses

Introduction

There is an overall mindset among practioners that soft lenses are not viable option for fitting keratoconus and keratoectasia because they do not correct the optical aberrations from the irregular corneal shape. Some believe that the geometries do not match the anatomy of most irregular corneas close enough to achieve a good fit. In reality, soft toric lenses are viable options for correcting residual refractive error in many patients with keratoconus and keratoectasia. Advancements in custom prolate and oblate aspheric soft lenses can better compensate for irregular corneal shape and yield a better fit and vision.[1]

There are many manufacturers of soft lenses. There are two main categories: simple toric designs and complex aspheric designs. If the cone apex was not too steep, a simple high modulus soft toric lens often provided good optics and a comfortable fit. Frequency 55 (CooperVision, Inc.), Hydrosoft Toric XW (CooperVision, Inc.), and Preference Toric XR (CooperVision, Inc.) have yielded good results in keratoconus with or without Intacs. Hydrosoft Toric XW and Preference Toric XR are preferred if astigmatism is greater than 3.5 D. For keratometry values over 52 D, Hydrosoft Toric XW is preferable. Although the Hydrosoft Toric XW and Preference Toric XR may be considered "out-dated" lenses by some practioners, these lenses have stood the test of time and proven themselves to fit well with minimal lens rotation. The Frequency 55 lens has the advantage of a faster turnaround time from order to delivery than the other two lenses.

Depending on degree of keratoconus, some patients after Intacs placement can expect to eventually be fit with a hybrid SynergEyes® lens or a rigid gas permeable (RGP) lens to maximize vision. It is recommended that after Intacs, patients wait 1 to 3 months before being fit with SynergEyes® lenses and wait 6 months before being fit with RGP lenses to avoid "lens sensitivity syndrome". This is the recommended wait time to allow the corneal nerves to recover before placing SynergEyes® or RGP lenses, respectively. The soft toric lenses discussed above can be very useful during the interim wait time as they can be fit as soon as 2 weeks after Intacs.[2]

New custom soft lenses such as Hydrocone (Medlens Innovations, Inc) with steep aspheric optical curves can provide stability, centration, and comfort on eyes which have apical asymmetry (which makes fitting symmetrical gas permeable lenses or piggyback systems difficult). These lenses can be fitted to very steep corneas; they also come in a large range of powers. Base curve, optical zone and diameter can be adjusted to improve the fit and vision. Patients with very sensitive eyes or who have a low comfort threshold are also good candidates for custom aspheric soft lenses.[3] Understanding the back surface geometry of a soft lens is as important to fitting these lenses as it is with a gas permeable lens. Custom aspheric soft lenses can be ordered with prolate or oblate aspheric curves. Using decision tree **(Table 15-1)** can help predict if a soft contact lens is appropriate and which type to trial. **Table 15-2** summarizes soft contact lenses that have proven useful for keratoconus.

Table 15-1: Soft lens decision tree

Lens	*Anatomical characteristics*	*Physiological characteristics*	*Lifestyle*
Soft toric	1. Central apex 2. Symmetrical geometry 3. Average apical radius	Accepts higher sensitivity to mechanical irritation	1. Lower visual needs and expectations 2. Better for more complicated work environments
Soft aspheric	1. Steep prolate or flat oblate geometry 2. Asymmetric geometry	Accepts higher sensitivity to mechanical irritation	1. Lower visual needs and expectations 2. Better for more complicated work environments

Case Report

A 22-year-old patient with advanced keratoconus in both eyes had been unsuccessful with gas permeable lens designs as well as a piggyback lens system. Attempts at fitting gas permeable lenses resulted with lenses that popped out and would not center on the cornea. Glasses did not provide adequate vision.

Corneal Topography

Right eye:	Steep topography, and central K measured 75.00 D
Keratometry:	70.87 @68
	64.00 @158
Left eye:	Steep topography and central K measuring 72.00 D
Keratometry	68.00 @52
	61.12 @142

Slit Lamp Evaluation

Right eye: Dense stromal staining present in the central cornea extending to the surface
Left eye: Dense stromal staining present in the central cornea extending to the surface

Refraction

Right eye: –5.00 –4.00 × 75	20/80
Left eye: –7.50 –2.75 × 110	20/80

Contact Lens Selection for Evaluation

Based on the patient's previous history of lens decentration, a lens design that would allow for corneal centration and comfort was the goal. Hydrokone is an alternative lens design, which is the latest option for keratoconus and can be fitted after Intacs and other procedures. It uses a steep aspheric central curve, flatter para-central curve, with a center thickness between 0.35 mm and 0.55 mm for minus lenses to provide stability.

Contd....

...Contd

Hydrokone Evaluation

	Diagnostic lens parameters	Over refraction
Right lens:	5.30 / 8.60 / –26.00 / 14.8	+2.25 – 1.00 × 15 20/50–2
Left lens:	5.70 / 8.60 / –24.00 / 14.8	+8.25 – .50 × 137 20/30–

Note: Over-keratometry was used to determine how well the lens contours over the surface topography.

Final Hydrokone Lens Order

	Final Hydrokone Lens Order	Acuity
Right lens:	5.30 / 8.60 / –25.00 / 14.8	20/40+
Left lens:	5.70 / 8.60 / –15.00 / 14.8	20/40

Table 15-2: Table of lens designs

Soft lens designs			
Lens type	Apical radii	Apical centration	Size of ectasia
Frequency 55	Mild to moderate	Centered	Small to moderate
Preference toric XR	Mild to moderate	Centered to moderate	Small to moderate
Harrison keratoconus	Mild to moderate	Centered	Small to moderate
Hydrasoft toric XW	Mild to moderate	Centered	Small to moderate
Hydrokone	Mild to advanced	Centered to moderate decentration	Small to moderate

Definitions				
Apical radii	Mild (<45.00)	Moderate (45.00 to 52.00)	Advanced (53.00 to 60.00)	Severe (>60.00)
Apical centration	Centered (within Central 3 mm)		Moderate decentration (Between central 3 and 6 mm)	Severe decentration (Outside central 6 mm)
Size of ectasia	Small (<3 mm)		Moderate (3 to 6 mm)	Large (>6 mm)

Note: This table is intended to be a general guide to some of the lens options and corneal characteristics. It is not a comprehensive list nor does it take all considerations into account.

Case Report

A 48-year-old patient had been unsuccessful with gas permeable lens designs as well as a piggyback lens system.

Corneal Topography

Right eye: Steep topography, inferior temporal K measuring 50.00 D.

Keratometry: 47.62 @152
43.50 @62

Left eye: Steep topography, inferior central K measuring 61.00 D.

Keratometry: 58.87 @44
51.50 @134

Contd....

...Contd

Slit Lamp Evaluation

Right eye: Clear cornea, no slit lamp signs of keratoconus present
Left eye: Stromal thinning present with Munson's sign

Refraction

Right eye: Plano –1.75 × 75	20/40 (ghosting)
Left eye: –.75 –3.50 × 90	20/100 (ghosting)

Contact Lens Selection for Evaluation

Based on the patient's previous history of lens decentration, a lens design that would allow for corneal centration and comfort was the goal. Hydrokone was selected for fitting.

Hydrokone Evaluation

	Diagnostic lens parameters	Over refraction	
Right lens:	8.50 / 8.60 / –3.50 / 14.8	+3.00 –2.50 × 75	20/25
Left lens:	5.70 / 8.60 / –11.00 / 14.8	+2.00 –1.50 × 110	20/25

Note: Over-keratometry was used to determine how well the lens contours over the surface topography. The decision was made to steepen the base curve of the right soft lens in order to reduce the fluctuating vision. The right lens was designed as a toric lens and the left was kept as a spherical design.

Final Hydrokone Lens Order

		Acuity
Right lens:	8.20 / 8.60 / Plano –2.25 × 75 / 14.8	20/40+
Left lens:	5.70 / 8.60 / –15.00 / 14.8	20/40

This patient was able to wear the contact lenses successfully with glasses over the soft lenses for reading. His wearing schedule was 12 hours a day and he reported that the vision was stable throughout the day.

When fitting custom soft lenses, there are two potential drawbacks. The first is these lenses are often quite thick. It is common to observe small lacy neovascularization at the limbus moving into the cornea with low DK lenses. Since custom soft torics and aspherics are often very thick, the oxygen getting to the cornea is significantly decreased. Neovascularization is particularly important to watch in patients who have had or are expecting PKP. The second disadvantage is fluctuation of vision. It is common for the vision to fluctuate during the day with this type of lens. Vision could vary two or three lines on an acuity chart. This may be related to lens hydration.

Conclusion

The ability to correct higher order aberrations with adaptive optics using soft contact lenses is new technology that is currently being studied. In the near future soft lenses should be available with adaptive optics which can provide optical correction for irregular corneas. These lenses do not rely on rigid surfaces and the post-lens tear film for correction. As higher order aberration refractions become more clinically available, the ability to correct difficult irregular corneas may make soft contact lenses the optical lens of choice as well as the comfort lens of choice.[4]

References

1. Lim L, Siow KL, Chong JS, Tan DT. Contact lens wear after photorefractive keratectomy: comparison between rigid gas permeable and soft contact lenses. CLAO J 1999;25(4):222-7.
2. Nepomuceno RL, Boxer Wachler BS, Weissman BA. Feasibility of contact lens fitting on keratoconus patients with INTACS inserts. Cont Lens Anterior Eye 2003;26(4):175-80.
3. Medlens Innovation Inc. Guidelines for Fitting the Hydrokone™ Lens. 1325 Progress Drive Front Royal, VA 22630. 877-533-1509. www.medlensinc.com
4. Marsack JD, Parker KE, Niu Y, Pesudovs K, Applegate RA., On-eye performance of custom wavefront guided soft contact lenses in one habitual soft contact lens wearing keratoconic. Journ Refract Surg, in press.

Robert Joyce, *OD*

16 Rigid Gas Permeable Lenses

Introduction

There are many manufacturers and types of rigid gas permeable (RGP) lenses available. Most RGP lenses fit into the categories listed below. **Table 16-1** is a list of lens distinguishing features of different lenses. RGP lenses can improve vision in patients of keratoconus and keratoectasia. As mentioned earlier, it is recommended to wait 6 months after Intacs prior to fitting RGP lenses as fitting earlier can result in the eye being too sensitive to wear the RGP lens.

Table 16-1: Rigid gas permeable lens characteristics

Base curve	Spherical, aspheric, asymmetric aspheric, toric
Optic zone	small, medium, large
Peripherial curves	Spherical, aspheric, multi-curve, toric, tangential
Overall diameter	intracorneal, mini-scleral, scleral
Blends	None to heavy
Fenestrations	Central, mid-peripheral

RGP Lens Catagories

In the past it was sufficient to think of the geometry of RGP lenses in multiple, spherical curves. Today there is the ability to create exact geometry on the back and front surface of lenses. This geometry is described by radii, eccentricity or conic constants and diameter. Most are familiar with radii either measured in millimeters from the center of the reference sphere or in diopters. The diameter or chord diameter is measured in millimeters. The eccentricity or conic constant describes the rate of change of the radius of the curve. If the conic constant is negative, the curve flattens as the chord diameter increases and is considered the prolate portion of the ellipse and if it is positive the curve becomes steeper as the chord diameter increases and is considered the oblate portion of the ellipses.

A way to categorize RGP lenses is by lens features or designs. **Table 16-2** is a list of lens categories with notable characteristics.

Table 16-2: Rigid gas permeable lens designs

Lens	*Ocular surface curves*	*Front curve*	*Design*	*Typical over-all diameter (mm)*
Standard spherical	Tri-curve, spherical, toric	Spherical, toric	Known	8.0-10.5
Multicurve	4 to 5 curves, spherical	Spherical	Both known, proprietary	<14
Aspheric	Aspheric	Spherical, aspheric	Both proprietary & known	Varies
Aspheric multi-curve	Multi-curve, spheric, aspheric	Spherical, aspheric	Both proprietary & known	Varies
Aspheric asymetric	Multi-curve asymetric asphericity	Spherical	Known	Varies
Mini-sclerals/sclerals	Spheric/aspheric	Spheric	Known, proprietary	≤18

Lens types are categorized here based on back surface geometry and overall diameter. Past limitations of the ability to cut lens surfaces gave rise to spherical lenses with multiple zones. Practitioners found that more peripheral curves with moderate to heavy blends between the zones would approximate the highly prolate geometry of the keratoconic cornea. Lenses can be designed and manufactured with greater complexity with the help of contemporary lathe technology and computer programs. Lenses can be produced with aspheric curves, asymmetric eccentricities and even decentered apices. Another advantage to creating lenses with specific geometry is that it decreases the need to blend and polish the ocular surface of the lens, thus making production more precise and repeatable.

Lens Design Characteristics

The goal in lens design is to create a lens architecture which provides optimal optics and fit. The purpose of applying a rigid lens to the irregular cornea is to cover the irregularity with a new optical surface. The underling tear lens has a close enough index of refraction, with respect to its thickness differential, to not cause noticeable optical aberration with a fit that bears on the apex or has little to no apical tear lens.

New fitting approaches which stress apical clearance or only feather apical touch provide a thicker tear lens which increases the likelihood of noticeable optical aberrations. One approach to correcting for optical aberrations introduced by the cornea/lens relationship is making the back surface of the lens optic zone aspheric. This approach can also help negate some of the negative spherical aberration induced by high minus prescriptions. Another approach to the correction of optical aberration in the cornea/lens system is to cut an asymmetric front surface. Both of these approaches are still new at this writing and future studies will provide answers on the efficacy of these approaches.

Asphericity cut into curves in lenses for fitting purposes can be cut into the base curve or into the peripheral curves or both. Creating oblate and prolate eccentricities in curves for the purpose of better peripheral alignment and vaulting the corneal apex equates to more precise control of the sagittal depth of the lens. Asymmetric designs are similar to back surface torics, but controlling the eccentricity of different quadrants of the lens can bring the lens into better alignment with a highly asymmetric cornea.

Asymmetric aspheric lenses have been designed to accommodate the occasion when the geometric apex of the irregular corneas is not at the geometric center of the cornea. Using spherical and symmetric aspheric lenses on a highly asymmetric cornea will tend to cause the lens to decenter if the overall diameter is small or may result in too much lift off in a certain quadrant if the overall diameter is large. It is also common to observe areas of heavy bearing accompanied with bubbles using symmetric designs on eyes with highly asymmetrical corneas. Steepening the base curve and increasing the eccentricity as well as changing the overall diameter to allow the lens to land on a more symmetric zone of the cornea can help. In some cases, peripheral toric designs or asymmetric aspheric designs are required. **Table 16-3** provides a summary of RGP lens designs.

Table 16-3: Table of lens designs

Rigid gas permeable lens designs

Lens types	*Apical radii*	*Apical centration*	*Size of ectasia*
Tri-curve	Mild to moderate	Centered to moderate decentration	Small to moderate
Aspherics (Aspheric secondary)	Mild to severe	Centered to moderate decentration	Small to moderate
Comfort cone oval, nipple	Moderate to severe	Centered to moderate decentration	Small to moderate
McGuire cone	Moderate to severe	Centered to moderate decentration	Small to large
Rose K2/ IC /PG	Moderate to severe	Centered to moderate decentration	Small to large
Dyna Z	Moderate to severe	Centered to moderate decentration	Small to moderate
Dyna Intra-limbal design	Moderate to severe	Centered to large decentration (depending on apical radii)	Small to large
I cone	Moderate to severe	Centered to large decentration (depending on apical radii)	Small to large
Jupiter (mini-scleral)	Moderate to severe	Centered to large decentration (depending on apical radii)	Small to large
Keratoconus biaspheric (KBA)	Moderate to severe	Centered to large decentration (depending on apical radii)	Small to large
QuadraKone oval	Moderate to severe	Centered to severe decentration	Small to large

Definitions

Apical radii	Mild (<45.00)	Moderate (45.00 to 52.00)	Advanced (53.00 to 60.00)	Severe (>60.00)
Apical centration		Centered (within Central 3 mm)	Moderate decentration (between central 3 and 6 mm)	Severe decentration (outside central 6 mm)
Size of ectasia		Small (<3 mm)	Moderate (3 to 6 mm)	Large (>6 mm)

Table 16-3 is intended to be a general guide to some of the lens options and corneal characteristics. It presents not a comprehensive list nor does it take all considerations into account.

The QuadraKone lens (Truform Optics) is an example of a new type of fitting system which allows the practitioner to control the asphericity of the lens geometry in each quadrant **(Figure 16-1)**. New technology in lens production allows for the production of lenses that are not only aspheric, but asymmetrical. Corneas with highly asymmetrical quadrants can be fit with closer alignment using this design. The lens is fitted by using the lens trial set and describing the needed change in eccentricity in the various quadrants. Usually only one or two quadrants need adjustment in the peripheral curve eccentricity.

The rate of flattening can be increased or decreased to best fit the cornea in each quadrant. For example, the superior quadrant of a contact lens will need to be much flatter to compensate for a more negative conic constant, while an eccentricity in the lower quadrant that is closer to a sphere is optimum if the conic constant is 0. Trying to fit a typical symmetrical multi-curve or even a symmetric aspheric lens design to this cornea

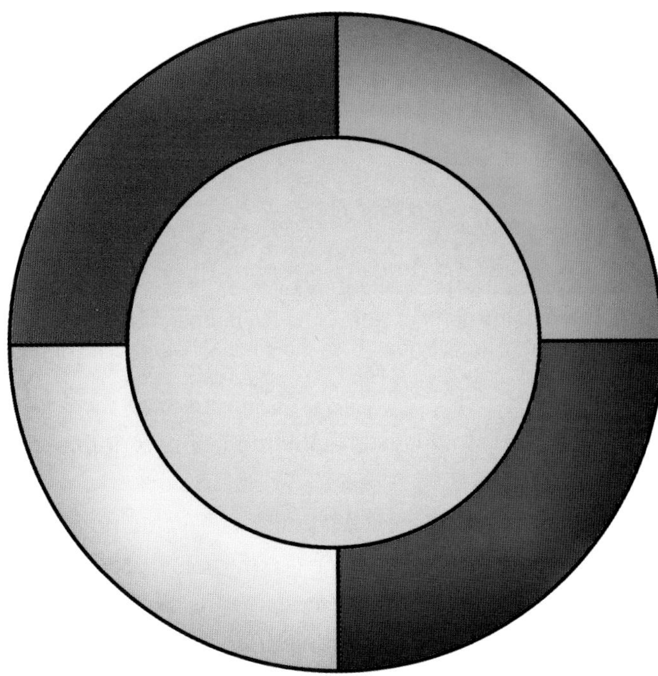

FIGURE 16-1: Schematic shows a contact lens with potentially different peripheral curves in quadrants.

could result in areas of unwanted bearing and mid peripheral air bubbles in the superior quadrant or excessive edge lift and peripheral bubbles in the inferior quadrant.

Lenses with proprietary curve systems can be spherical and aspheric or bi-aspheric. Typically "bi-aspheric" refers to a lens that has an aspheric zone or zones for fitting purposes and another aspheric zone for optical purposes. Proprietary lens designs have well defined fitting guides, trial lens sets and consultation support to help arrive at the best fit lens.

Mathematical Approach to Fitting Using Sagittal Height and Eccentricity

Using a purely mathematical perspective can aid in fitting lenses in keratoconus according to Randy Kojima (Precision Technology Service,Vancouver, BC, Canada). Every contact lens is fit by matching the sagittal height of the lens to the corneal sagittal height (sag). By creating the ideal peripheral angle (local slope) of a lens to the angle (local slope) of the peripheral cornea, the ideal centration, comfort and physiological response can be achieved.

The first step in fitting the irregular cornea is to determine the sag of the cornea. As sag is not routinely used, it is useful to review its definition. In measuring the sag of the cornea for contact lens fitting, the "chord of contact" should be determined, which is the diameter between the two points of contact lens/cornea touch, "Y" in **Figure 16-2**. From this point of touch or peripheral alignment, the height of the cornea from this reference marker is defined by "Z" in **Figure 16-2**. Imagine an island with a mountain in the center. If the diameter across the island is measured, this could be considered chord diameter. From sea level across that axis, the height of the mountain would be considered the sag.

The goal in keratoconus is to create a lens with a higher measured sag of lens than cornea. By creating a relationship with a tear layer cushion between the lens and cornea, we can protect the eye from bearing and possible scarring. This is only one consideration. An equally important factor is the relationship of the

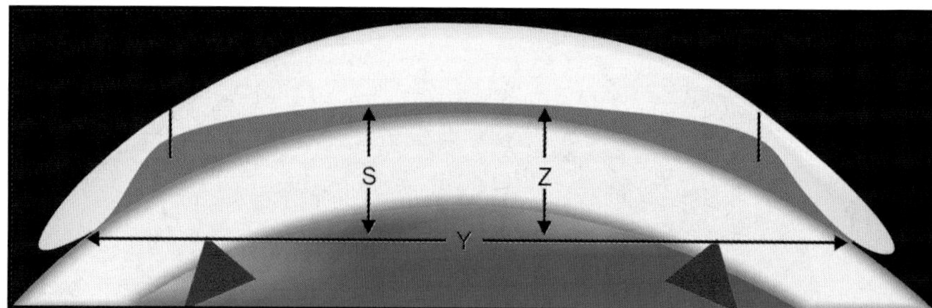

FIGURE 16-2: Chord of the contact lens. "Y" is the diameter of the chord of contact. "Z" is the sagittal height of the cornea. "S" is the sagittal height of the lens (Courtesy: Dr. John Mountford).

peripheral alignment of lens and cornea. How can a mathematical description of corneal shape and contact lens design be best matched?

Corneal topographers measure the rate of corneal flattening as E-value (Eccentricity), P-value (Shape factor) or Q-value (Asphericity). Eccentricity (E) may be the most commonly used. On any prolate cornea, E-value describes the rate of flattening of our cornea from the apex to the periphery. In the above island example, E describes the rate of flattening from the peak of the mountain (the visual axis) down to sea level (the periphery of the cornea where the contact lens touches cornea).

Corneal topographers indicate the rate of flattening for normal spherical or mildly astigmatic eyes as values between 0.60 and 0.65 E **(Figure 16-3)**. However, the average oval cone patient has E-values of 0.90 to 1.10 E and nipple cones typically measuring >1.20 E **(Figure 16-4)**. If a sphere is zero E-value, it is clear that keratoconic eyes significantly change in shape from the apex to the periphery. It is prudent to attempt

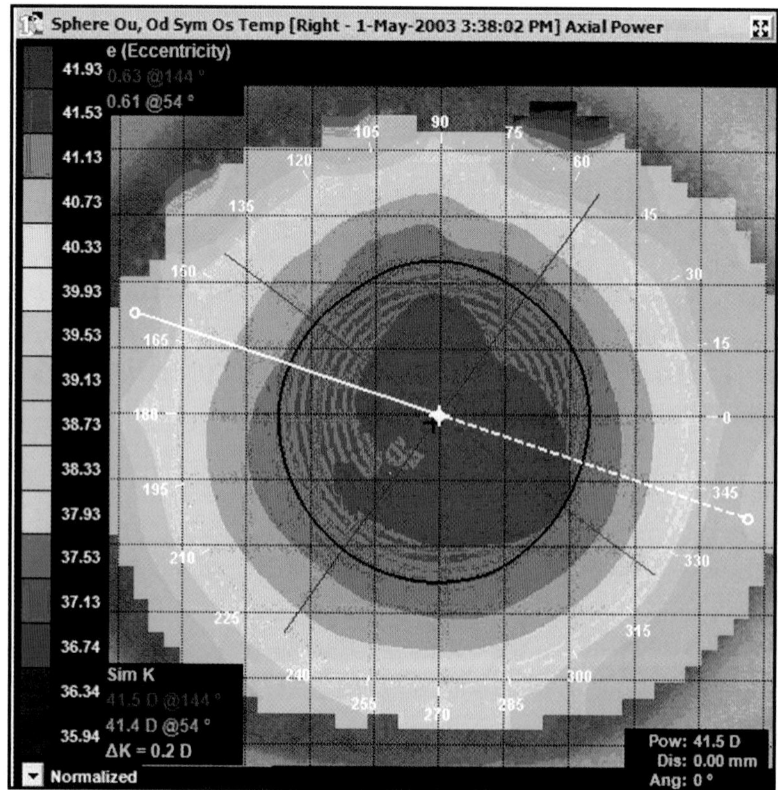

FIGURE 16-3: Corneal topography, normal eye. E-value of 0.61 is measured along the flat meridian which describes the rate of flattening of this normal spherical shape cornea.

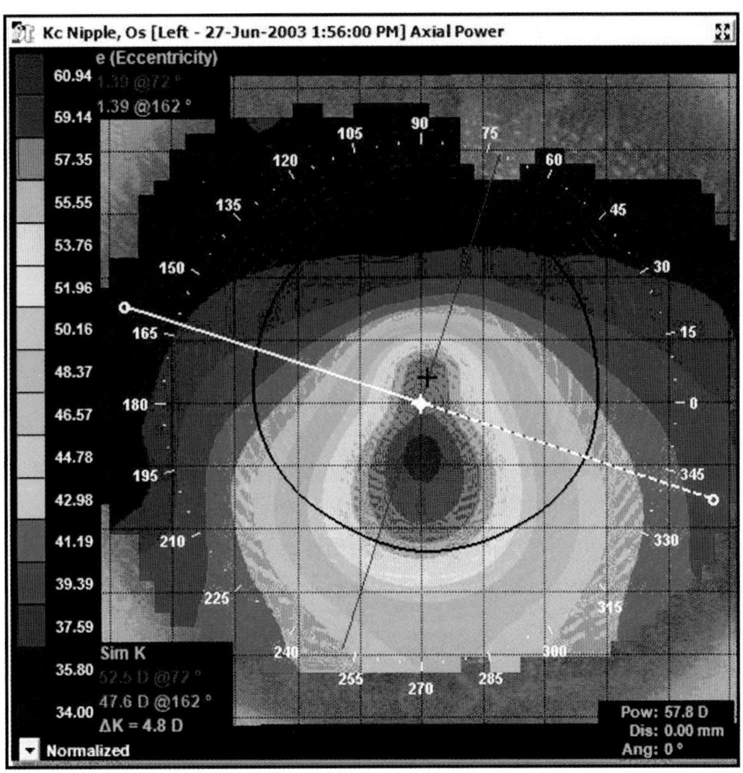

FIGURE 16-4: Corneal topography, central keratoconus. E-value of this nipple cone is 1.39 indicating a very high rate of change from the apex of cone to the periphery of the cornea.

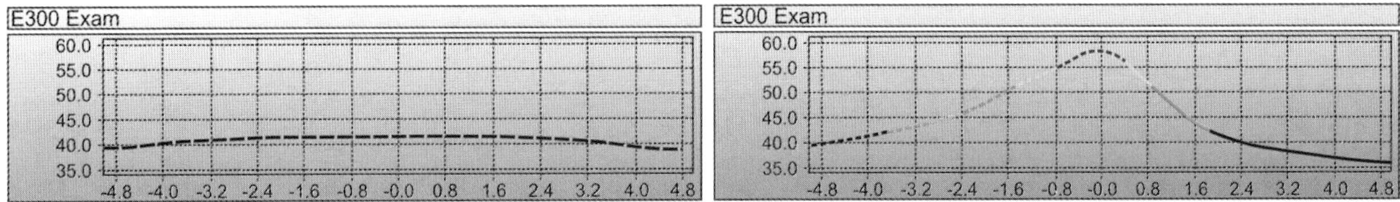

FIGURE 16-5: Comparison of the rate of curvature change. Along the flat axis between the normal spherical cornea (left graph) and the central cone (right graph). Note the significantly different rates of flattening between the normal eye and the keratoconic cornea. The X-axis indicates the distance along the flat axis with 0.0 mm corresponding to the visual axis; negative values (mm) and positive values (mm) correspond to nasal and temporal directions, respectively. The Y-axis indicates the radii of curvature represented along the length of the flat axis.

to match the rate of flattening of the lens to the high rate of flattening of the keratoconic cornea. It is also possible to analyze the cross-sectional curvature of the cornea **(Figure 16-5)**. One design that is fit solely on mathematical considerations (sag and E) is the keratoconus bi-aspheric (KBA) lens which was designed by John Mountford, OD and Don Noack, OD in Brisbane, Australia and manufactured by Precision Technology Services in Vancouver, Canada.

The KBA lens is a large 10.2 diameter lens which is designed to vault the cone (higher sag of lens than cornea) and align nearer to the corneal periphery where more symmetrical corneal shape may be found. Secondly, by manufacturing the entire back surface with an eccentricity value to match the corneal rate of flattening, the alignment relationship (angle) and surface area of contact can be optimized to create the ideal centration and comfort. Lastly, when creating a lens with a high back surface eccentricity or asphericity, radial astigmatism is induced. The KBA lens compensates for this by neutralizing the back surface asphericity with a compensating asphere on the front surface to eliminate this induced astigmatism, producing an optical sphere. The KBA lens design offers practitioners a logical and mathematic approach to fitting. Sag and E-values can be used to determine the parameters of a lens for a specific cornea.

A corneal topographer greatly aids the practitioner in determining the ideal trial and ultimately, final lens parameters. Many of the modern topographers efficiently incorporate contact lens software that suggests an initial lens. This mathematical method can be utilized without a corneal topographer. When a KBA lens is observed to bear on the cone, the sag is too low. The solution is to steepen the base curve. If the lens exhibits excessive apical clearance and generally associated reduced visual acuity, the sag is too high. The solution is to flatten the base curve. When there is excessive edge lift, the lens E-value is higher than the corneal E-value. The solution is to lower the lens E-value. When the edge appears very tight and/or the lens positions low, the E-value of the lens is lower than the corneal E-value. The solution is to increase the lens E-value.

The KBA lens is a specific lens design based on qualifying and quantifying the shape of the keratoconic cornea. One can apply the same sagittal height and eccentricity concepts to other contact lens designs. It is recommended to understand how the different parameters affect the sagittal depth of the lens. **Table 16-4** describes how the sagittal depth changes with lens parameter changes.

Table 16-4: Sagittal depth and lens parameter

Lens property	*Overall sag*
Increased radius of curvature	Decrease
Decreased radius of curvature	Increase
Increase chord diameter	Increase
Decrease chord diameter	Decrease
Prolate or negative eccentricity	Decrease
Oblate or positive eccentricity	Increase

Mini-scleral and Scleral Designs

Mini-scleral and scleral gas permeable lenses are another lens modality. Scleral lenses have existed since the beginning of contact lenses, but the modality was unsuccessful due to the materials that were used at that time. Today with the use of high DK materials and improved methods of lens fabrication, prescribing scleral and mini-scleral lenses are viable options **(Figure 16-6)**.

When considering a scleral lens modality, please review the decision tree (Chapter 14) to determine which patients will be the best candidates. The following is a list that represents those who would be the best candidates for mini-sclerals:

1. Patients with irregular corneas who have epithelial breakdown.
2. Steep cones on topographies where other lens modalities do not allow for lens centration.
3. Patients who are sensitive to the movement of the contact lens.
4. Individuals who work in a dusty environment.
5. Dry eyes and keratoconus.
6. Highly toric corneal transplants.

Fitting Process for Mini-scleral Lenses

Topography is a necessary tool in order to fit mini-sclerals. Information derived from the map is helpful to select the first diagnostic lens. Christine Sindt, OD recommends using the shape factor and reference sphere. This information is available from elevation map of a corneal topographer.

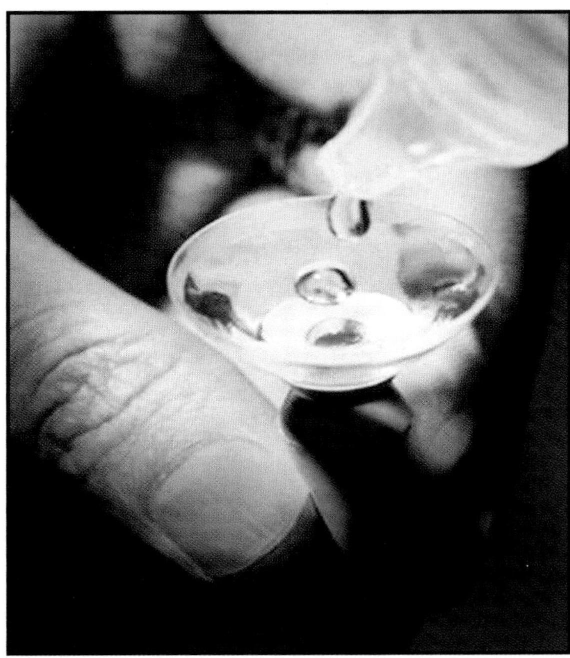

FIGURE 16-6: Preparing mini-scleral lens for insertion. The bowl of the lens is filled with saline solution to prevent bubbles from forming and to keep fluid underneath the lens.

Shape Factor

Shape factor is a measure of corneal asphericity and a derivative of eccentricity, defined as "e2".[1,2] Shape factors differ from eccentricity in that it is possible to describe prolate corneas as positive values and oblate corneas as low positive or negative values. In normal corneas, the steepest radius is near the center while the flattest curvature is toward the limbus. This is the definition of a prolate cornea. Patients with keratoconus have highly prolate corneas with high positive shape factor values. Less commonly, the cornea may display flatter radii centrally and steeper radii peripherally. This defines an oblate cornea. Examples of oblate corneas are seen in post-refractive surgical cases and in most cases of pellucid marginal degeneration.

Reference Sphere

Reference sphere is a measurement of the radius of curvature that best matches the average curvature of the cornea as measured by the elevation map on a corneal topographer. [1,2] The reference sphere is also referred to as the "fitting sphere" or "best fit sphere" and is the means by which the elevation map defines the height of the cornea.

Elevation is measured in microns and can be positive or negative. Positive elevation measurements at a certain point indicate that the corneal surface is above the reference sphere at that point, and negative elevation measurements indicate that the cornea falls below the reference sphere at a given point. [3,4]

To calculate the first diagnostic contact lens, simply use the following formula:

Reference sphere – Shape factor = Base curve of the mini-scleral trial lens.

Example

- Reference Sphere is 43.50
- Shape Factor is +.37 (prolate)
- Diagnostic base curve is 43.13

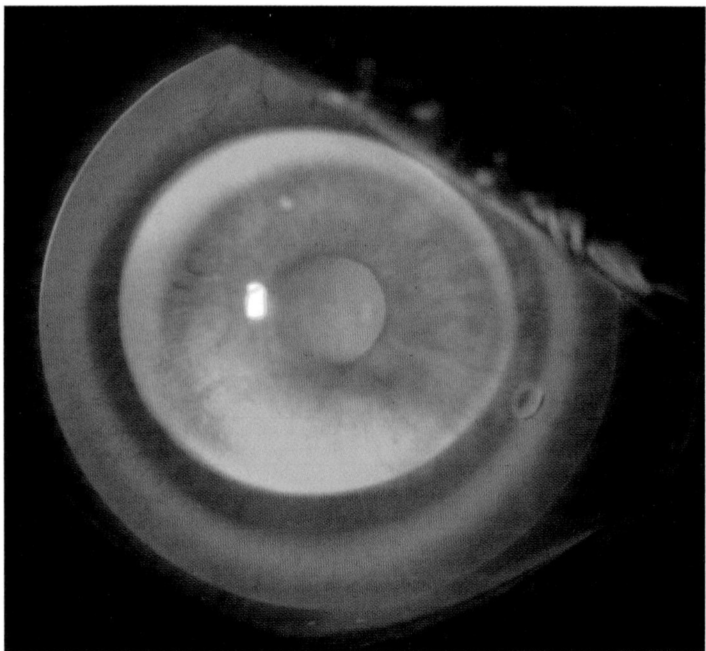

FIGURE 16-7: Ideal fit for a Jupiter mini-scleral design. Note the fluorescein pattern that shows diffusion inside the lens margin (Courtesy: Christine Sindt, OD).

The characteristics of an ideal fit for a mini-scleral would include at least 10 microns of tear film clearance over the entire corneal surface. In addition, increased clearance at the limbus is necessary to avoid impingement. The third element is scleral alignment with the edge just above the scleral epithelium. These lenses do not move when the patient blinks; however, this is not a closed system. There is some circulation of tears that occurs in the lens periphery due to forces on the surface of the contact lens with blinking action. In order to access a good fit in the periphery instill fluorescein and have the patient blink. After five or six good blinks some fluorescein should be observed permeating under the periphery of the lens **(Figure 16-7)**. If this is not seen, the lens is too tight. Flattening the peripheral curve system will solve this problem and allow diffusion. Conversely, fluorescein should not instantly enter from the periphery because then the lens may be too loose or show peripheral edge lift-off. This will cause discomfort for most patients.

Overall lens diameter is determined based on the patient's horizontal visible iris diameter (HVID) **(Table 16-5)**.

Table 16-5: HVID to lens diameter

HVID	*Lens diameter*
10.7 to 11.4	14.4
11.4 to 12.0	15.0
12.1 to 12.7	15.6

All of the curves on the mini-scleral lens can be specified when the lenses are ordered. Various fitting sets are available from Medlens innovations. This is truly a custom designed lens and a great adjunct to our armamentarium.

Conclusion

Fitting RGP lenses in patients with keratoconus and keratoectasia has become more complex due to greater options available to the practitioner. There are many types of base curves, optical zones, peripheral curves, overall diameters, blends, and fenestrations. A variety of lens designs offers a multitude of ways to further customize lenses. RGP lenses can also be modified in individual quandrants. Mini-scleral and scleral lenses are also viable options.

References

1. McKay T. A clinical guide to the Humphrey corneal topography system. Dublin, CA:Humphrey;1998.
2. Medmont International Pty Ltd. Medmont E300 corneal topographer user manual.Australia:Medmont Intl; 2006; March:43.
3. Caroline P, Andre M. Elevating our knowledge of the corneal surface. CL Spectrum 2001;16:56.
4. Roberts C. A Practical Guide to the Interpretation of Corneal Topography. CL Spectrum 1998;13: 25-33.

Dianne Anderson, *OD, FAAO,* ***Robert Joyce,*** *OD*

17 Hybrid Contact Lenses

Introduction

First generation hybrid contact lenses had a history of low oxygen transmission, being difficult to produce, separations at the junction of lens materials, causing neovacularization, and inconsistent optical quality. Notwithstanding these limitations, many practitioners believe the hybrid lens is an excellent platform for improving vision in keratoconus and keratoectasia. For some patients after Intacs, the goal is to switch from a RAP lens to SynergEyes® lens.

In 2005, SynergEyes®, Inc. has introduced a new hybrid lens in a high DK material. The lens has a low incidence of separation at the junction and is offered in a much larger variety of base curves and designs than its predecessor lens. There are currently has two basic hybrid designs available. The SynergEyes® A lens has a spherical base curve (BC) and a spherical peripheral or skirt curve. The SynergEyes® KC lens has a prolate ellipsoid optic zone and a spherical skirt curve **(Table 17-1)**. This lens can improve vision in patients with keratoconus and keratoectasia. This lens can be fit as soon as 1 to 3 months after Intacs placement.

When selecting a patient for a hybrid lens, all the factors of the decision tree apply (Chapter 14). The corneal anatomy that best fits the current SynergEyes® designs are corneas with low oblate and prolate eccentricities for the A lens and moderately prolate, central and slightly asymmetric ectasias in the KC lens. This lens seems appropriate to consider when a patient needs better optics than provided in a soft lens and better comfort than with a gas permeable lens. Caution should be used with this lens when a patient has increased mechanical sensitivity, a very steep corneal apex or very asymmetric (decentered) corneal apex. As fitting hybrids can sometimes seem counterintuitive, it may be very useful for practitioners with questions to call SynergEyes®, Inc. for consultation.

Fitting the SynergEyes® Hybrid Lens

Many challenges of achieving the optimal contact lens fit in cases of keratoconus, keratoectasia, and pellucid marginal degeneration may be overcome or at least diminished with hybrid lenses. Although counterintuitive, steeper base curves are required to achieve a healthy vault over the irregular corneal surface. A base curve that is too flat creates an undesirably tight lens on the cornea, which results in irritation at the junction and

Table 17-1: Table of lens designs

Hybrid lens designs

Lens type	Apical radii	Apical centration	Size of ectasia
SynergEyes A	Mild	Centered to moderate decenteration	Small to large
SynergEyes KC	Mild to advanced	Centered to moderate decenteration	Small to moderate

Definitions

Apical radii	Mild (<45.00)	Moderate (45.00 to 52.00)	Advanced (53.00 to 60.00)	Severe (>60.00)
Apical centration	Centered (within central 3 mm)	Moderate decentration (between central 3 and 6 mm)		Severe decentration (outside central 6 mm)
Size of ectasia	Small (<3 mm)	Moderate (3 to 6 mm)		Large (>6 mm)

Note: This table is intended to be a general guide to some of the lens options and corneal characteristics. It is not a comprehensive list nor does it take all considerations into account.

decreased wearing time for the patient.[1] The skirt curve helps maintain centration and is fit to match the eccentricity of the cornea. Eccentricity (E) values can be measured via topography or estimated from the horizontal visible iris diameter (HVID) measurement. Corneas with high E-values flatten at a greater rate from the apex to the periphery. Corneas with lower E-values are more spherical and demonstrate less flattening in the periphery. Corneas with an HVID greater than standard average of 11.8 mm usually require a steeper skirt curve to match the increased sagittal height of the cornea. Conversely, flatter skirt curves may be necessary to match the lower sagittal height of corneas with HVID less than 11.8 mm. [2]

Determining the Base Curve

With SynergEyes® lenses, the best fit is achieved using the "Total clearance technique." [3] This is defined as the optimal apical clearance fit rather than an alignment fit **(Figure 17-1)**.

Initial steps for apical clearance fitting in keratoconus have been suggested as follows:

1. A base curve approximately 1 D steeper than the average sim K reading,
2. A base curve approximately 1 D flatter than the cone apex. The cone apex is best measured via topography with the cursor placed over the steepest area on the cone. The radius of an inferior cone can be estimated via keratometry with the eye in upward gaze.
3. Base curves should be modified via diagnostic fitting. Optimal apical clearance is achieved when there are no bubbles or central bearing beneath the GP center.

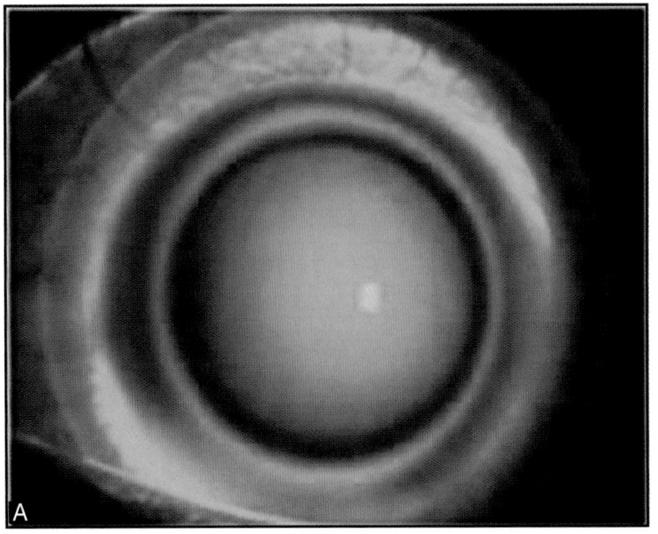

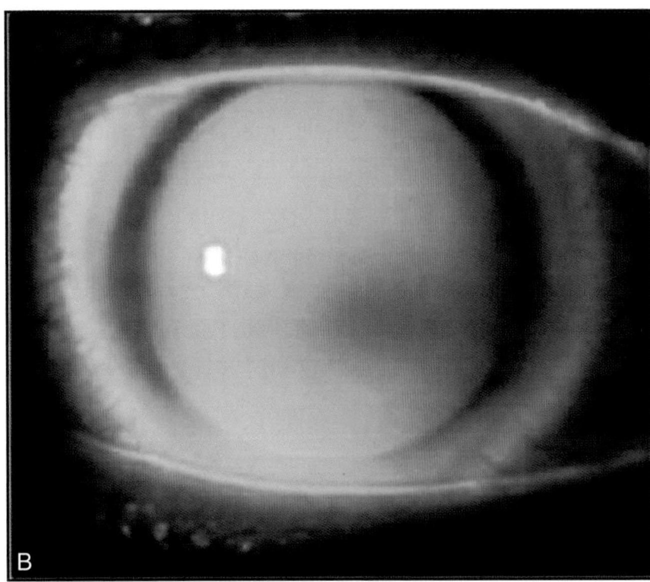

FIGURE 17-1: Fluorescein patterns with SynergEyes® lens. Apical clearance in normal cornea (A) and apical touch in keratoconus (B) is shown.

Determining the Skirt Curve

Initial skirt curves are chosen according to the following guidelines: [1]

1. Flatter skirt curves are recommended for corneas with greater E-values and/or smaller HVIDs.
2. Steeper skirt curves are recommended for corneas with lower E-values and/or larger HVIDs.
3. Skirt curves should be modified via diagnostic fitting. The appearance of bubbles beneath the skirt indicates the need for a flatter radius. The appearance of a ring of bearing in the gas permeable periphery requires a steeper skirt curve to achieve total clearance and maintain the optimal sagittal height relationship **(Figure 17-2)**. Edge fluting also requires a steeper skirt curve **(Figure 17-3)**.

Straight forward keratoconic fits require steeper base curves with flatter skirt curves to match the prolate ellipse corneal shape. More challenging fits such as global cones require flatter base curves with steeper skirt

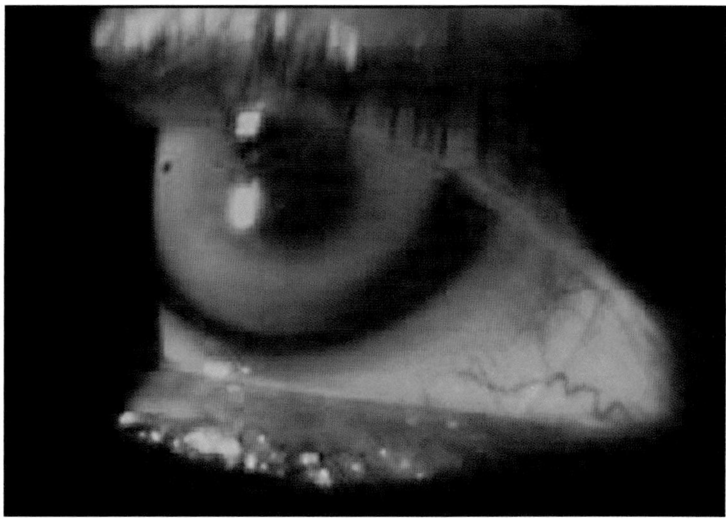

FIGURE 17-2: Fluorescein pattern with SynergEyes® lens with peripheral ring of bearing.

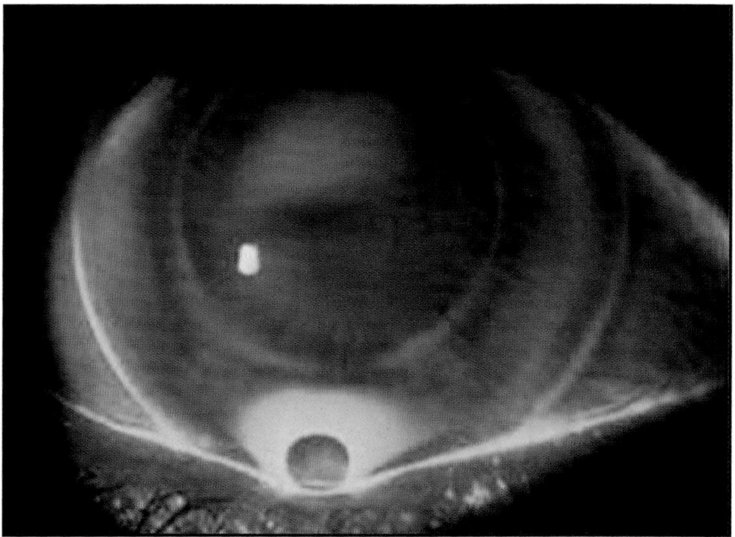

FIGURE 17-3: Fluorescein pattern with SynergEyes® lens with edge fluting.

curves. This helps eliminate apical bubbles and peripheral bearing beneath the gas permeable portion and simulates a reverse geometry fit.

Particular attention should be given to the architecture of the ectatic cornea. This is best achieved with corneal topography. Axial maps give a good overview while tangential maps give a more concentrated view of the cone apex. The SynergEyes® A lens is used to fit corneas with cone apices flatter than 47.50 D and the SynergEyes® KC lens is used to fit corneas with apices steeper then 47.50 D. The KC lens has an aspheric back surface that flattens from the center toward the periphery. This works exceptionally well on corneas with steep cone apices and high eccentricity.

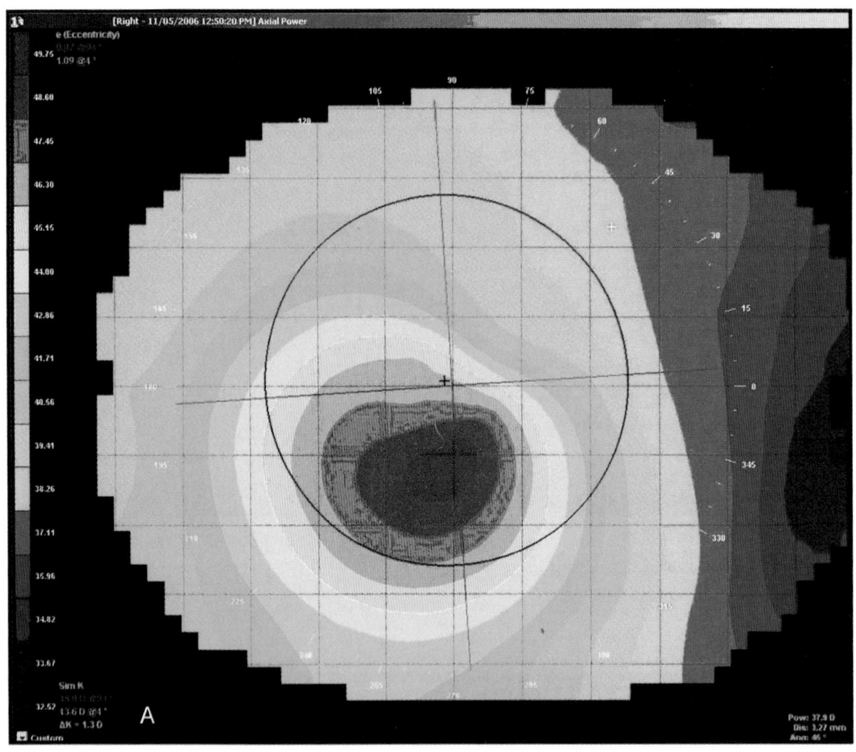

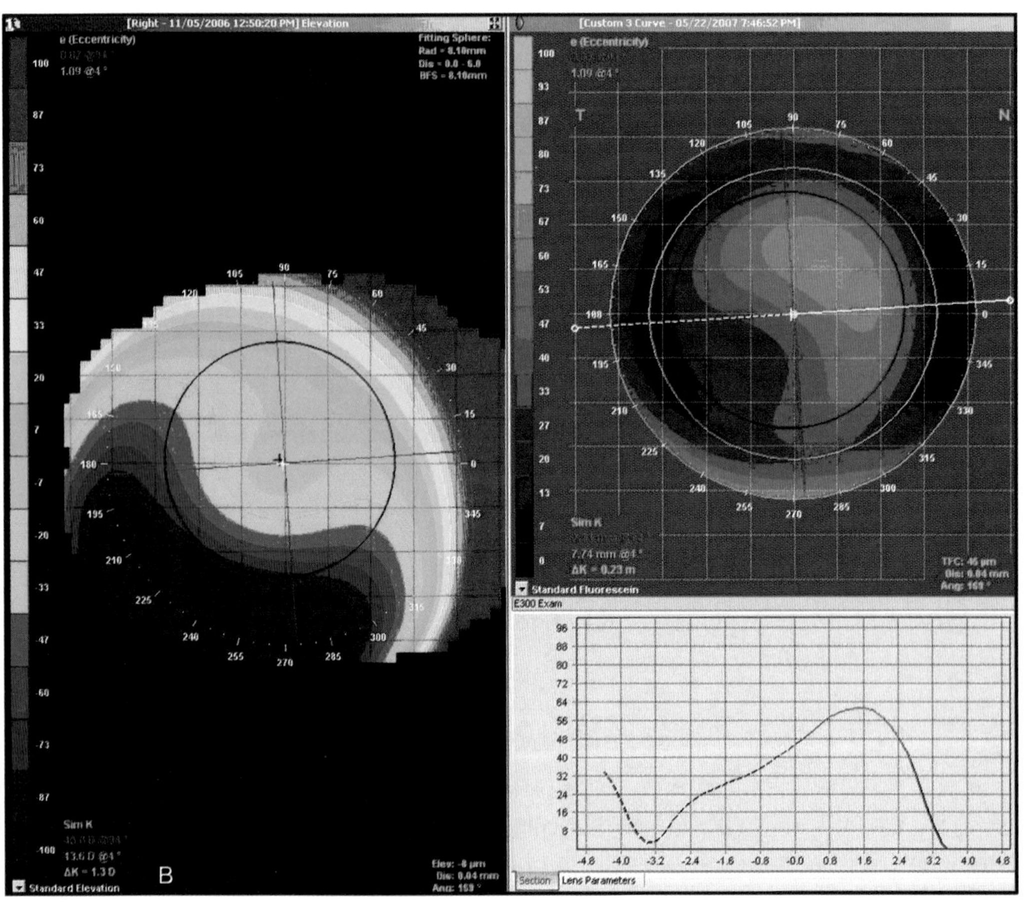

FIGURE 17-4: SynergEyes® A lens fitting for keratoconus. Corneal topography (A) and fitting profile (B) are displayed.

Case Reports

Keratoconus

A patient with keratoconus **(Figure 17-4)** was fit with SynergEyes® A. Ave Sim K=44.30 D, fit with SynergEyes® A, 7.5 (45.00) / –6.50/ 8.5, 0.70 D steeper than Ave Sim K

Another patient was fit with SynergEyes® KC lens. Ave Sim K=48.15 D

Fit with SynergEyes® KC 6.7 (50.50)/ -5.00 / 8.5, 2.35 D steeper than Ave Sim K.

Pellucid Marginal Degeneration

Many pellucid marginal degeneration (PMD) corneas may be fit well with the SynergEyes® A lens. The goal is to fit the base curve just steep enough to clear the steepest portion of the cornea without inducing a large bubble over the superior flat portion. The elevation map helps determine the best fit sphere as a starting point for diagnostic trials. It also helps predict the fluorescein pattern with that sphere. In many cases of PMD, a spherical lens pattern is not acceptable. The highly oblate shape of a PMD cornea may require and oblate geometry lens such as the SynergEyes® PS.

A patient with PMD and Ave Sim K= 42.2 D Fit with SynergEyes® A 7.9 (42.75)/ -3.25/ 8.9. The steeper skirt curve fits best on this oblate PMD cornea which steepens in the periphery **(Figure 17-5)**.

Post-penetrating Keratoplasty

Many post-penetrating keratoplasty (PKP) corneas have large amounts of irregular cylinder. These irregularities can be vaulted nicely with the SynergEyes® A lens. Another advantage to fitting the hybrid is ease of centration. Due to the high level of toricity of these corneas, it may be difficult to achieve adequate centration even with large diameter RGP lenses. Many of these patients would otherwise require a piggyback system. It is vital to maintain proper fit and oxygen permeability (Dk/t) of any lens on a post-PKP cornea. Neovascularization or irritation at the host/graft junction must be avoided. Start with a base curve close to the average Sim K reading when fitting the SynergEyes lens on post-PKP corneas.

A patient with PKP. Ave Sim K=42.8D, fit with SynergEyes® A 7.9 (42.75)/ –5.00 / 9.2.

It is difficult to achieve a desirable lens-to-cornea relationship in a PKP eye with excessive astigmatism **(Figure 17-6)**The SynergEyes® A lens centered well and vaulted the irregular surface nicely. The lens was fit very close to the Ave Sim K.

Conclusion

Hybrid lenses have come along way in manufacturing technology and in understanding of fit characteristics. As important as the changes that have been made in materials and production of new hybrid lenses is the understanding of how to fit them. The decision tree (Chapter 14) will help rule out patients who may not be good candidates for SynergEyes lenses. Ensuring that this lens vaults over the cornea and has sufficient sagittal depth will solve many fitting problems. Inspection for lens flexure will help understand when the expected visual results are not achieved. Understanding the counterintuitive fitting parameters will increase over-all fit success.

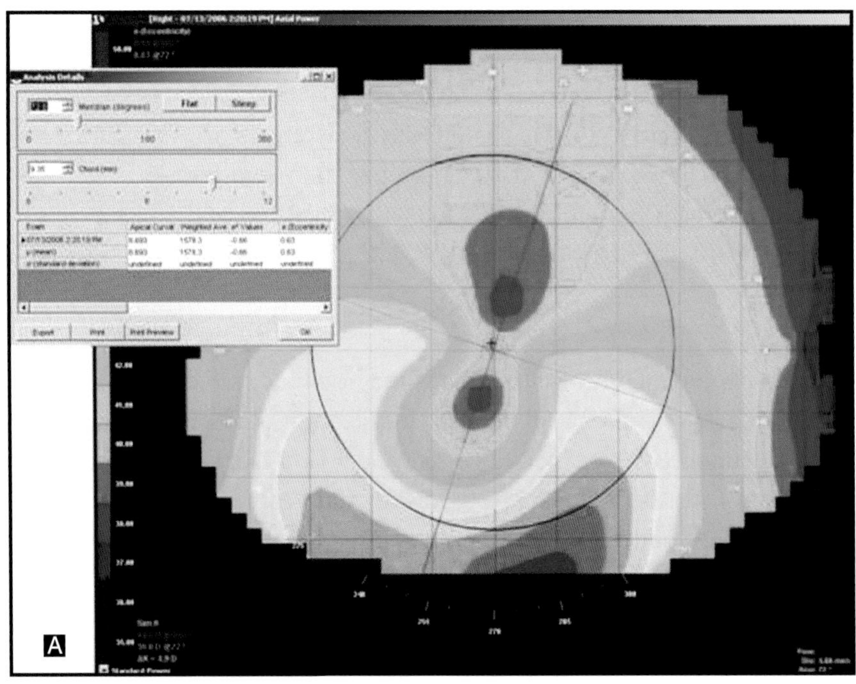

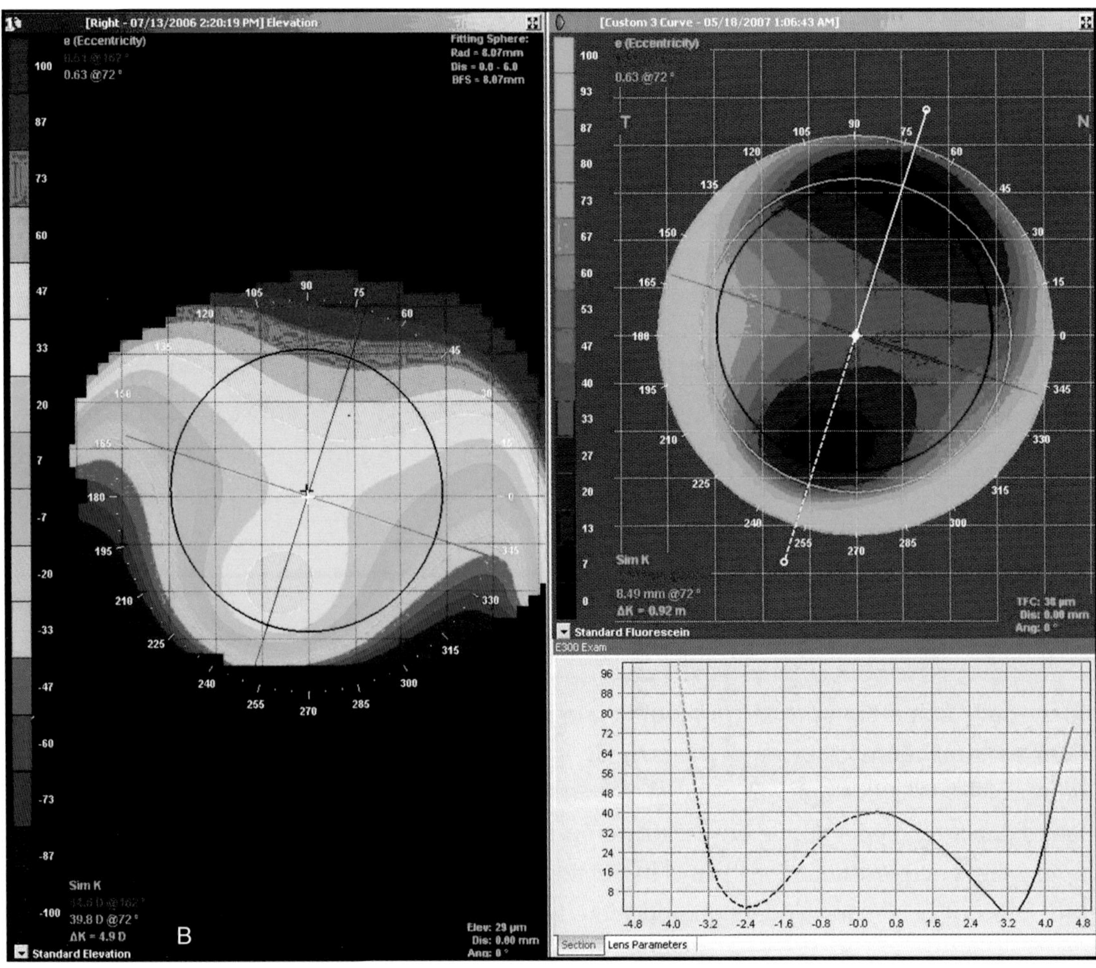

FIGURE 17-5: SynergEyes® A lens fitting for pellucid marginal degeneration. Corneal topography (A) and fitting profile (B) are displayed.

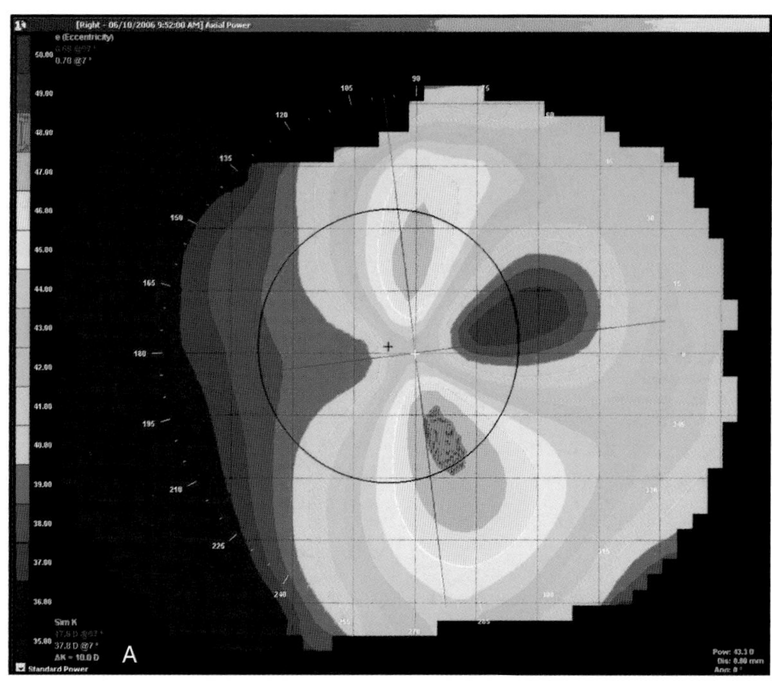

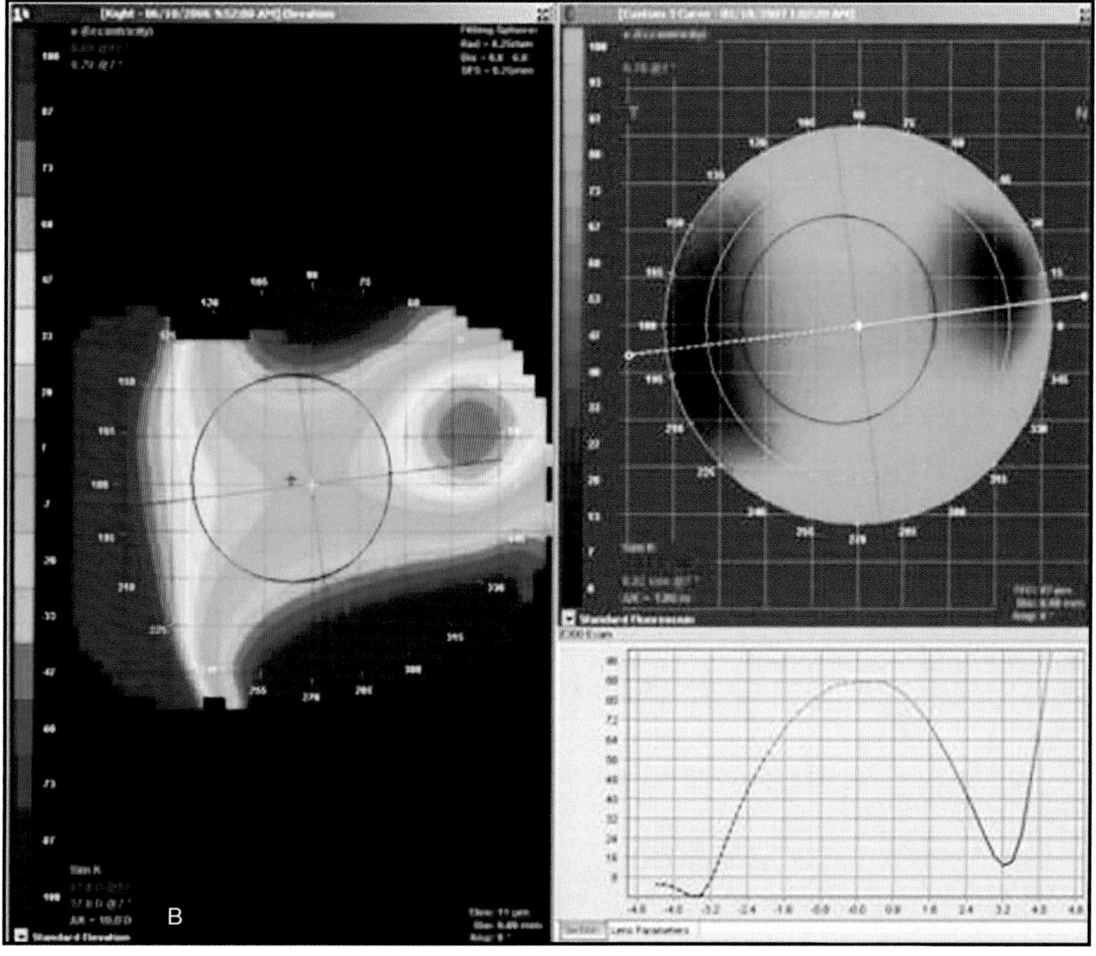

FIGURE 17-6: SynergEyes® A lens fitting for post-penetrating keratoplasty. Corneal topography (A) and fitting profile (B) are displayed.

References

1. Bergenske P. Prescribing soft toric contact lenses. CL Spectrum 2005;20:34-9.
2. Caroline P, Andre M. Correcting irregular astigmatism with the new SynergEyes® hybrid contact lens. Refr EyeCare 2006; Oct. Available at refractive eyecare.com/archive/oct 2006; Accessed Aug 3,2007.
3. DePaolis M, Beeman J, Ryan R. Fitting irregular corneas with a hybrid lens. CL Spectrum 2006;21:42-5.

Section 6

Toward the Ultimate Goal of Reducing Need for Glasses and Contact Lenses

Brian S Boxer Wachler, MD, **Shawn Jalali,** MD

18 Visian ICL and Verisyse Insertable Lenses

Visian ICL

The Visian ICL (Implantable Collamer Lens, Staar Surgical, Monrovia, CA) is a thin, foldable intraocular lens made from Collamer, a biocompatible lens material that blocks ultraviolet light **(Figure 18-1)**. The soft ICL lens is placed within the eye and behind the iris, in the posterior chamber. The ICL vaults over the crystalline lens **(Figure 18-2)**. The procedure is a painless, easy, and quick experience for patients. The lens can be placed in about 10 minutes. Since the Visian ICL is a thin and foldable lens, only a small (3 millimeters) incision is required to insert this lens. Once the lens is in place, sutures are typically not needed to close the incision. Patients do not feel the ICL. It is like a dental filling in that it is there, but one does not know that it is there. The ICL is not visible to other people, only to eye doctors who examine the patient with a microscope.

The goal of the Visian ICL is to improve uncorrected vision without the use of contact lenses or glasses. Patient with keratoconus may benefit from the Visian ICL as keratoconus is more mild without needing Intacs

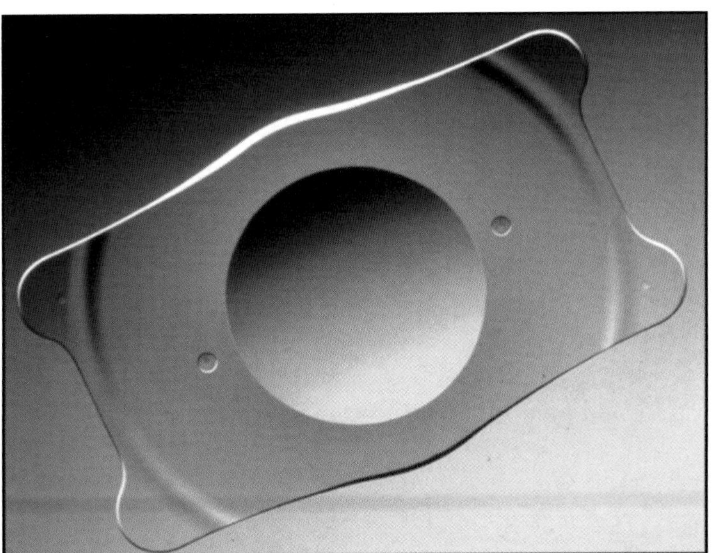

FIGURE 18-1: The Visian ICL.

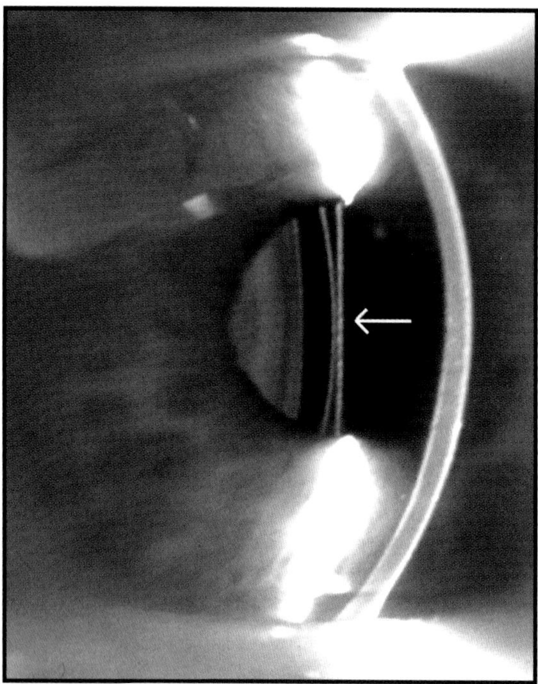

FIGURE 18-2: Visian ICL (arrow) vaulting over crystalline lens as shown with Scheimpflug imaging.

prior to Visian ICL, while other patients will need Intacs and/or other corneal procedure first before being able to consider Visian ICL. The above goal also applies to Verisyse lens which is discussed later in this chapter.

The Visian ICL has been proven to be safe and effective. The ICL is approved by the Food and Drug Administration (FDA) in the United States for correction of myopia in healthy eyes. The ICL has a long 14-year track record in Europe. The toric ICL and hyperopia ICL are available outside the United Stated and are presently under FDA studies in the United States. As many patients with keratoconus also have myopia, the ICL is well-suited to be considered in these patients. The ICL is available in powers between –3 D and –15.0 D with less than 2.5 D of astigmatism in the United States for the correction of myopia in adults and from –15.0 D to –20.0 D with less than 2.5 D of astigmatism for the reduction of astigmatism. Internationally, ICL is available in powers up to –23 D with up to 6 D of astigmatism for the correction of myopic astigmatism and from +3.0 D to +21.0 D for the correction of hyperopia.

Visian ICL has proven to be an important addition to vision correction options, especially for patients with keratoconus who have had corneal rehabilitation with Intacs, C3-R®, and/or CK. The Visian ICL has the advantage of correcting residual refractive error that often accompanies keratoconus and keratoectasia.

Advantages of the Visian ICL

1. Wide range of refractive correction
2. Small incision entry
3. Very high quality of vision and gain of best-corrected spectacle acuity
4. Safety and stability
5. Removable
6. Superb cosmetic results
7. Few complications

Quality of Vision

In our experience, Visian ICL often produces superior vision quality compared to the traditional corneal refractive surgery. After Visian ICL is implanted, many patients report a significant improvement in the quality of vision. It is common for patients to describe the quality of vision as "high definition vision" or say "this is the best I've ever seen in my life." This is likely the result of the lens position. The ICL is in the posterior chamber behind the iris and is closest to the nodal point (plane at the posterior lens capsule) than any other vision correction procedure.

Removable

It is natural for some patients to have apprehension about surgery. The ICL offers an advantage over laser vision correction in that there is a piece of mind for patients knowing that the ICL is potentially removable, although removing an ICL is rarely indicated. A major benefit of Visian ICL is that in the event that a patient experiences negative side effects, the lens can be removed or replaced, if needed.

Although meticulous preoperative measurements are taken to determine the power of the lens for each case, over- and undercorrection can occur. Options for under- or overcorrection are glasses, contact lenses, and ICL for residual refractive errors.

Safety and Stability

Many recent research studies show that the Visian ICL for correction of moderate and high myopia is a safe and effective procedure.[1-2] The multi-center FDA Visian ICL clinical trial with three-year follow-up concluded that the Visian ICL was safe, effective, and predictable to treat myopic errors. The three-year data of this study, based on the assessment of 526 eyes of 294 patients, produced the following results:

- 99 percent of patients were satisfied/very satisfied with their results
- 95 percent of patients had uncorrected visual acuity of 20/40 or better
- 59 percent of patients had uncorrected visual acuity of 20/20 or better
- Once vision was corrected, the correction was stable and did not change over the follow-up period
- Additionally, the incidence of glare, halos, double vision, night vision problems, and night driving difficulties decreased or remained unchanged from before surgery
- No change in glare (78.3%), no change in halos (79.4%), and no change in night driving difficulties (76.1%)
- No change in double vision (97.2%)
- No change in night vision (76.0%)
- No endophthalmitis, hypopyon, iritis, IOL dislocation, pupillary block, cystoid macular edema or hyphema was reported in any of the patients
- Raised IOP requiring intervention (3.8%)
- Retinal detachment (0.6%)
- Anterior subcapsular opacities (2.7%). Only 0.4% progressed to clinically significant opacities.
- Surgical reintervention (0.8%)

Halos and Night Glare

Because there is no ablation or any other changes to the cornea involved with this procedure halos and glare around lights at night are not commonly reported after this procedure. Patient with larger pupil sizes (over 7.5 mm) should be counseled that there could be a higher risk of experiencing halos or glare at night.

Trauma to the Crystalline Lens

Since the Visian ICL is placed behind the iris and in front of the crystalline lens, potential trauma to the crystalline lens may result. Fortunately, the final version of the ICL that is commercialized (V4 model) provides excellent vault over the crystalline lens. Trauma to the crystalline lens could be minor and cause only a small anterior subcapsular opacity which usually does not affect the outcome of the operation. If subcapsular opacities develop and become large they may be visually significant and require a phacoemulsification with intraocular lens implantation. This is very rare. Identifying that there is no vault (ICL touching crystalline lens) appears to be a risk factor. If no vault is present and a small subcapsular opacity if developing, the ICL can be exchanged for a longer lens that will provide appropriate vaulting over the crystalline lens.

Peripheral Iridectomy

It is recommended that beginning ICL surgeons make the peripheral iridectomies (PIs) with a Nd:Yag laser 2 weeks prior to ICL implantation. This allows the new ICL surgeon to focus on ICL placement on the procedure day. Two laser PIs should be made superiorly several clock hours apart. It is important to confirm the PIs are patent by visualizing anterior capsule through the opening. Merely observing a "red reflex" through the iris is not a guarantee of patency as the thin, intact iris posterior pigment epithelium allows a red reflex, but the PI is not patent. Non-patent PIs have the risk of elevated intraocular pressure (IOP) postoperatively. It is worth reiterating that the anterior capsule should be visualized to confirm the posterior pigment epithelium of the iris is not intact which will allow aqueous to flow through the PI. It can be a challenge to visualize capsule through the iris opening since pigment is often floating in the anterior chamber during the laser PI procedure which may obscure the view. If IOP remains elevated in the postoperative period after ICL placement, the surgeon should have a high level of suspicion of non-patent PIs and consider repeat Nd:Yag PI.

Experienced ICL surgeons may consider surgical PIs that are made on the day of ICL insertion. Here the surgeon can perform a surgical iridectomy in the operating room immediately after ICL implantation following instillation of an intracameral miotic. We perform a surgical vacuum iridectomy after implantation of the lens in the same session after the Visian ICL is implanted.[3] This techniques avoids patients needing the laser PI two weeks in advance. Vacuum PI side effects are rare. One possible side effect is self-limited iris bleeding into the anterior chamber which resolves within a few days without any consequences. In sum, laser and surgical PIs are safe.

Increased Postoperative IOP

As discussed above, some patients might experience an increase in IOP. On the first day, the cause is usually retained to viscoelastic. If elevated increased IOP persists at 1 week, the cause may be: (i) early steroid response, (ii) non-patent PIs, or (iii) angle crowding from iris due to excessive vault. Inspection of angle, vault, and PIs allow the etiology to be identified. IOP reducing medication should be considered until the cause is resolved.

Case Reports

Case 1

43-year-old patient with keratoconus, high myopia and irregular astigmatism was referred to us for vision correction. Patient had prior surgical history of double segment Intacs implantation in March 2004 in the right eye which were explanted in August 2004 due to halos. The patient had pupils greater than 8 mm. Topography shows degree of keratoconus **(Figure 18-3)**. Preoperative manifest refraction (MRx)

Contd....

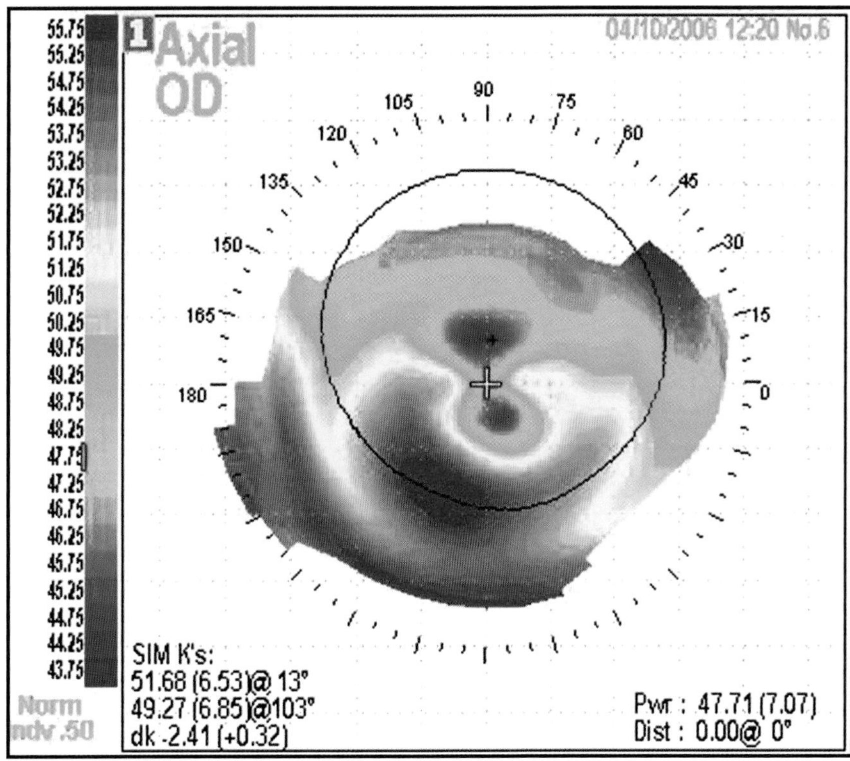

FIGURE 18-3: Pre-ICL topography of case 1.

....Contd

in the right eye was –10.75 –3.75 × 60 yielding 20/60. Uncorrected visual acuity (UCVA) was count fingers. A Visian ICL with a lens power of –15.5 D was implanted in the right eye. On first postoperative day, UCVA was 20/30 and MRx was plano –1.50 × 100 yielding 20/25+2. At 1 month postoperative visit, UCVA was 20/30 and MRx was +0.75 –2.25 × 85 producing 20/20+1. At 3 months postoperative visit, UCVA was 20/30 and MRx was +1.0 –1.50 × 075 giving 20/20.

Case 2

41-year-old patient with keratoconus and high myopia was referred to us for vision correction. Topography indicates inferior steepening in the right eye **(Figure 18-4)**. Preoperative MRx was –12.75 –1.50 × 165 yielding 20/40 and UCVA was count fingers. A Visian ICL with a lens power of –14.0 D was implanted in the right eye. On the first postoperative day, UCVA was 20/25. At 3 months postoperative visit, UCVA was 20/25. MRx was plano –0.75 × 160 yielding 20/25.

Verisyse lens

The Verisyse lens also known as Artisan lens (Ophtec, Groningen, Netherlands) is a single-piece intraocular lens manufactured from ultraviolet light absorbing polymethylmethacrylate (PMMA) **(Figure 18-5)**. It is known in the United States as Verisyse lens and in Europe as the Artisan lens.[4-6] The lens is inserted through either a 6.5 or 5.5 mm incision depending on the optic selected. The incision often requires sutures due to incision length. Within the anterior chamber, the lens is secured to the anterior iris by attaching the haptic to the iris **(Figure 18-6)** through a process called enclavation. The procedure takes about 20 to 30 minutes, but a newer foldable model will make the procedure faster as a smaller incision is used. Like the Visian ICL, the patients cannot feel the Verisyse lens.

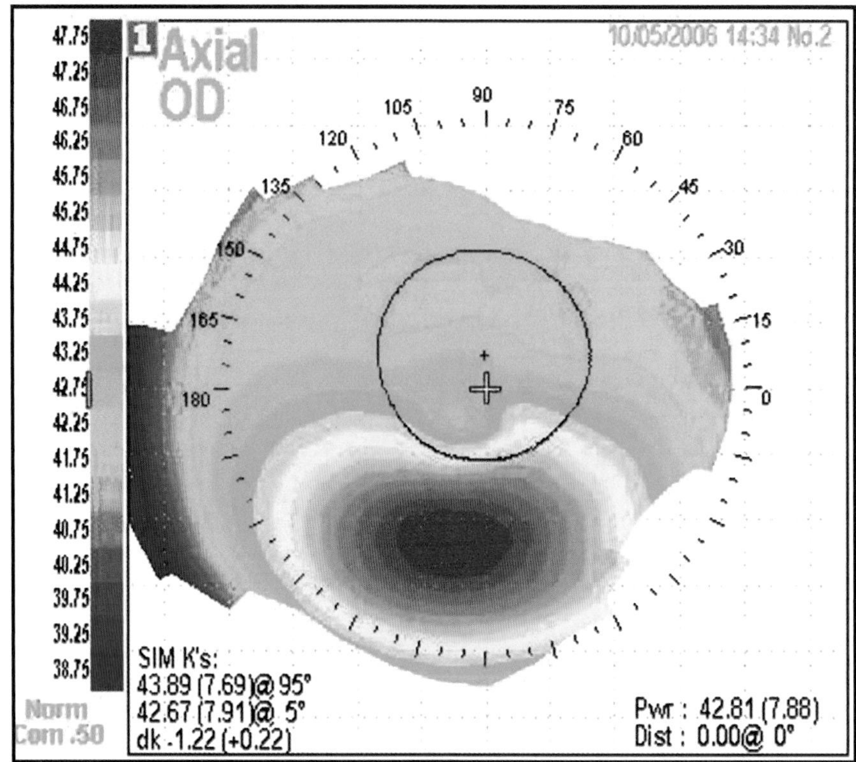

FIGURE 18-4: Pre-ICL topography of case 2.

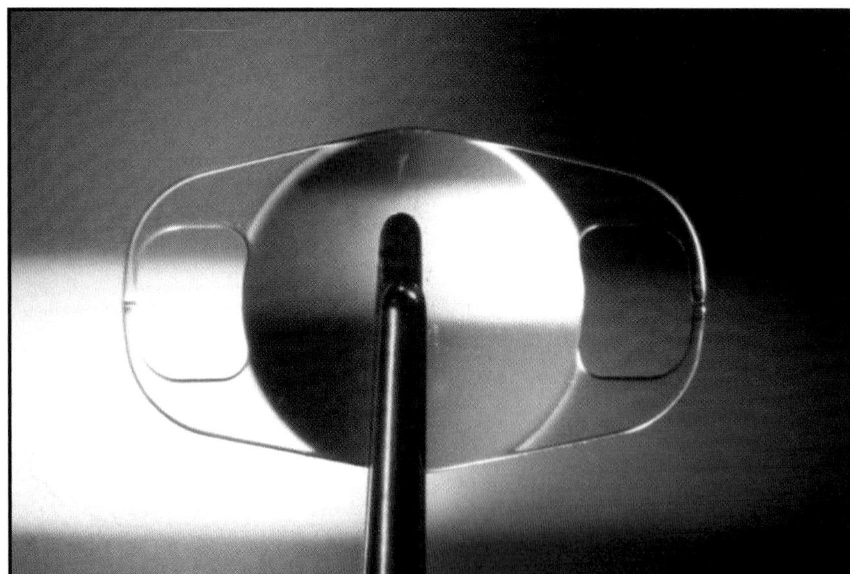

FIGURE 18-5: The Verisyse (Artisan) Lens. The lens is being held by a forceps.

The Verisyse lens has been proven to be safe and effective. It is FDA approved in the United States for correction of moderate to severe myopia in two different models: 5 mm optic for –3.0 to –20.0 in 0.5 diopter steps with astigmatism less than 2.5 D, and the 6.0 mm optic for –3.0 to –15.50 diopters in 0.50 diopter steps and astigmatism less than 2.5 D. Verisyse lens is intended for patients with pupil sizes up to 6.5 mm in low light, as larger pupils are at risk of glare and halos. The Verisyse lens has a 16-year track record in Europe under the trade name Artisan lens. The toric and hyperopic Verisyse lenses are under FDA study and

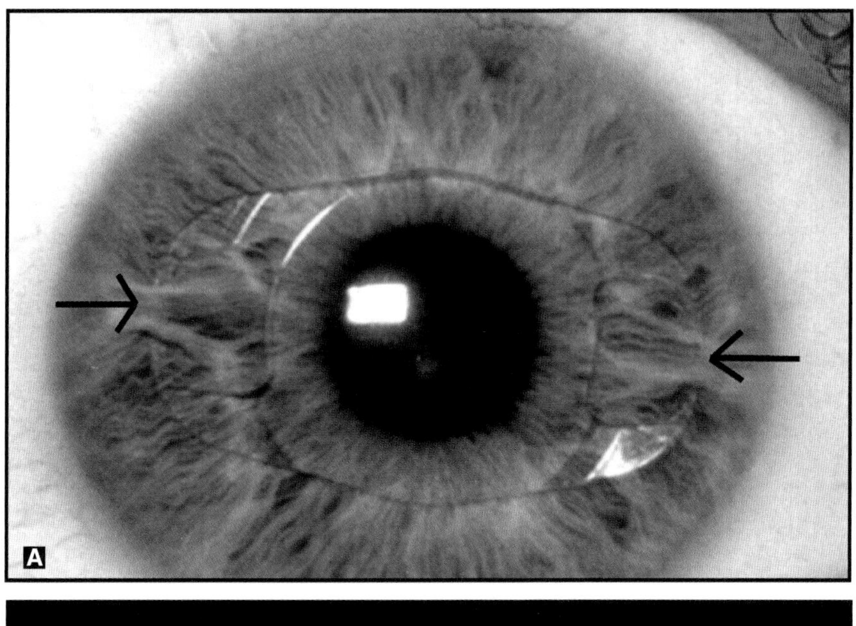

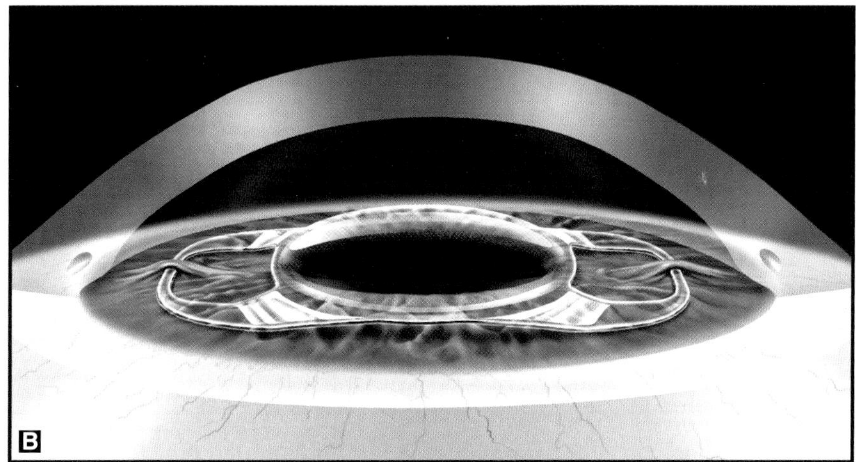

FIGURE 18-6: The Verisyse lens is attached to the iris (arrows) by peripheral clips on the lens (A) and it is positioned within the anterior chamber (B).

are available outside the United States. In Europe the Artisan lens can correct from +2.0 to +12 D of hyperopia and –2.0 to –7.5 D of astigmatism.

The Verisyse lens has helped many patients with keratoconus who have myopia. The Verisyse lens is an important option for patients with keratoconus who have had corneal rehabilitation with Intacs, C3-R®, and/or CK. As with the Visian ICL, the Verisyse can correct residual refractive error from keratoconus and keratoectasia. Over- and undercorrection can occur and can be treated with glasses, contact lenses, or Verisyse exchange.

Advantages of Verisyse Lens

1. Wide range of refractive correction
2. High quality of vision and gain of best-corrected spectacle acuity
3. Safety and stability
4. Removable
5. Few complications

Safety and Stability

In the FDA clinical study of 662 patients implanted with the Verisyse Lens, three years after the operation produced the following results:

- 100 percent had an uncorrected visual acuity of 20/40 or better
- 78.9 percent had an uncorrected visual acuity of 20/20 or better
- The majority of the patients reported no night visual symptom change
- No change in night glare (73.6%), no change in halos (72.0%) nor in starburst (78.5%)
- No endophthalmitis, hypopyon, no pupillary block , no raised IOP requiring treatment
- Retinal detachment (0.6%)
- Iritis (0.5%)
- IOL dislocation (0.8%)
- Anterior subcapsular opacities (0.7%). Only 0.25% progressed to clinically significant opacities.
- Surgical reintervention (4.2%)

Removable

As with the Visian ICL, the Verisyse lens is removable. It does require a larger incision as the lens is not foldable. A future foldable version will eventually reduce the incision size. To remove the lens, the haptics are de-enclavated, a process by which the iris is removed from the haptics, and the lens is removed from the anterior chamber.

Infection

Endophthalmitis has been reported after the Verisyse lens. Fortunately, this is very rare. Early intervention is important.

Trauma to the Crystalline Lens

During the surgical insertion of the lens, it is possible to inadvertently touch the crystalline lens with the Verisyse lens. Small numbers of crystalline lens opacities occurred in the FDA study with the Verisyse lens and the Visian ICL. Once the Verisyse lens is inserted and positioned, lens opacities should not occur to due the distance between the Verisyse lens and the crystalline lens.

Halos and Glare

Patients with larger pupils seem more prone to halos and glare with the Verisyse lens compared to Visian ICL. We suspect it is because the former is farther from the nodal point as it is in front of the iris, where the latter is behind the iris. It seems prudent to counsel patients with pupils greater than 6.5 mm about this risk.

Peripheral Iridectomy

A Nd:Yag or surgical PI can be performed as described above in Visian ICL section.

Increased IOP

On the first postoperative day, increased IOP can be elevated due to retained viscoelastic. Elevated IOP after 1 week may be due to a steroid response or unknown causes. There was a case in the FDA clinical trial of a patient with elevated IOP that required IOP lowering drops and eventually had the Verisyse lens removed in order to normalize IOP. This is a rare side effect. The Verisyse lens is not as sensitive to non-patent PIs compared to the Visian ICL as the former is positioned in the anterior chamber.

Case Reports

Case 1

A 53-year-old patient with keratoconus and high myopia was referred to us for vision correction. Topography shows keratoconus in the left eye **(Figure 18-7)**. Preoperative MRx was –15.50 –0.50 × 180 yielding 20/30-2 and UCVA was count fingers. A Verisyse lens with a lens power of –15.50 D was implanted. On the first postoperative day, UCVA was 20/50–1. At the 1 month postoperative visit, UCVA was 20/40–1 and MRx was +0.75 –0.25 × 0 yielding 20/40.

Case 2

A 25-year-old patient with keratoconus, high myopia and irregular astigmatism was referred to us for vision correction. Topgraphy shows keratoconus in the right eye **(Figure 18-8)**. Preoperative MRx was –7.25 – 6.25 × 20 producing 20/30–2 and UCVA was count fingers. A Verisyse lens with a lens power of –12.0 D was implanted. On the first postoperative day, UCVA was 20/50. At the 3 months postoperative visit, UCVA was 20/40–2 and BSCVA was 20/40+1 with MRx of plano –0.50 × 130.

Comparison of Visian ICL and the Verisyse Lens

Both Phakic Intraocular Lenses

- Are able to correct a wide range of myopia and astigmatism
- Correct vision by complementing the crystalline lens

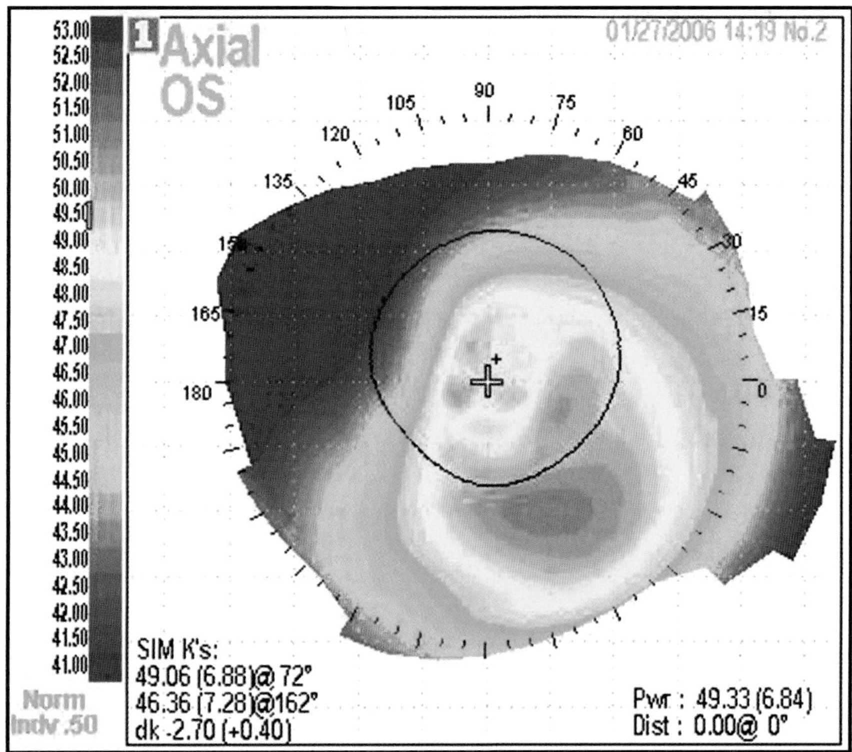

FIGURE 18-7: Pre-Verisyse topography of case 1.

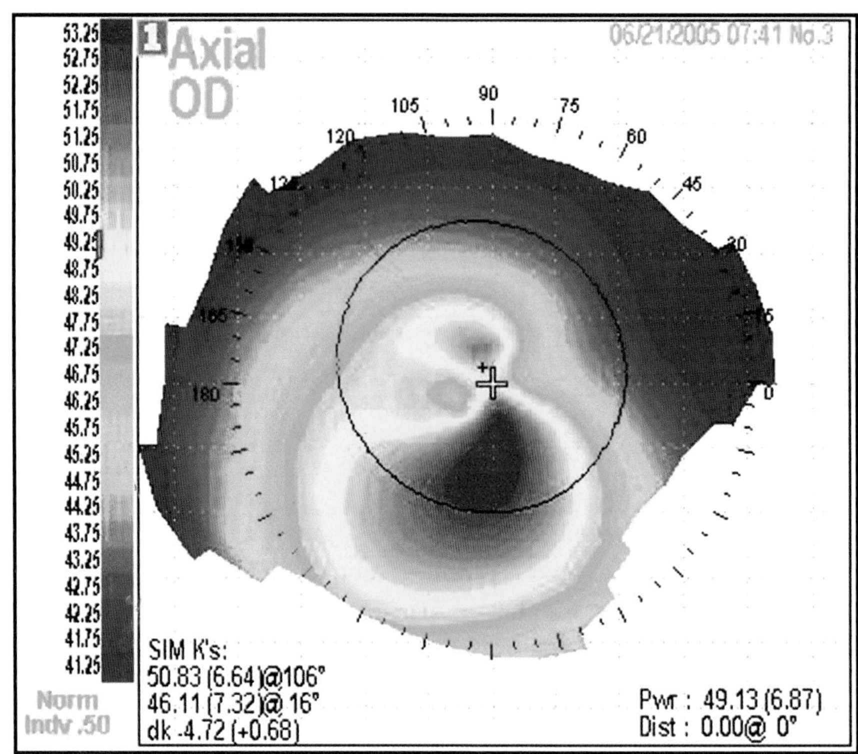

FIGURE 18-8: Pre-Verisyse topography of case 2.

- Are removable, if necessary
- Contain an ultraviolet filter

Differences between the Visian ICL and Verisyse Phakic Intraocular Lens

There are several differences between these lenses. These include:

- The Visian ICL is a foldable lens, therefore a smaller incision is used for the implantation of this lens. The small incision can correct small degrees of astigmatism and therefore we place this incision in the steep axis of manifest refraction. The Verisyse lens is not foldable and requires larger incision. Sutures are necessary to close the incision and there is a higher chance for inducing astigmatism. We also place the incision in the steep axis. With the Verisyse lens, if there is 2 to 3 D of astigmatism, we make a clear corneal incision; for less than 2 D of astigmatism, we make a scleral tunnel. The Veriflex (foldable Verisyse) allows for a smaller incision than presently used.
- The Visian ICL procedure is performed in 10 to 15 minutes, including surgical PI. The Verisyse IOL requires 20 to 30 minutes since it requires a larger incision with suturing. The Veriflex will enable shorting operating times.
- The Verisyse lens clips onto the iris and the light reflex off the lens can be visible to the patient in the mirror or an observer, while the Visian ICL is placed in the posterior chamber making it invisible to the casual observer.

On balance, both lenses are excellent. We have extensive experience with both lenses and conducted a retrospective study of two groups of patients who were treated for myopia. Keratoconus was not present in these groups. In the Visian ICL group, average myopia was –11.0 D ranging from –3.5 D to –20.0 D while the Verisyse group had average of 10.69 D ranging from –5.50 D to –18.0 D. Average age was 40 years

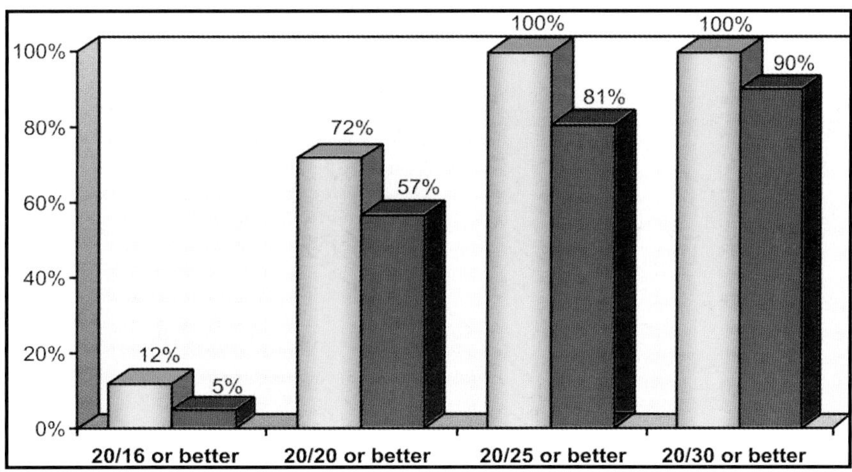

FIGURE 18-9: Comparison of UCVA in Visian ICL and Verisyse groups. The Visian ICL (yellow bars) showed better UCVA than Verisyse lens (pink bars).

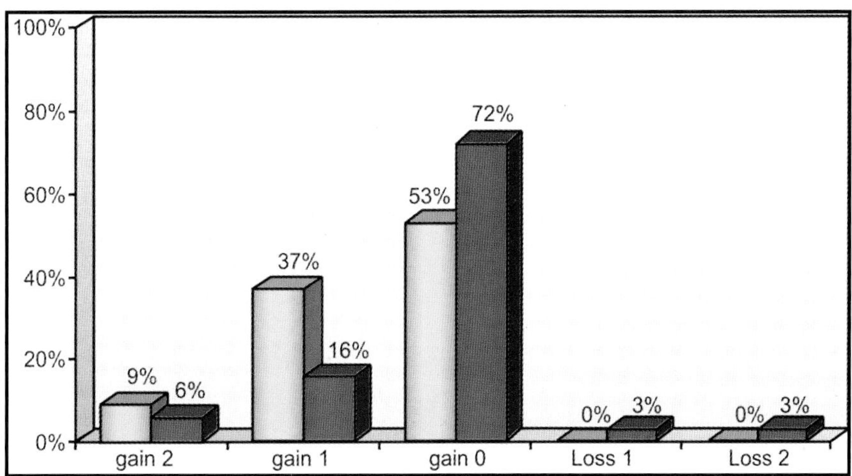

FIGURE 18-10: Comparison of BSCVA changes in Visian ICL and Verisyse groups. The Visian ICL (yellow bars) showed greater gain lines of BSCVA than the Verisyse lens (pink bars).

in ICL group and 41 years in Verisyse group. We found both UCVA **(Figure 18-9)** and BSCVA **(Figure 18-10)** improvement was greater in the Visian ICL than the Verisyse lens. We believe the greater gain in BSCVA in the ICL group results from the ICL being closer to the nodal point than the Verisyse lens. In addition, we found the Visian ICL to be more accurate. Deviation from target in the ICL group was only 0.003 D +/– 0.40 and in the Verisyse was –0.35 D +/– 0.88. The lower standard deviation in the ICL group reflects greater accuracy. The scattergrams also show the difference in accuracy **(Figures 18-11 and 18-12)**.

Conclusion

The Visian ICL and Verisyse lenses provide the ability to significantly improve uncorrected visual acuity without altering the corneal shape. Often after correction of a significant amount of myopia and astigmatism, BSCVA can improve compared to preoperative values. This likely reflects the benefit of the lens position being behind the cornea.

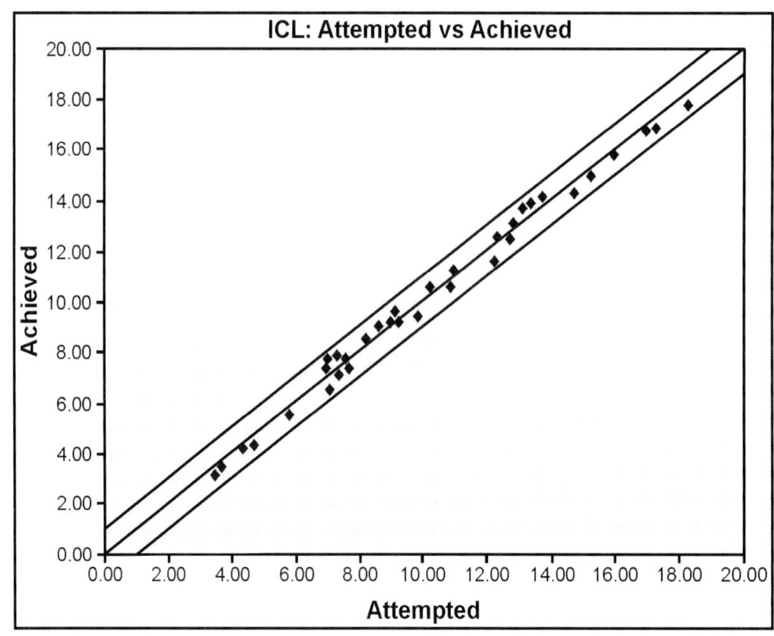

FIGURE 18-11: Scattergram of attempted vs achieved correction for Visian ICL group.

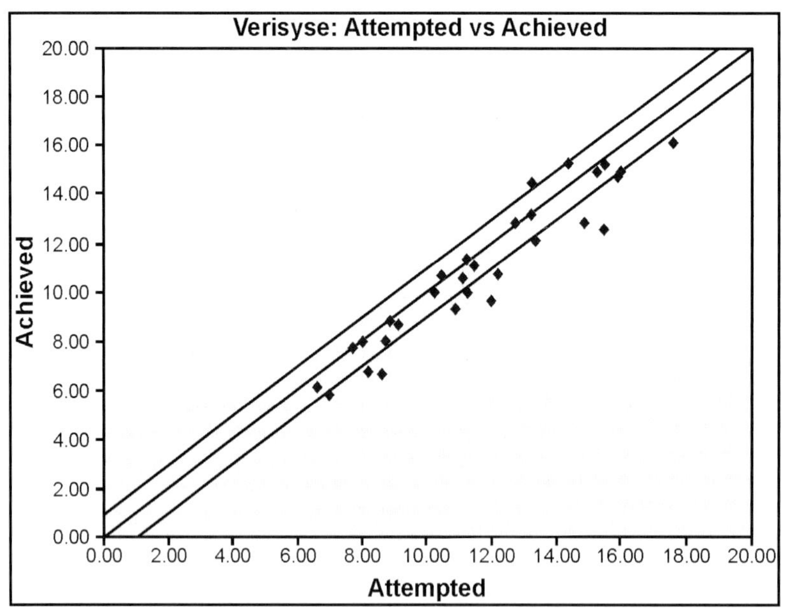

FIGURE 18-12: Scattergram of attempted vs achieved correction for verisyse group.

References

1. Pineda-Fernández A, Jaramillo J, Vargas J, Jaramillo M, Jaramillo J, Galíndez A. Phakic posterior chamber intraocular lens for high myopia. J Cataract Refract Surg 2004; 30:2277-83.
2. Lackner B, Pieh S, Schmidinger G, Hanselmayer G, Dejaco-Ruhswurm I, Funovics MA, Skorpik C. Outcome after treatment of ametropia with implantable contact lenses. Ophthalmology 2003; 110:2153-61.
3. Hoffer KJ. Pigment vacuum iridectomy for phakic refractive lens implantation. J Cataract Refract Surg 2001;27:1166-8.
4. Moshirfar M, Grégoire FJ, Mirzaian G, Whitehead GF, Kang PC.Use of Verisyse iris-supported phakic intraocular lens for myopia in keratoconic patients. J Cataract Refract Surg 2006;32:1227-32.
5. Coullet J, Guëll JL, Fournié P, Grandjean H, Gaytan J, Arné JL, Malecaze F. Iris-supported phakic lenses (rigid vs foldable version) for treating moderately high myopia: randomized paired eye comparison. Am J Ophthalmol. 2006;142:909-16.
6. Tehrani M, Dick HB. Short-term follow-up after implantation of a foldable iris-fixated intraocular lens in phakic eyes. Ophthalmology 2005;112:2189-95.

A John Kanellopoulos, MD

19 PRK and C3-R®

Introduction

In 1988, LASIK was born in the laboratories of the University of Crete in Greece under the direction of Ioannis Pallikaris, MD. Throughout the years, refractive surgeons have gained tremendous insight in LASIK. It is now understood that there is a limit to the amount of laser ablation that the human cornea can undergo before changing its biomechanical properties. Years ago, keratoectasia has emerged as a serious potential LASIK complication.[1] In most cases, a thin stromal bed combined with a preoperative irregular corneal topography such as forme fruste keratoconus are usually the isolated contributing factors.[2] Chapter 3 describes in detail the current understanding of risk factors for keratoectasia. For some patients it may be a challenge to explain how they developed keratoectasia in the context of normal preoperative topography and well-documented sufficient residual stromal bed thickness.

In the 1990s, penetrating keratoplasty was used to treat keratoectasia when vision could not be rehabilitated with RGP contact lenses.[3] In the early 2000s, Intacs® became a viable option. While Intacs® alone can improve the irregular corneal shape in ectasia, they cannot stabilize a destabilized cornea.[4] In 2002, The author became involved with C3-R® (corneal collagen crosslinking with riboflavin) which involved the use of UVA irradiation and topical riboflavin (see Chapter 7 for more details) which has been shown to be safe and effective for stabilizing corneas.[5-8] As discussed earlier (Chapter 8), Intacs can be combined with crosslinking.

In Chapter 18, Visian ICL and Verisyse lenses were discussed for improvement of uncorrected vision in keratoconus. For select patients after C3-R®, it may be possible to improve uncorrected vision with custom surface photorefractive keratectomy (PRK). It is important to keep in mind, this is a new area of investigation with relatively few patients treated. Long-term results will be important to analyze as they become available. The first case we treated is presented below.[9]

Case Report

A 29-year-old patient underwent LASIK in one eye for myopic astigmatism 3 years earlier. Before LASIK, his initial uncorrected visual acuity (UCVA) was 20/80 and his best spectacle-corrected visual acuity (BSCVA)

Contd....

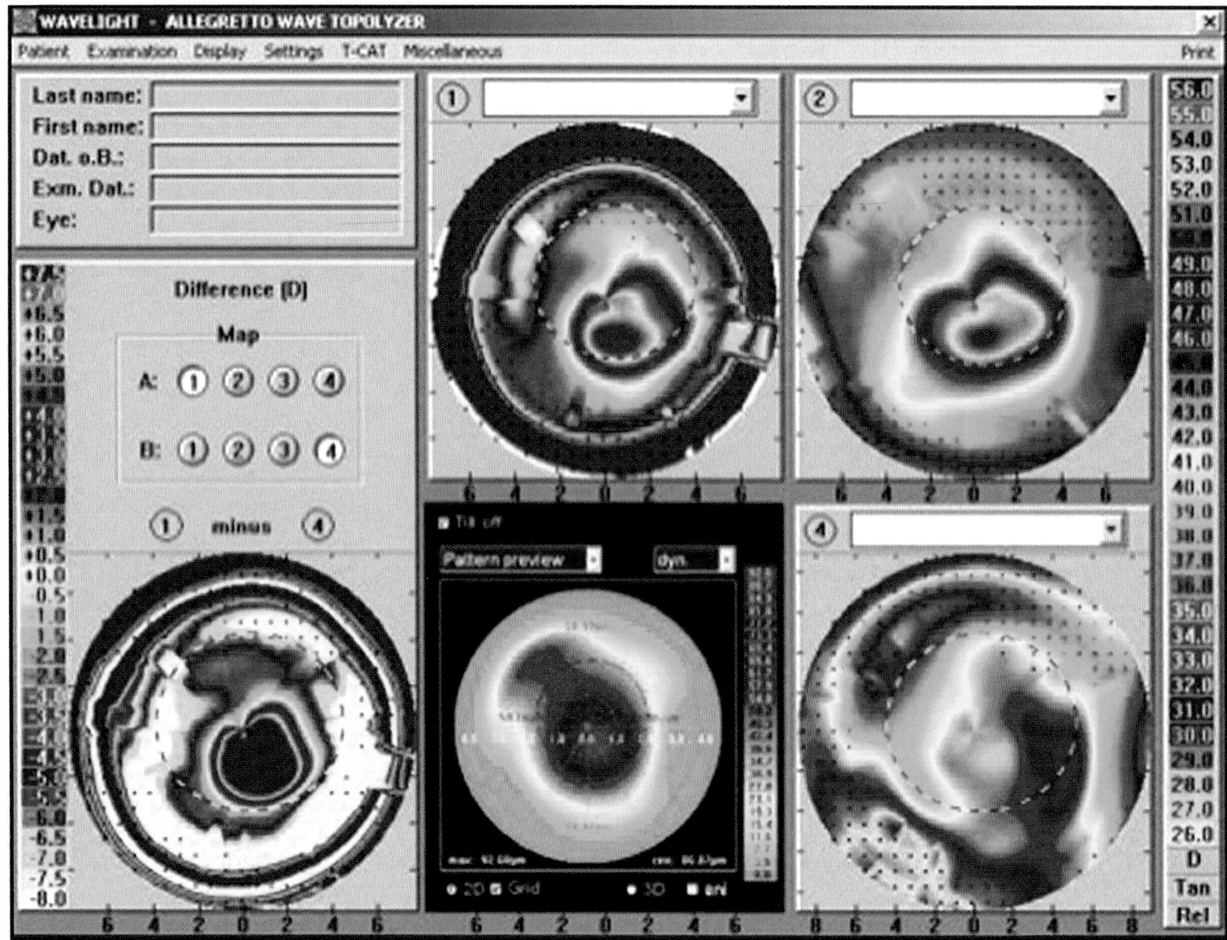

FIGURE 19-1: This display of topographies depicts the mapping of patient's cornea over course of treatment. 1 (upper left): The cornea topography of this case when first seen by the author with central cornea ectasia and mid-periphery flattening as an effect of the Intacs® that were present. 2 (upper right). Cornea topography is 2 months following the removal of Intacs® and 1 month following C3-R®. The central steepening increased after Intacs® explant (periphery changed from blue to green color). 3 (lower middle): The cornea topographic ablation pattern is shown that was used for PRK. It is notable that this ablation pattern is highly irregular with deeper ablation plan inferiorly and right to the center, which matches location of the central cornea irregularity in the previous topographies. 4 (lower right): Cornea topography was 6 months after topography-guided PRK. The central cornea appears more regular and much flatter. 5 (lower left): This map depicts the difference by subtracting the cornea topography 4 (final result) from the cornea topography 1 (our initial map). The difference reflects the topography-guided ablation pattern (lower middle map).

....Contd

was 20/20 with a refraction of –2.00 –175 × 85. Three months post-LASIK he began experiencing regression with myopia and astigmatism and UCVA decreased to 20/200 and BSCVA was 20/80 with –3.50 –2.00 × 120. The treating physician diagnosed keratoectasia based on irregular topography and the loss in BSCVA. The physician inserted double segment Intacs® which were significantly decentered. The patient's UCVA remained 20/200 and BSCVA was 20/100. The treating surgeon recommended cornea transplantation as the next step. I evaluated the patient 11 months after LASIK and 3 months after decentered Intacs® implantation **(Figure 19-1)**. Pachymetry by Orbscan (Bausch & Lomb, Rochester, NY) and ultrasound pachymetry was 410 μm at the thinnest point, and the endothelial cell count was 2,750 cells per mm^2 (Noncon Robo; Konan Medical, Hyogo, Japan).

Contd....

....Contd

The patient and I discussed the benefits and risks of corneal transplant, as well as C3-R® in order to biomechanical stabilize the corneal ectasia. The decision was made to explant the decentered Intacs®. One month later the patient was then treated with C3-R® using standard settings: ultraviolet A light at 3 mW/cm^2 for 30 minutes combined with topical 0.1% riboflavin ophthalmic solution applied every 2 minutes throughout the 30 minutes period. We used a 2-minute pre-soak of riboflavin before starting the treatment. This treatment was performed with "epi-off" (removal of the corneal epithelium after applying 20% alcohol on the surface for 30 seconds). A bandage contact lens was placed on the cornea for 5 days, and the patient was treated with topical ofloxacin 1% (Ocuflox; Allergan, Irvine, Ca) and prednisolone acetate 1% (Predforte, Allergan) four times a day for 10 days. The bandage contact lens was removed at day 4, following complete re-epithelialization.

At 3 months postoperatively, the patient's UCVA improved from 20/400 to 20/70 and his BSCVA improved from 20/200 to 20/40. The refraction changed from –4.50 –4.50 × 120 to –4.50 –4.00 × 115, and a corneal topography changed was noted **(Figure 19-1)**. The stability of these parameters and the corneal topography between months 1 and 3 of this treatment encouraged us to proceed with topography-guided PRK. Because there was not a significant amount of tissue to be removed, our goal was to reduce the irregular astigmatism and attempt to provide the patient with visual acuity not requiring spectacle or soft contact lens correction. Because the patient's corneal thickness was 410 μm, we were able to treat his full spectacle correction using the Allegretto Wave excimer laser (Wavelight, Erlangen Germany) with topography-guided customized ablation treatment (T-CAT) software. After placing 20% dilution of alcohol on the corneal surface for 30 seconds and subsequent epithelium removal, PRK was performed. A bandage contact lens was placed for 5 days and the patient was treated again with ofloxacin and prednisolone four times a day for 10 days. The bandage contact lens was removed at day 4, following complete re-epithelialization. One month after topography-guided treatment, the patient's UCVA was 20/20- and BSCVA was 20/20 with a refraction of +0.50 –0.50 × 160. The corneal endothelium count remained stable at 2,700. The patient complained of night vision symptoms of halos and ghosting. The patient is now at 34 months postoperative with UCVA of 20/20 with some mild night vision problems and corneal topography irregularity **(Figure 19-1)**. One can also appreciate the difference map between pre- and postoperative topography-guided treatment as well as the actual ablation profile that was used for the treatment **(Figure 19-1)**.

During the past 3 years, we have had experience with customized topography-guided excimer ablations which we have presented and reported.[10,11] This customized approach can help the cornea irregularity in select cases and may enhance visual rehabilitation. This was the first report of keratoectasia treatment using a combination of collagen crosslinking to stabilize the corneal biomechanics followed by surface PRK for visual rehabilitation. Corneal stabilization combined with together with full visual rehabilitation leads us to believe that this approach may have a wider application in the near future. We feel that the combined procedure discussed here may be a valuable alternative to cornea transplantation in select patients. As only a relatively small number of patients have been treated with C3-R® followed by customized PRK, we look forward to further study with longer follow-up to be done in this area.

In patients with keratoconus and keratoectasia, PRK should not be considered as a procedure to attempt emmetropia with goal of UCVA 20/20 as one uses LASIK or PRK routinely for primary cases. The treatment should be directed toward "normalizing" the cornea surface and allowing for improvement of BSCVA. There is an obvious danger in thinning these corneas too much by attempting to correct the total refractive error.

There is a limit of how much cornea tissue can be safely removed by PRK before the cornea is biomechanically weakened again. This critical amount would be the threshold at which going beyond it would undo the benefit of C3-R® and trigger active ectasia again At present, no one knows what the maximum amount of safe tissue ablation is. This is an important question to answer in the future. In the meantime, we do not ablate more than 50 microns with PRK. This is an arbitrary number that we believe is conservative, but long-term follow-up is necessary to verify how stability is maintained.

Case Report

A 28-year-old male physician underwent LASIK in November 2002. Preoperatively, his manifest refraction was –5.50 –1.50 × 015 20/20 and –4.25 –1.25 × 0168 20/20 in right and left eye, respectively. Four months following surgery, the uncorrected vision was 20/25 in both eyes. The manifest refraction was +0.25 –1.25 × 090 yielding 20/20 in the right eye and was +0.25 –0.25 × 110 produced 20/15 in the left eye, but the topography suggested the early development of ectasia in the right eye. The keratometry readings were 38.75/39.25 × 22 in right eye and 38.50/39.00 × 162 in left eye. The pachymetry readings were 375 microns and 407 microns, in right and left eyes, respectively which suggested a deeper than expected laser ablation of 154 μm (vs 105 μm planned) and 138 μm (vs 140 μm planned) in right and left eyes, respectively.

Two years later, the patient returned with of 20/40 UCVA in the right eye and 20/20 UCVA in the left eye. Manifest refraction in the affected right eye was –0.75 –3.50 × 091 with 20/30, and +0.75 –0.50 × 128 was 20/20 in the left eye. The topography suggested the presence of ectasia only in the right eye **(Figure 19-2)**. In the right eye, keratometry readings were 43.25/40.75 × 157 and the pachymetry readings were 383 μm. The next month, the patient underwent C3-R® in the right eye.

Two years after C3-R® and four years following LASIK surgery, the uncorrected vision in the affected right eye was 20/30, with a manifest refraction of –1.50 –1.75 × 073 which yielded 20/20. The uncorrected vision in the unaffected left eye was 20/20 with a manifest refraction of +0.75 –0.50 × 0128 producing 20/20. The keratometry readings were 42.75/40.62 × 163 in the right eye. Central thickness in the right eye increased from 375 μm to 416 μm.

Nomogram Adjustments

For PRK after crosslinking, the laser treatment must be applied with caution because more rigid, crosslinked, corneas may have a different ablation depth/pulse than the untreated corneas. Crosslinked corneas appear to result in overcorrections after PRK versus PRK on a normal cornea. For this reason, we recommend to use 75 to 80% of the measured sphere and cylinder as a correction parameter when planning the ablation with T-CAT software.

Can LASIK "Regressions" be a Form of Ectasia?

Case Report

Six years ago, a 34-year-old female underwent LASIK for –11.00 D of myopia **(Figure 19-3)**. A Moria M2 (Moria, Antony, France) microkeratome was used to create a 125 μm flap (calculated with subtraction pachymetry) and an Allegretto laser with a 6 mm optical zone was used to conserve tissue. The ablation

Contd....

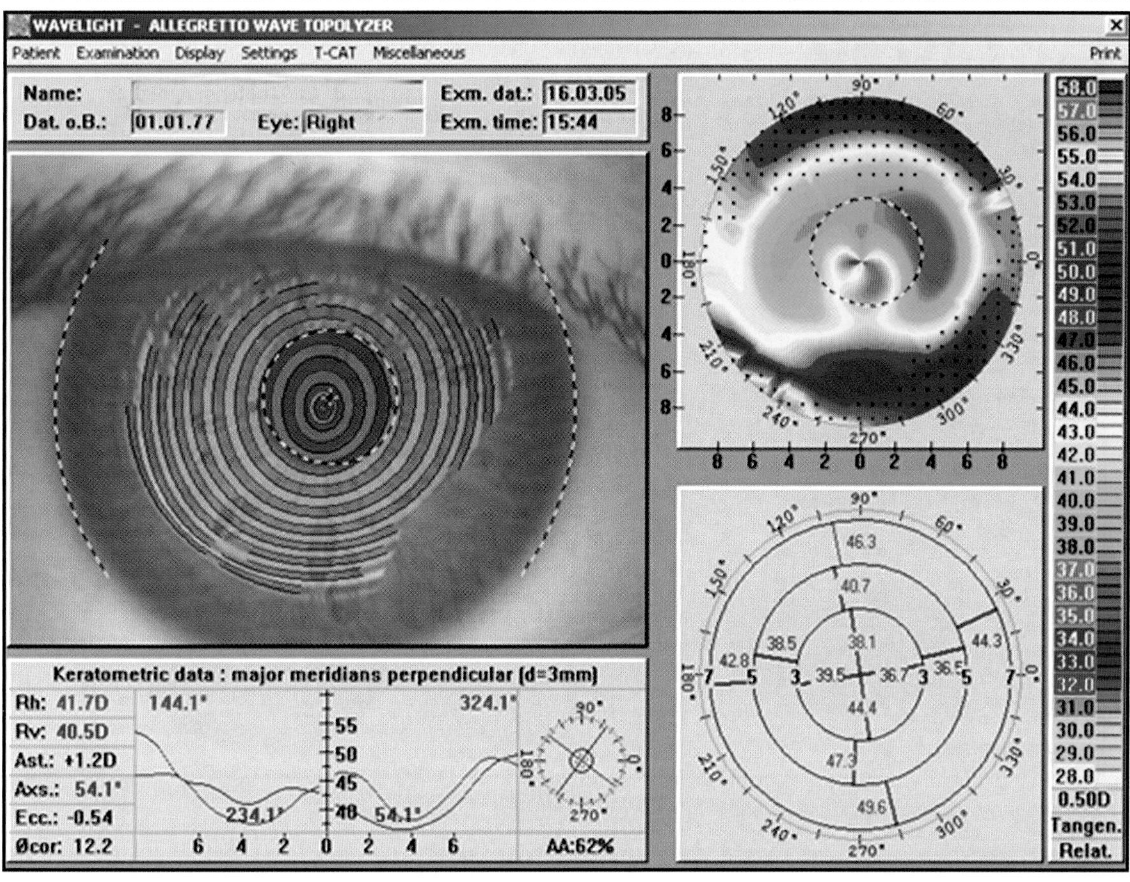

A

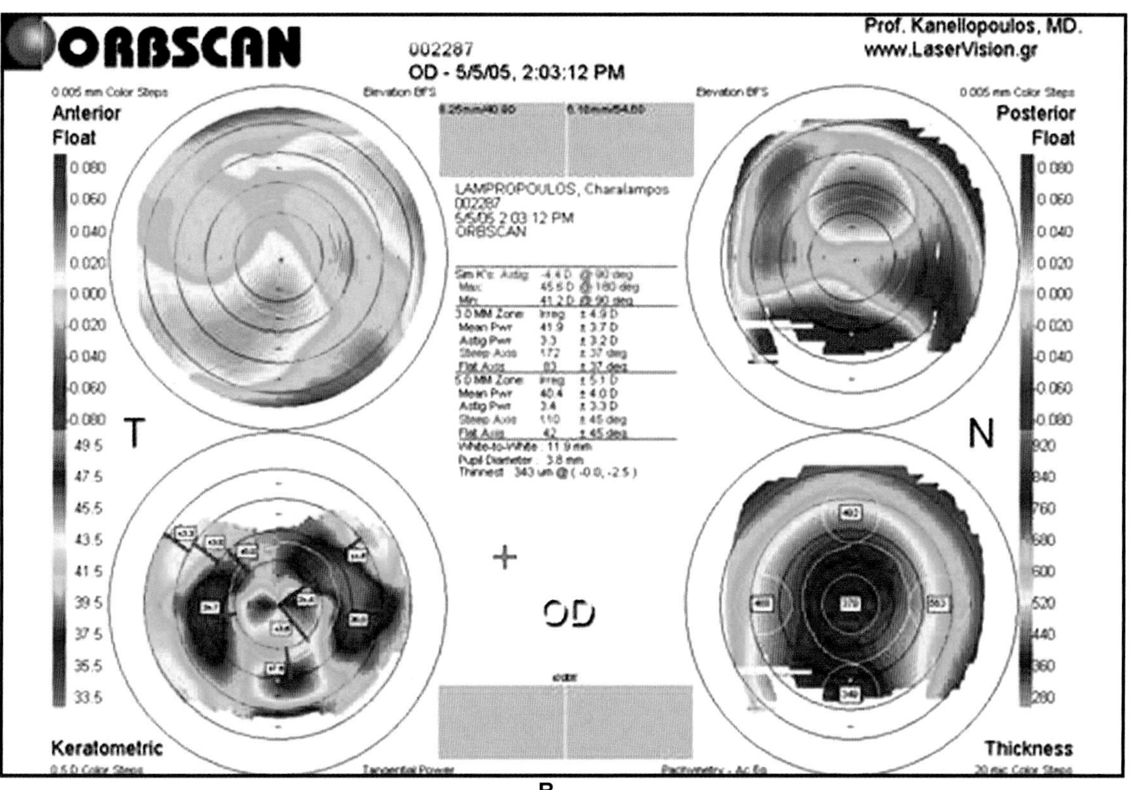

B

FIGURE 19-2A and B: Keratoectasia after LASIK. The topography at this point suggested the presence of ectasia only in the right eye (A) and Orbscan (B).

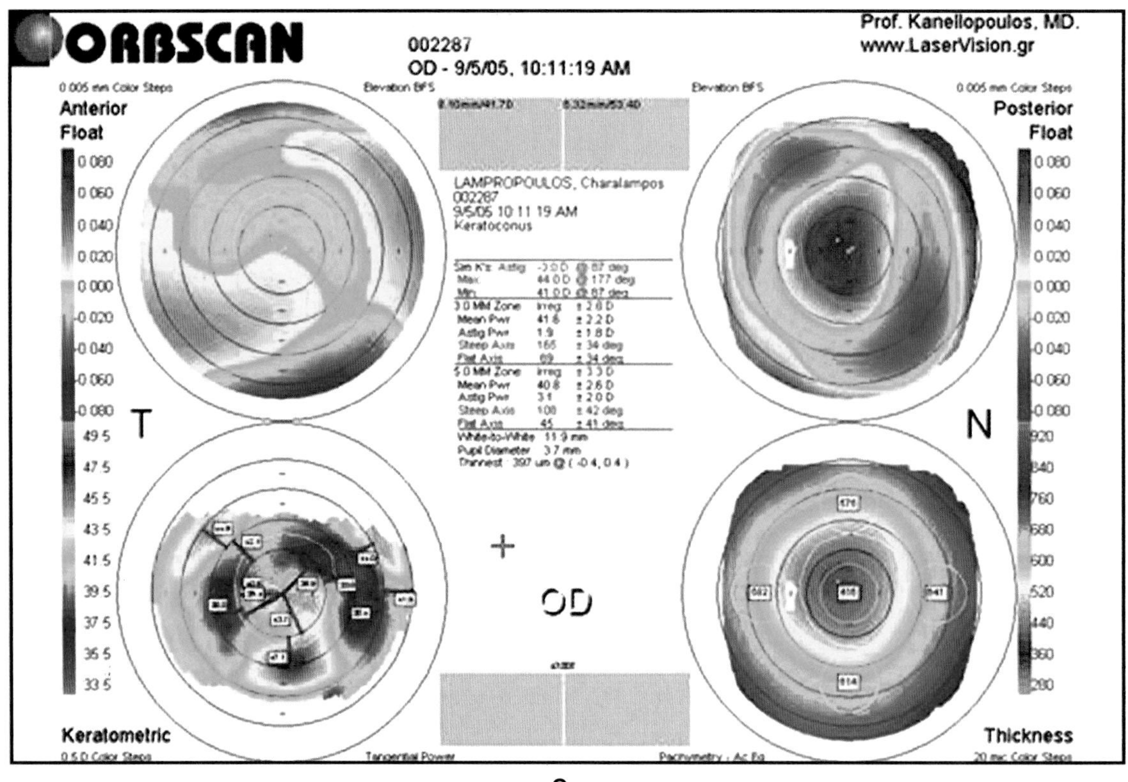

C

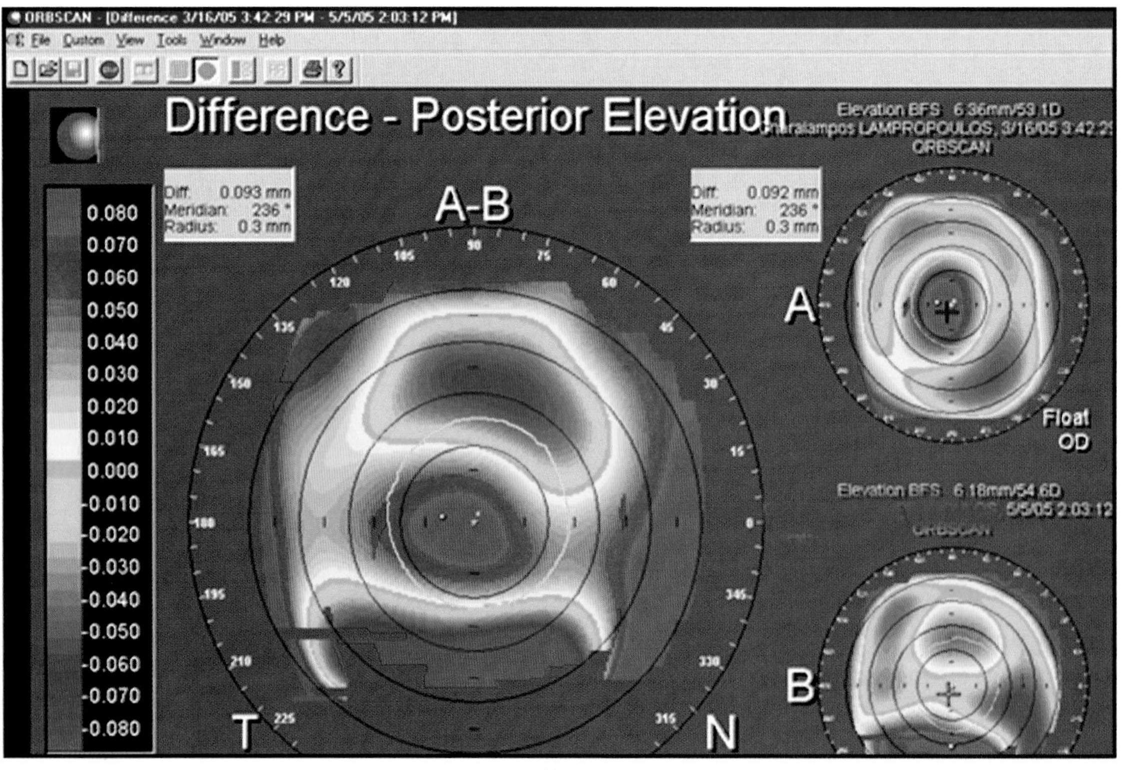

D

FIGURE 19-2C and D: Keratoectasia after LASIK: Flattening occurred post-crosslinking (C) which is evident on the difference of the elevation maps (D).

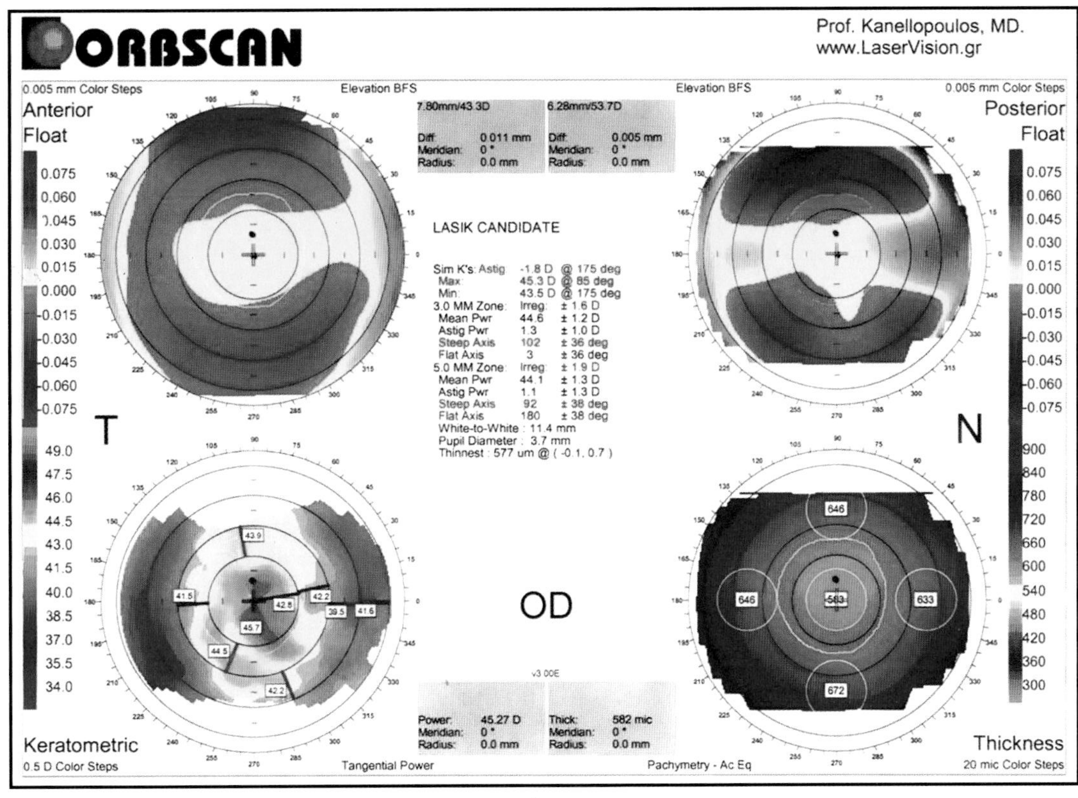

A

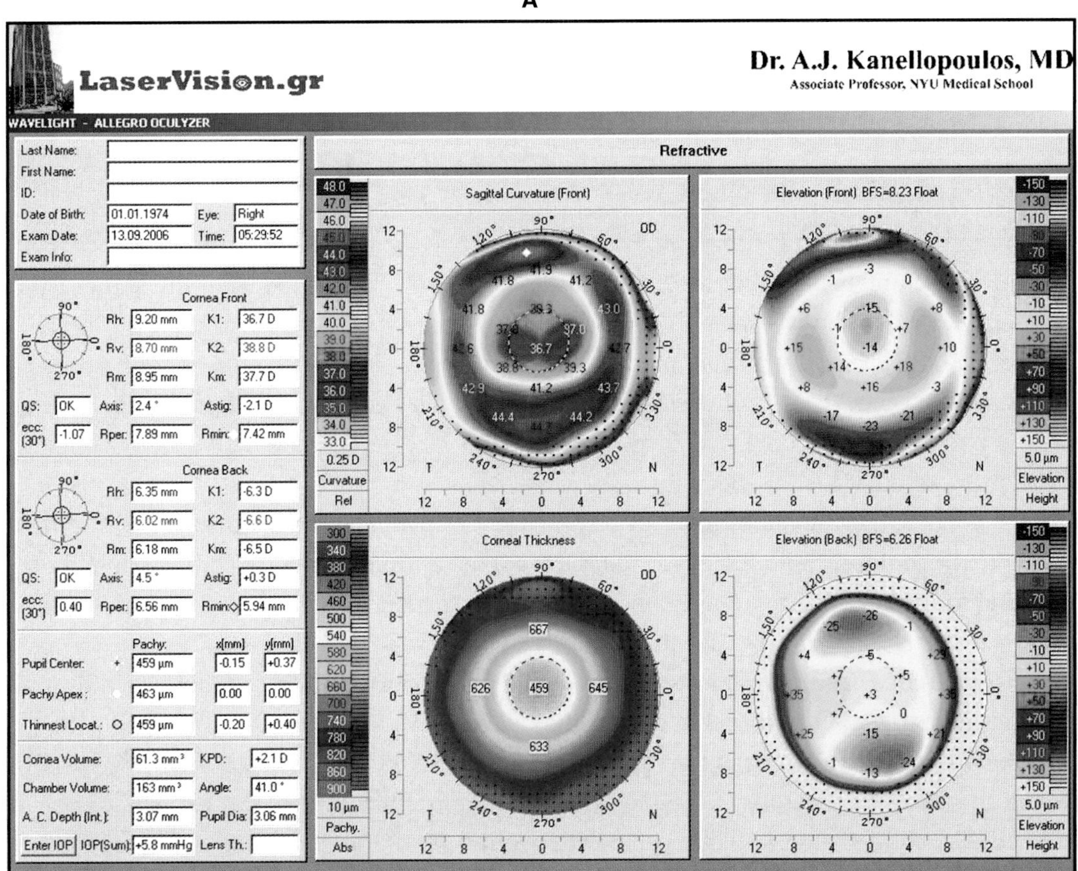

B

FIGURE 19-3A and B: Preoperative Orbscan of the right eye (A) and postoperative Pentacam (B) after LASIK for high myopia. Pentacam images of the same cornea show biomechanical flattening after crosslinking.

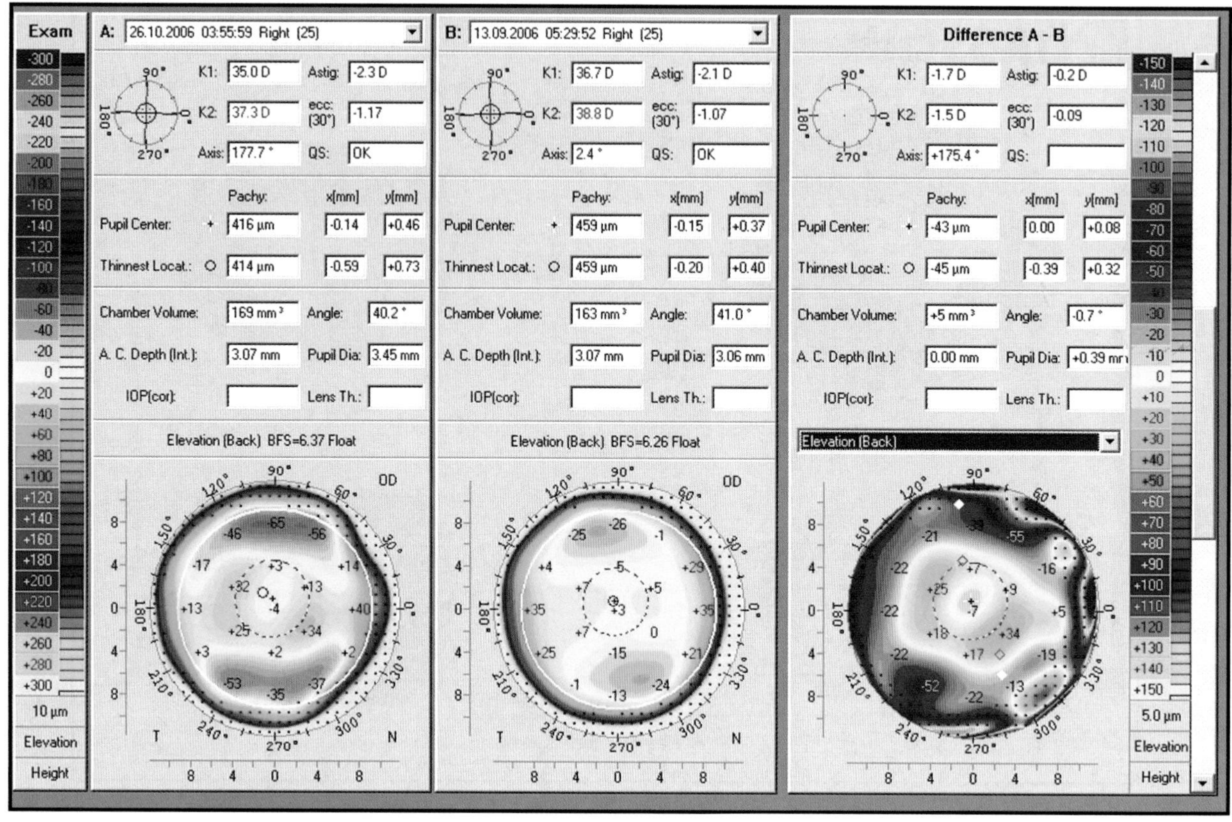

C

FIGURE 19-3C: (c) Pre-crosslinking posterior cornea surface does not show any signs of ectasia (middle) . One month after crosslinking, the posterior surface shows mild flattening (left). It is evident that flattening has occurred which is more obvious in the difference map (right), This effect corrected late regression of –1 diopter.

....Contd

depth was 130 μm and residual cornea bed measured 320 μm. For 5 years after the surgery, the patient was satisfied and refraction was plano OU and UCVA 20/20 OU. The patient then presented with 20/40 UCVA and 20/20 BSCVA, with eyes measuring –1.50 D and –0.75 D, in right and left eye respectively. No keratoectasia was evident on the topography and Oculus Pentacam. Preoperatively, central cornea thickness is approximately 563 μm **(Figure 19-3)**.

There are three options for this patient:

1. *Conventional LASIK enhancement:* In some cases, I have lifted the flap for LASIK enhancement. For these procedures, I intraoperatively measure cornea and stromal bed in order to avoid significantly reducing the residual stromal bed. Since 2000, I have tried to adhere to the guideline of 270 μm for residual stroma following LASIK.
2. *Wavefront-guided LASIK enhancement:* It could be performed with asphericity adjustment with Allegretto Wave Eye-Q laser with a treatment goal of –0.50 D for the Q value (asphericity), in order to reduce spherical aberrations that are typically induced by correction of high myopia. The hope is that the post-enhancement Q value would be less positive. Through past experience, we have learned that correction of –10.00 D shifts the asphericity of the cornea an average –0.30 D to ±2, therefore inducing significant spherical aberrations.

Contd....

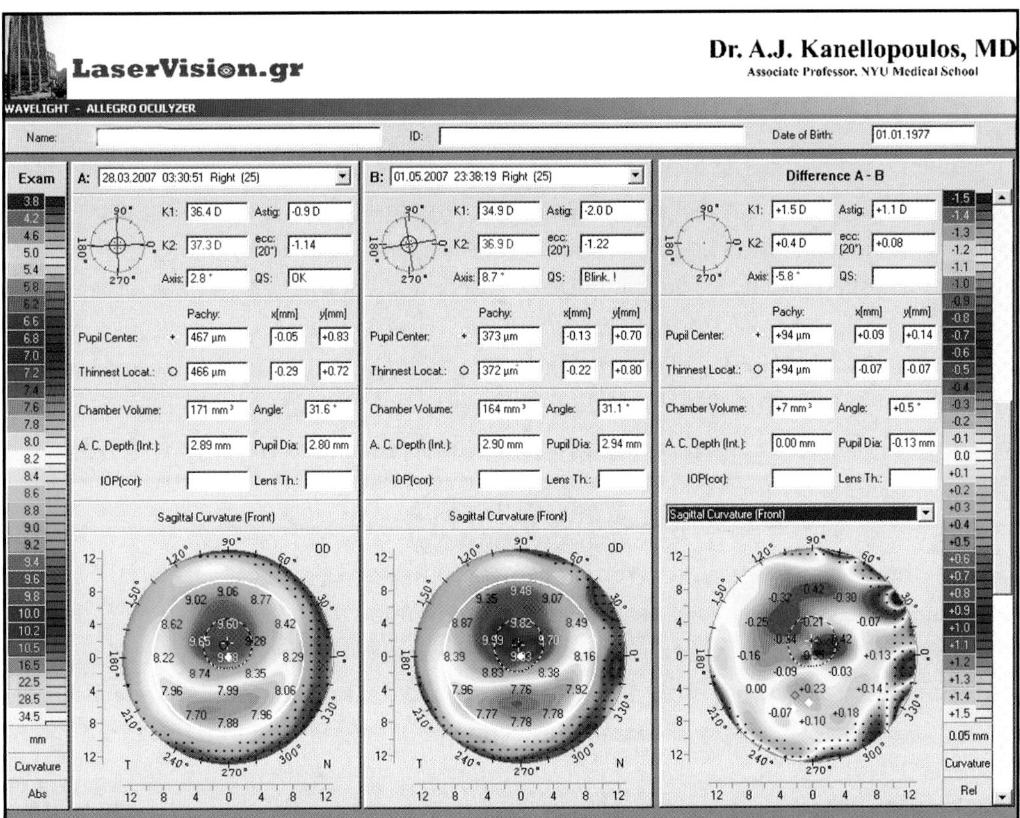

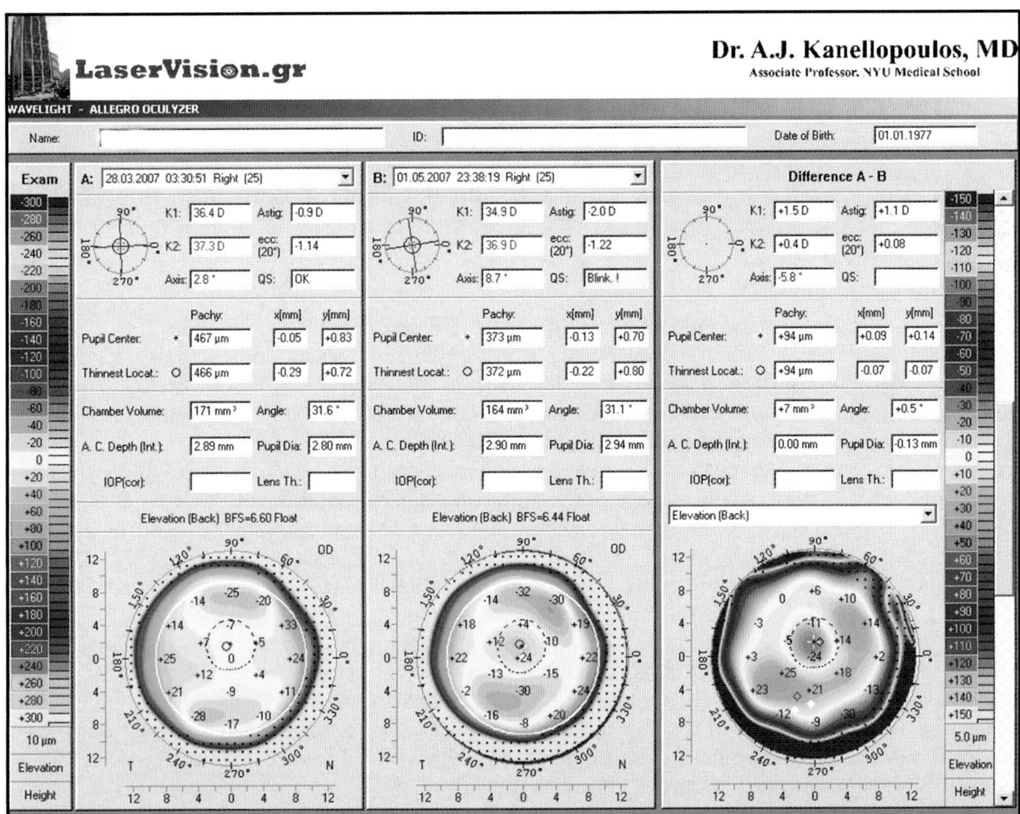

FIGURE 19-4: Pentacam maps. The sagittal curvature front (A) and posterior cornea elevation (B) show the biomechanical change of crosslinking that produced the regression reversal.

....*Contd*

3. *C3-R®*: The goal of crosslinking in this case would be to cause further flattening to correct residual myopia.

For this patient, I proposed that the patient was experiencing a late biomechanical shift of the thinned cornea, but not keratoectasia. The patient understood the nature of the crosslinking procedure and that laser enhancement may still be needed afterwards. The patient elected to have epi-off C3-R®. Initially the patient was unsatisfied and experienced pain and discomfort for the first 10 days while the epithelium healed. At 1 month follow-up, UCVA was 20/20 and her refractive error was –0.25 D in each eye. She eventually achieved 20/15. This case is consistent with previous reports on the biomechanical changes that occur following LASIK. Crosslinking in this case led to a significant biomechanical effect reflected by a change in the posterior cornea contour centrally and paracentrally **(Figure 19-3)**.

Case Report

A 27-year-old female was status post-LASIK for –10 D in each eye five years ago. She had LASIK enhancement for -1.00 D in each eye 3 years ago and deteriorated again to refraction of –1.50 D. Instead of another LASIK enhancement, she underwent corneal crosslinking. The refraction reversed to plano in each eye. The Pentacam comparison of pre- and post-C3-R® for the anterior sagittal curvature and posterior cornea elevation shows the biomechanical change of crosslinking that produced the regression reversal **(Figure 19-4)**.

Conclusion

These cases show that any surprise regression noted, even years after LASIK, could be biomechanical changes of the cornea. Such cases may be treated by this minimally invasive alternative. Other causes of regression should be ruled out such as early nuclear sclerotic lens changes. Further work in this area will determine how predictable crosslinking for refractive regression along with the limits of correction that is achievable.

References

1. Binder PS. Ectasia after laser in situ keratomileusis. J Cataract Refract Surg 2003;29:2419-29.
2. Randleman JB, Russell B, Ward MA, Thompson KP, Stulting RD. Risk factors and prognosis for corneal ectasia after LASIK.Ophthalmology 2003;110(2):267-75.
3. Klein SR, Epstein RJ, Randleman JB, Stulting RD. Corneal ectasia after laser in situ keratomileusis in patients without apparent preoperative risk factors Cornea 2006;25(4):388-403.
4. Kanellopoulos A, Pe L, Perry H, Donnenfeld E. Modified intracorneal ring segment implantations (Intacs) for the management of moderate to advanced keratoconus: efficacy and complications. Cornea 2006,25: 29-33.
5. Wollensak, G, Spoerl, E, and Seiler, T. Riboflavin/ultraviolet -a-induced collagen cross linking for the treatment of keratoconus. Am J Ophthalmol 2003;135: 620-7.
6. Seiler T, Hafezi F. Corneal cross-linking-induced stromal demarcation line. Cornea 2006; 25: 1057-59.
7. Spoerl E, Huhle M, Seiler T. Induction of cross-links in corneal tissue. Exp Eye Res 1998; 66: 97-103.
8. Hafezi F, Mrochen M, Jankov M, Hopeler T, Wiltfang R, Kanellopoulos A, Seiler T. Corneal collagen cross linking with riboflavin/UVA for the treatment of induced kerectasia after laser in situ keratomileusis. J Refract Surgery 2007. In press.
9. Kanellopoulos A. Post-LASIK ectasia. (Letter-to-the-editor). Ophthalmology 2007;114:1230-1.
10. Kanellopoulos AJ. Topography-guided Custom re-treatments in 27 symptomatic eyes. J Refract Surg 2005; 21:S513-8.
11. Kanellopoulos AJ, Pe L. Wavefront-guided enhancements using the wavelight excimer laser in symptomatic eyes previously treated with LASIK. J Refract Surg 2006; 22: 345-9.
12. Kanellopoulos AJ , Binder PS. Collagen cross-linking (CCL) with sequential topography-guided PRK. A temporizing alternative to penetrating keratoplasty. Cornea. In press.

Index